OTOLARYNGOLOGY RESEARCH ADVANCES

HANDBOOK OF MODERN TECHNIQUES IN AUDITORY CORTEX

OTOLARYNGOLOGY RESEARCH ADVANCES

Additional books in this series can be found on Nova's website under the Series tab.

Additional e-books in this series can be found on Nova's website under the e-book tab.

OTOLARYNGOLOGY RESEARCH ADVANCES

HANDBOOK OF MODERN TECHNIQUES IN AUDITORY CORTEX

DIDIER A. DEPIREUX
AND
MOUNYA ELHILALI, PH.D.
EDITORS

NOVA BIOMEDICAL
New York

For permission to use material from this book please contact us:
Telephone 631-231-7269; Fax 631-231-8175
Web Site: http://www.novapublishers.com

Additional color graphics may be available in the e-book version of this book.

Library of Congress Cataloging-in-Publication Data

ISBN: 978-1-62808-894-6

Library of Congress Control Number: 2013947634

Published by Nova Science Publishers, Inc. † New York

Contents

Preface

Physics is mathematical not because we know so much about the physical world, but because we know so little; it is only its mathematical properties that we can discover.

Bertrand Russell

Auditory cortex occupies the central stage in the auditory pathway. Upon this stage, neural input from the cochlea, heavily processed by nuclei of the brainstem, auditory midbrain and auditory thalamus, converge. Auditory cortex is composed of a variety of fields, which vary in number depending on the species. The most studied part is Primary Auditory Cortex, denoted **AI** and implicitly the main source of recent progress as evidenced in this book. Input into auditory cortex gets redistributed, in part for more abstract, categorical processing and in part to multisensory areas. A large number of projections loop back towards thalamus and midbrain.

While its location was already established by direct physical stimulation by Ferrier in 1873, its inner workings or even its role is still very much under study. Suffice it to say that we still have more questions about auditory cortex than we have answers. In particular, the main method used to unravel the inner workings of (mostly primary) auditory cortex employed pure tones and click trains. While both of these types of stimuli are easy to generate, neither represent natural sounds. Some notable early exceptions to the exclusive use of tones and clicks were the use of broad-band, noisy sounds, described in the first chapter by Eggermont. Following up on the work of Eggermont and his colleagues, simultaneously building on techniques developed in the maturing field of visual physiology, and with the advent of fast computers which allowed detailed signal processing, it became possible to use and have better control over complex stimuli used to probe the auditory pathway. This confluence of opportunities made possible the developments presented in this book.

In this volume, we aimed to provide a user's guide for techniques that have been developed and have particularly blossomed since the mid-1990's. This book is intended as a resource in the use of complex broadband and natural sounds to study and characterize cortical responses, and in the technique of spectro-temporal receptive fields, or **STRF** as a method to characterize neural properties. Given the blossoming of such techniques in the field of auditory physiology, the editors felt the time was auspicious to present tutorials on these topics in order to widen their appeal to the physiology community and provide a primer for researchers interested in the topic.

In Chapter 1, Dr Eggermont provides a personal *history and chronological introduction* to the spectro-temporal receptive field (STRF). This chapter provides the background that led to many aspects of the STRF in its current form. By now, STRF-based analyses have been used in many species. In mice, STRFs have been employed to measure differences in sound perception between pregnant and non-pregnant females, and in rats STRFs have been used to assess changes associated with tinnitus. In ferrets, STRFs have facilitated an understanding of the coding of speech. Cats, bats, macaques, humans, and songbirds are examples of other species in which STRFs have been utilized to characterize cortical responses. Most importantly, the STRF has been used very effectively to characterize responses to sound, and by its very nature, more closely approximates complex sounds present in natural environments.

In Chapter 2, Drs Elhilali, Shamma, Simon and Fritz present the *basis for the derivation of the linear STRF*: its construction, elementary characterization (rank, SVD, □'s), and dual time- and Fourier-domain representation (STRF/MTF). This chapter is conceptually the simplest but also the most relevant for understanding current literature. It details the mathematical foundation of the STRF, outlines of its limitations and describes a rosetta stone of how to decipher and interpret STRFs and their implications in understanding cortical processing.

In Chapter 3, Drs Atencio and Schreiner consider the effect of *stimulus choice* on the derivation and analysis of the receptive field. Over the years, different types of stimuli have been developed and used, with each having its strengths and deficiencies. From the early "Biotope" of Smolders and Aertsen, to the auditory gratings or ripples, both fixed and continuously changing, dynamic chords, random spectral shape stimulus, Poisson distributed tones and natural stimuli, it can be daunting to choose the most appropriate stimulus!

In Chapter 4, Drs Depireux and Shechter delve into *phenomenological extensions* of the linear STRF. One of the challenges in analyzing data collected from in vivo preparations, and applying formal theoretical models, stems from the fact that neural data obtained in the awake animal is usually very noisy. This is due in part to the nature of neural firing, and in part to changes in attentional and behavioral states of the animal during a recording session. Whether the animal is passively listening or actively engaged in a behavior, the experimenter has at most a few hours to obtain all recordings. While more data might reduce experimental noise and variability, in practice such data are not always obtainable. Thus, this chapter explores the addition of intuitive and manageable non-linearities, including the coding of contrast and the uncovering of complex cells in auditory cortex.

In Chapter 5, Dr Marmarelis establishes more formal foundations for nonlinear dynamical modeling, and introduces a *general modeling framework for the nonlinear spectro-temporal processing* in the auditory system. In non-linear systems, it is customary to use Volterra and Wiener kernel models with suitable customized bases, as they offer a general model for a nonlinear dynamic system with finite memory. Here, a variant of this nonlinear modeling methodology is presented, which utilizes the novel concept of Principal Dynamic Modes to obtain efficient models of the input-output relationship between multi-dimensional sets of signals and neural responses, including complex interactions between neural ensembles.

In Chapter 6, Drs David, Oliver, Gallant and Theunissen detail new approaches for computing and *validating linear and higher order response functions.* While a reverse correlation will always result in some STRF (or higher order function), this chapter delves into whether the obtained *receptive field is statistically significant* and meaningful. It also addresses the limitations of different STRF implementations and the (equivalent) challenge of choosing the most appropriate analytical approach, thus providing the theoretical counterpart to Chapter 4. A cross-validation framework for testing predictive power provides a useful tool for a relatively unbiased comparison of models that might differ substantially in their underlying structure. Similarly, since estimation data are usually limited because of recording time constraints, this chapter explains how model performance can be improved by imposing prior assumptions on the fits, but cautions that these biased approaches many not generalize across data sets and can confuse the interpretation of results. Also addressed in this chapter is the well-known fact that certain aspects of the auditory input such as loudness or bandwidth can influence the response of a neuron. By construction, these aspects cannot be modeled by the linear STRF. They summarize various *adaptations of classical models* that have been used as possible approaches for integrating stimulus context and transient changes into the neural models. STRF models that incorporate contextual influences into their structure promise new insights into higher-order representation of auditory stimuli.

Finally, in Chapter 7, Drs Sahani, Williamson, Ahrens, and Linden, delve further into the use of *probabilistic methods for linear and multilinear models.* Moving away from the receptive field *characterization* that has been the approach utilized in the previous chapters (except to some extent Chapter 6), this chapter presents a methodology that is more focused on system *identification.* A predictive approach, generally speaking, concentrates less on describing the neurons and their coding using receptive fields, and more on the ability to predict the neural response to new stimuli. This chapter focuses on the mathematical methods that underlie this predictive probabilistic approach, including multi-linear formulation, in which representations that contain both nonlinear transforms of sounds and spectrotemporally local contextual interactions can be studied.

We hope these chapters will help the curious reader to understand and forge their own path towards developing modern methods for functional exploration of auditory cortex and understanding its role and inner workings. We have barely begun to understand how and why the many stations along the auditory pathway - from the cochlea to the auditory nerve, cochlear nucleus, superior olive, lateral lemniscus, inferior colliculus, and auditory thalamus - prepare the neural input necessary for the various fields of auditory cortex, so as to allow the brain to extract sound source localization, pitch, and timbre in a very efficient and noise-robust way, often in the presence of competing sound sources and noise.

We just know that much is yet to come!

A thousand paths are there which have never yet been trodden; a thousand salubrities and hidden islands of life. Unexhausted and undiscovered is still man and man's world.

Awake and hearken, ye lonesome ones! From the future come winds with stealthy pinions, and to fine ears good tidings are proclaimed.

Friedrich Nietzsche, in Thus Spake Zarathustra The Bestowing Virtue,

Didier A Depireux and Mounya Elhilali, Ph.D.
University of Maryland and Johns Hopkins University
May, 2013.

In: Handbook of Modern Techniques in Auditory Cortex ISBN: 978-1-62808-894-6
Editors: Didier A. Depireux and Mounya Elhilali

Chapter 1

The STRF: Its Origin, Evolution and Current Application

Jos J. Eggermont
Department of Physiology and Pharmacology and Department of Psychology,
University of Calgary, Calgary, AB, Canada

1. Introduction

The most used stimulus in auditory research is the single tone, and except for threshold estimation has fairly little to contribute to our understanding of hearing. As Schnupp et al. (2010) put it:

> "Real-world sounds, like those we just described, are immensely rich and complex. But in sharp contrast to these "natural" sounds, the sounds most commonly used in the laboratory to study hearing are by and large staggeringly dull. The most common laboratory sound by far is the sine wave pure tone, a sound that most nonscientists would describe, entirely accurately, as a "beep" – but not just any beep, and most certainly not an interesting one. … A pure tone is, indeed, so bare as to be almost 'unnatural': pure tones are hardly ever found in everyday soundscapes, be they manmade or natural."

In contrast, broadband stimuli may allow, by using only one stimulus, to probe the neuron on: excitation, (lateral) inhibition, their interaction, post-activation suppression, latency and frequency-tuning information, and for some stimuli ('ripples') also modulation transfer functions. Responses to broadband stimuli are more level invariant than those to tone pips, and reflect what the neuron is doing under natural stimulation. This may be more relevant for studying the ecological aspects of communication. This book covers the use of broadband dynamic stimuli to probe the processing power of neurons, and to derive useful predictors of what the neuron will do under varied environments. It all started with changes in the philosophy behind the way experiments need to be conducted as expressed in Eggermont et al. (1983c):

> "We will call this [old] approach the *experimenter-centred* approach; the experimentally observed variable is the occurrence of action potentials (spikes), commonly expressed as a firing rate. One may also use criteria as just detectable changes in firing rate, e.g. in the construction of frequency-tuning curves, and more recently also changes in synchrony between the occurrence of the spikes and the stimulus. The stimuli used in this approach are the familiar ones such as clicks, tone- and noise-bursts or continuous tones of various frequencies. ... One calculates the occurrence of spike activity as a function of time, τ, *after* the onset of stimulus presentation. The experimenter-centred approach is therefore a method of *forward correlation.* The second [new] approach, pioneered by De Boer (1967, 1968), ... may be called a *subject-centred* approach. This way of thinking considers the occurrence of an action potential (event) as a sign or as an indication that something particular happened with the stimulus preceding that action potential. Each action potential is considered as signalling a stimulus that was of interest to the neuron and may be even to the animal. For this type of approach the stimulus preferably is diverse in nature, and the pioneering papers reported results based on Gaussian wide-band noise as a stimulus. By correlating the events with the stimulus in a given interval prior to the event one obtains an estimate of the average stimulus that caused the spikes. This correlation procedure where one looks at the average stimulus as a function of time, τ, prior to the spike is therefore a method of backward- or *reverse-correlation* (De Boer, 1968)."

It has been more than 30 years since the spectro-temporal receptive field (STRF) was first used to describe the joint sensitivity to the spectral and temporal dimensions of a Gaussian white-noise (GWN) stimulus in the auditory midbrain (Aertsen and Johannesma, 1981b; Eggermont et al., 1981; Hermes et al., 1981). The STRF was specifically associated with stimuli characterized by randomly varying spectro-temporal features, and was calculated using a generalization of reverse correlation (or spike-triggered averaging; de Boer and de Jongh, 1978). The STRF of a neuron can be interpreted as the best linear model that transforms a time-varying stimulus into a prediction of the firing probability of a neuron. In spectro-temporal reverse correlation, the spectrograms of the sound that precede the spike in a given time window (typically up to 100 ms before the spike) are averaged (cf Figure 6). Parts of the sound that consistently activate the neuron, that is, frequency components to which the neuron is tuned and occur at a more or less fixed time before the spike (determined by the spike latency), will add up more than frequency components that fail to activate the neuron but reflect the background activity within the analysis window. After the neuron has fired it will be temporarily less sensitive (because of short-term synaptic depression, feedforward inhibition, and/or after-hyperpolarization) and the average spectro-temporal energy in the excitatory frequency band will be less than the background activity. Because we are considering the average spectrogram preceding the spikes, this postactivation suppression will show up in the spectrogram preceding the excitatory part. By contrast, lateral inhibitory areas, if present, typically flank the excitatory ones at approximately equal latencies (deCharms et al., 1998; Valentine and Eggermont, 2004).

The STRF is based on time-frequency analysis (Eggermont and Smith, 1990) and nonlinear systems theory (Eggermont 1993). The general methodology is known as the white-noise approach (Marmarelis and Marmarelis, 1978), closely related to the cross-correlation method (Palm and Pöppel 1985) for developing a Wiener series model of a nonlinear system. It was very early on recognized that the reverse-correlation function between spikes and the GWN waveform (De Boer, 1967; 1969) is basically identical to the first-order Wiener kernel of the system (Eggermont et al. 1983c). Therefore, the reverse-correlation function does not just reflect linear processing but instead should be considered the best linear fit to the observed input–output transformation (Palm and Pöppel 1985; Eggermont 1993). However, if the response of a neuron is not phase locked to fine details of the stimulus waveform the first-order Wiener kernel cannot be recovered from the noise. Given that in central parts of the brain phase locking is present only at low frequencies (Wallace et al., 2000, 2011), one could consider the dynamic spectrum or spectrogram rather than the waveform as the effective stimulus. The parallel auditory processing along the tonotopically organized afferents, separates the dynamic spectrum into energy fluctuations within discrete frequency bands, e.g., one-third octave bands (Aersten and Johannesma, 1980). The STRF can then be interpreted as the first-order Wiener kernel of a multiple-input system, composed of the system's impulse responses to these different narrow-band inputs. Note, however that these narrow-band filters are not independent (Gourévitch et al., 2009). It is important to note that spectro-temporal reverse correlation (with an appropriate time-frequency representation) is equal to the single Fourier transform of the second-order Wiener kernel (Eggermont et al. 1983c; Eggermont 1993).

I will now retrace the steps that led to the origin of the STRF. It all started in the Netherlands, initially in the lab of Egbert de Boer in Amsterdam (mid 1960's) and coalesced in the theoretical work of Pim Johannesma and Ad Aertsen in Nijmegen (in the 1970's). Egbert de Boer was one of the two supervisors for my Doctoral Thesis (1972), and I was familiar with his ideas when I started my thesis work in 1969. In 1978 I joined the Nijmegen lab as the new Head of the Biophysics Department and started electrophysiological recordings from the frog midbrain using STRFs for characterizing these neurons. My experimental collaborators in this work were initially Dik Hermes, who had already set up experimental equipment by the time I arrived, and later Willem Epping with whom I also worked on cross-correlations of neural spike trains, as well as linear and non-linear analysis of temporal modulation transfer functions.

2. Reverse Correlation in Amsterdam

The spirit of the time at the introduction of the reverse correlation (revcor) function can best be illustrated by a few quotes:

> "Responses of single fibres in the cat's auditory nerve due to white-noise stimulation were recorded on magnetic tape. The stimulus and the series of action potentials (spikes) were subsequently analyzed with the help of an "average-response computer". Matters were arranged in such a way that the computer averages the noise-waveshape fragment during a certain period prior to each spike. In this way the causative phenomena behind the excitation of the auditory neuron reveal themselves and can be further analyzed. … after all these nerve spikes have been processed, we have the average waveshape of the noise *just prior to a nerve spike.* It gives a picture of those portions of the stimulus that have–on the average–-given rise to the action spikes. The function so computed, actually is the CCF [cross-correlation function] of the input-noise and the output-spike signal. This function is a good representation of the cross-correlation function taken across the cochlear filter." (De Boer and Jongkees, 1968).

> "The method involves stimulation of the ear of an experimental animal (cat) with white noise, recording of the train of action potentials from a single fiber of the auditory nerve, and computation of a specific type of cross-correlation function. For each fiber the result comes in the form of a time function, which can be associated with the nerve fiber studied. That function is known as the "revcor function" (reverse-correlation function) of the fiber. The Fourier transform of a revcor function has the character of a bandpass-filter frequency response; the corresponding frequency response function has extremely steep slopes and, in fact, is very similar to the pure-tone tuning curve" (de Boer, 1973).

De Boer and his student de Jongh started recordings from cat auditory nerve fibers around the time that I was working on my Ph.D. thesis (in a different lab and on a different topic). It took them a while to obtain long-term stable recordings that could be fed into the "Average Response Computer" as triggers for the GWN and to obtain the revcor functions for individual fibers. The results were only published in 1978. I quote:

> "For the case of stimulation with wide-band signals the process of excitation of a primary auditory neuron can be split up into two parts, one involving linear filtering of the acoustical stimulus and the second one representing the generation of a stochastic series of pulses. The impulse response of the linear filtering stage can be measured with the reverse-correlation method. Revcor functions have very little phase modulation in their waveform and a gradual phase spectrum in the region of resonance (within 20 dB from the top). The output signal of the linear filtering stage—the excitatory signal--is a good predictor of firing probability. Positive values give rise to increased firing probability, negative values produce suppression, even of spontaneous activity. For wide-band stimuli, the spectral content–as measured from the autocorrelation function–of the firing probability is indistinguishable (within 1 dB) from that of the excitatory signal. That is, no trace of frequency-selective nonlinearity is observed. This holds for the range within 12-15 dB from the top of the power spectrum, and for the great majority of neurons tested. Neurons with resonance frequencies above 2.5 kHz show characteristic waveform differences between the firing probability and the --rectified-- excitatory signal. Nevertheless, the conclusion above on the power spectrum remains valid. When stimulus intensity varies rapidly over a large range, adaptation effects can be observed. These do not affect the timing pattern of the neuron's action potential but appear to control the (instantaneous) rate of firing in relation to the excitatory signal." (De Boer and de Jongh, 1978).

The limitations of the revcor technique, its insensitivity to nonlinearities and its limited dynamic range, were clear from the beginning:

> "The results presented illustrate the predictive power of the revcor function and confirm the validity of the associated simple linear model [for the peripheral auditory system]. … In view of known data on combination-tone generation and two-tone suppression we would have expected more evidence of nonlinearity, particularly of nonlinear filtering. … For these stimuli a linear transform of the stimulus is the principal controller of firing probability: the principle of specific coding (de Boer, 1973). Expressed in another way, this principle states that the components of a stimulus partake in the excitation of a neuron in relative proportions that are given by the neuron's revcor amplitude spectrum. … In this respect the revcor function has advantages over conventional descriptors of the response pattern observed in auditory nerve fibers, like the tuning curve or the click PST histogram. The method of reverse correlation has the additional advantage that it reveals details of frequency selectivity around the resonance

frequency which are difficult to get otherwise. However, the method is not suited to reveal details about the skirts of the frequency response curve far from the top. In particular, the resolving power is not sufficient to assess the presence or absence of the low-frequency "tails" of the tuning curve in the revcor spectrum." (De Boer and de Jongh, 1978).

3. The Pre-Event Stimulus Ensemble

Johannesma (1972) generalized the interpretation of the revcor function into the pre-event stimulus ensemble (PESE) and so ultimately paved the way for the STRF. The first experimental steps were made by van Gisbergen et al. (1975) with single-cell recordings from the ventral cochlear nucleus (VCN) in cats.

They stated clearly how the PESE concept was used in practice:

> "The usual approach in sensory neurophysiology is to present a well-determined stimulus and to investigate its effect on the neuronal firing pattern. De Boer changed this direction of view with his reverse correlation method (de Boer, 1967, 1969; de Boer and Kuyper, 1968). He set out to analyze which stimuli out of gaussian white noise induce the neuron to generate spikes. ... Inspired by this work, Johannesma (1972) has introduced the concept of the pre-spike or the pre-event stimulus ensemble (PESE). The stimulus which is relevant for the generation of a spike is a segment of the whole stimulus which precedes the spike and which has a limited duration T. Therefore if a spike is generated at time t_o the pre-spike stimulus of that spike is the stimulus extending between t_o and (t_o – T). The PESE is the ensemble of the stimuli of duration T which each precede a neural event, a spike of the response. The average of the PESE is identical with the cross-correlation function between input and output of the neuron (de Boer and Kuyper, 1968). For this to be valid it is not necessary to make assumptions about the linearity of the system. For the first and second order neurons in the auditory system under stationary stimulus conditions T appears to be smaller than 20 msec." (Van Gisbergen et al., 1975).

A great variety of temporal response patterns is found in the VCN, among these are the primary-like pattern, the chopper, build-up and complex patterns. Van Gisbergen et al. (1975) could, however, not demonstrate any relation between the reverse correlation function and the PST histogram to tone bursts. It was concluded that the reverse correlation function solely reflects the frequency selectivity of the neuron.

An alternative method to reveal the power-spectrum of the filter characteristics of the neuron for wide-band stimulation is by computing for each part of the signal preceding a spike (PESE) the power spectrum and subsequently averaging these power spectra. A difference between the average PESE power spectrum and the power spectrum of the wide-band stimulus ensemble (SE) indicates a stimulus response relation. Figure 1 shows two examples from neurons in the VCN of the cat. One unit shows a reverse correlation function for which also the average temporal intensity and the average spectral intensity of the PESE are shown. The right-hand column shows the overall stimulus ensemble using random events (spontaneous activity) as triggers for averaging. The middle column shows results for a unit where no reverse correlation could be obtained, but nevertheless the average temporal intensity as well as the average spectral intensity differed from those for random triggers. This method therefore can give both the latency (based of the temporal intensity) and the best frequency (based of the spectral intensity). In a time window closely before the spike event, one observes in both units on average more spectral energy than in the SE, reflecting an excitatory frequency component. It may happen, though, that there is an appreciable amount of post-activation suppression. This will cause the average PESE power spectrum to contain less energy than the SE in the excitatory band in the time window of the suppression. Averaging over a large time-window, then, may result in no apparent difference between the power spectra of the PESE and the SE. A sign of this phenomenon is present in the first unit (left-hand column) in Figure 1.

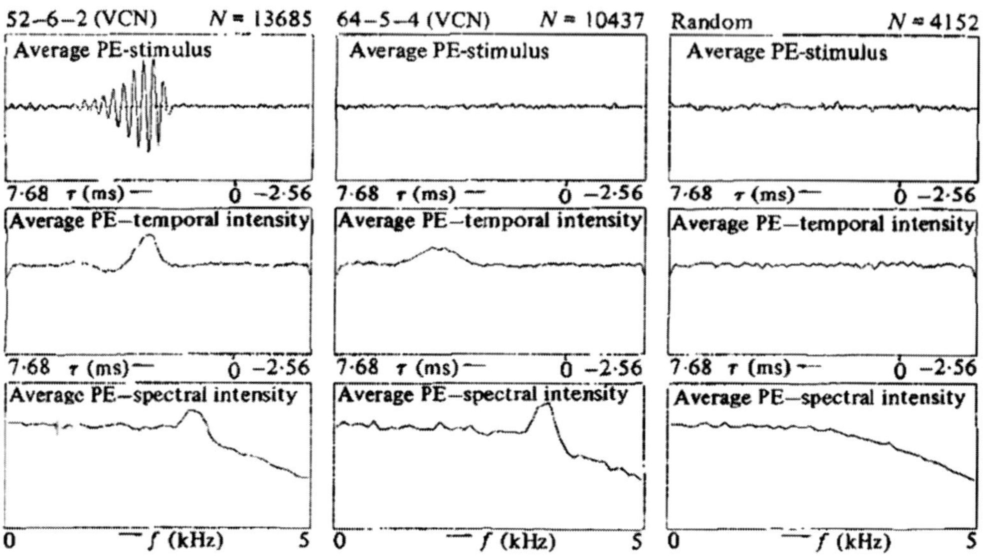

Figure 1. The effect of phase locking upon the revcor function (top row). The results for two neurons from the VCN in the cat (Johannesma and Aertsen, unpublished) are shown; they had nearly the same characteristic frequency namely about 3 kHz. One of the units, left column, shows a clear revcor function (note that the time axis runs from 7.56 ms before a spike to 2.56 ms after a spike), the other unit represented in the middle column shows no sign of a reverse correlation. For comparison the right column shows the results for spontaneous activity correlated with the noise stimulus. In the second row the average temporal intensity of the noise preceding the spikes is shown, both units show a peak superimposed upon the average noise level (cf. the right column) at about 3 (respectively 5) ms. before the spike. In the bottom row, the average spectral intensity of the noise preceding a spike is shown: again both units show a clear peak around 3 kHz superimposed upon the noise spectrum. The lack of phase locking for the second unit abolishes the reverse correlation function but relevant response properties can still be obtained using spectral and temporal intensity averaging. From Eggermont et al. (1983c) reprinted with permission from Cambridge University Press.

4. The First STRFs in Nijmegen

4.1. The Dynamic Spectrum Analyzer

In the mid 1970's Aertsen joined Johannesma as his Ph.D student and started to put some theoretical and computational meat on Johannesma's ideas for a spectro-temporal representation of neural responses. This resulted in an impressive series of papers in the journal Biological Cybernetics that methodically laid out the concept, computation and interpretation of the STRF. Because sufficient computer power (PDP 11/45) at the time was only available off-line, a real-time "Dynamic Signal Analyzer" was built. This provided the electrophysiologists, i.e., me and my students, with real-time feedback on the spectro-temporal properties of the neurons in the auditory midbrain of the grass frog. Aertsen and Johannesma (1980) wrote:

> "The main point of interest in the present paper is the *spectro-temporal characterization* of acoustic stimuli. For narrowband signals a parametric description in terms of *instantaneous amplitude* and *instantaneous frequency* appears to be attractive. A more general approach, also covering wideband signals, is a description by means of the *dynamic power spectrum.* Both types of analysis are described. Mathematically they can be based on the theory of *analytic signals.* The basic principles of this theory are summarized."

The first STRF-like representations were made using a Dynamic Spectral Analyzer (DSA). The stimulus (tone pips, natural sounds or noise) was continuously passed through a set of 1/3rd octave filters, entered a delay line that was read out whenever a spike was recorded from a neuron and averaged across spikes. This method obviously had different temporal resolution for different center frequencies of the filters, but was corrected to some extent by compensating for the frequency-specific filter delays. The papers by Johannesma et al. (1981) and Aertsen and Johannesma (1981a) suggest that the STRF is a second-order (i.e., non-linear) property of the stimulus. In their words:

> "In the present paper the STRF is considered in the general framework of nonlinear system theory, especially in the form of the Volterra integral representation. The STRF is proposed to be formally identified with a linear functional of the second order Volterra kernel. The experimental determination of the STRF leads to a formulation in terms of the Wiener expansion where the kernels can be identified by evaluation of the system's input-output correlations. For a Gaussian stimulus ensemble and a nonlinear system with no even order contributions of order higher than two, it is shown that the second order cross correlation of stimulus and response, normalized with respect to the spectral contents of the stimulus ensemble, leads to the stimulus-invariant spectro-temporal receptive field. ... Having discussed the existence and possible determination of general stimulus-invariant system characteristics we now return to the original question regarding the concept of the STRF. By the choice of the dimensions of frequency and time the STRF clearly is a second order system characteristic. In view of what has been said about stimulus-dependence we propose to let the *second order Volterra kernel*, or rather its single Fourier transform be the source of the STRF. This choice implies that a stimulus-invariant STRF of a neuron can be defined, i.e. it *exists,* provided that the neural system function meets the conditions of a convergent Volterra series expansion." (Aertsen and Johannesma, 1981a).

Others emphasized the notion that the STRF is linear in the spectro-temporal intensity density of the stimulus, i.e., the result of a cross-correlation with the stimulus (Blake and Merzenich, 2002; Valentine and Eggermont, 2004), where the STRF is the result of a linear operation on stimulus level and frequency of random tone pips. In essence, the operations on the independent linear filters in the DSA also suggest a linear relationship. This was controversial among the members of the Nijmegen group, some advocating the STRF as resulting from a non-linear analysis of the input signal, others maintaining that the STRF was just a linear correlation with a transformed input signal.

Stimulus normalization of the DSA output was obtained using the following steps (Aertsen and Johannesma, 1981b): The subtraction from the average pre-event stimulus (APES) of the a priori expected average spectrogram (AS) of the overall stimulus ensemble. This lead to the *Difference Spectrogram* DS = APES-AS. The division of each separate channel in the DS by the filter-dependent constant resulted in the *Equalized Difference Spectrogram* (EDS). The division (in the frequency domain) of the EDS by the shifted spectrum demodulated the various channels in the EDS with respect to the spectral composition of the SE at the various frequencies within the pass-band region of the corresponding DSA-filter and resulted in the *"Normalized" Pre-Event Spectrogram.* This "stimulus-equalized" average pre-event dynamic spectrum gives a first indication of the "spectro-temporal receptive field" of a neuron under natural stimulus conditions. Results for a limited number of recordings were presented (Aertsen et al., 1981) and, in general, were comparable to the outcome of an analogous analysis of experiments with tonal stimuli.

Arriving at the theoretical STRF from the experimental results by application of a formal normalization procedure was effectively hindered by the nature of the spectrogram analysis as performed in the DSA. An approximate "normalization" procedure was applied to a number of single unit recordings from the grassfrog's auditory midbrain and suggested that spectrogram analysis had fundamental shortcomings (Aertsen and Johannesma, 1981b).

For 12 neurons recorded from the midbrain in the grass frog stimulated with Gaussian wide-band noise the STRF was estimated using the DSA (Eggermont et al., 1983a). A quantitative procedure was developed to predict the neuron's response as far as it could be derived from the DSA-STRF. Adopting a linear interpretation of the DSA-STRF, this procedure basically consisted of a convolution between DSA-STRF and the spectrogram of the stimulus for each 1/3rd octave frequency band followed by a summation over the various frequency bands. In this way we estimated to what extent the DSA-STRF characterized the neuron's firing behavior. Heuristic approaches, in which the neuron was modeled by a parallel series of band-pass filters, summation across frequency bands and processing via a static nonlinearity (either a linear half-wave rectifier or a quadratic half-wave rectifier), representing a spike-generating mechanism, resulted in a considerable improvement of the characterization. Eggermont et al. (1983b) subsequently tested the usefulness of the estimated DSA-STRF for predicting responses to other stimuli such as noise with different frequency content or species-specific vocalizations. It appeared that the predicted response to vocalizations was at best in qualitative agreement with the actual response. Clearly, the STRF as a linear description of the neurons response is incomplete for characterizing the neuron's response to a wide variety of signals.

4.2. Computing Frequency-Time Distributions

A necessary part in the calculation of the STRF is the availability of a spectro-temporal representation of the stimulus and the PESE. The choice was an easily computable, albeit complex-valued spectro-temporal representation originally designed by Rihaczek (1968). The effectiveness for computation arose from the fact that this representation is separable in a spectral part and a temporal part; both simple to compute and easily cross-multiplied

(Johannesma et al., 1981; Johannesma and Aertsen, 1982). Johannesma liked to invent new words and acronyms as illustrated in the following quote (Johannesma et al., 1981):

> "Representation of simple stationary sounds can be given either in the temporal form by display of the waveform as function of time or in the spectral form by intensity and phase as function of frequency. For complex nonstationary sounds, e.g. animal vocalisations and human speech, a combined spectra-temporal representation is more directly associated with auditory perception. The well-known sonogram or dynamic power spectrum has a finite spectra-temporal resolution and neglects phase relations of different spectral and temporal sound components. In this paper the complex spectra-temporal intensity density (CoSTID; Rihaçzek, 1968) is presented as a coherent spectra-temporal image of a sound, based on the analytic signal representation. The CoSTID allows an arbitrary form of the spectra-temporal resolution and preserves phase relations of different sound components. Since the CoSTID is a complex function of two variables, it leads naturally to the use of colour images for the spectra-temporal representation of sound: the phonochrome. The phonochromes are shown for different technical and natural sounds."

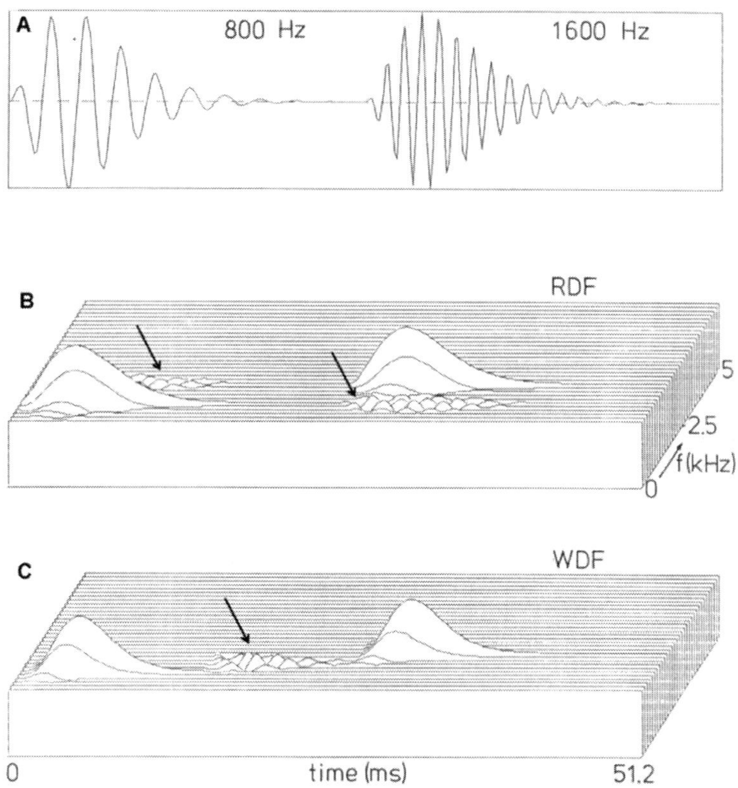

Figure 2. Rihaczek (RDF) and Wigner (WDF) distribution functions for an 800-Hz tonepip followed by a 1600-Hz tone pip as shown in (a). Interaction products occur between the two signals present within the analysis window and that do not have to be simultaneous, nor do they have to be harmonically related. These "ghosts" (indicated by arrows) are clearly visible in the RDF (b) and the WDF (c) but occur in a different place for both functions. Reprinted from Hearing Research, Vol 271, J.J. Eggermont, Context Dependence of Spectrotemporal Receptive Fields with Implications for Neural Coding, Pages 123-132, (2011), with permission from Elsevier.

Eggermont and Smith (1990) later expanded on its use and described the similarities and differences of the Rihaczek distribution (RDF) and the Wigner distribution (WDF) functions. The latter has the advantage that it is real valued and with improved processing speed compared to the RDF used in the 1980's that was a clear advantage. We also showed that a simple transformation of the real-valued WDF results in the complex RDF (see also Aertsen et al., 1984). We found no appreciable differences between the shapes of the WDF and RDF for narrow-band signals; however, the differences became obvious for signals with increasing bandwidth. For midbrain neurons under GWN stimulation, the WDF-based STRF had a smaller bandwidth than the RDF-based STRF. Thus, the analysis technique is one of the first aspects to consider when comparing STRFs across studies. The WDF of the sound-pressure waveform is correlated with the neural response by reverse correlation (Eggermont et al., 1983c). Thus, the STRF is a linear estimate of the neuron's frequency-time-filter function. For theoretical reasons, an STRF based on the Wigner distribution has many appeals (Eggermont and Smith, 1990; Kim and Young, 1994). However, the STRF based on the WDF (or the RDF) has a representation that includes "ghosts" related to the interaction between frequency components in the analysis window (Figure 2). These "ghost-like" interactions represent phase relationships of the signal components (in Figure 2 the two-tone pips) in the analysis window for the WDF or RDF (Eggermont, 2011).

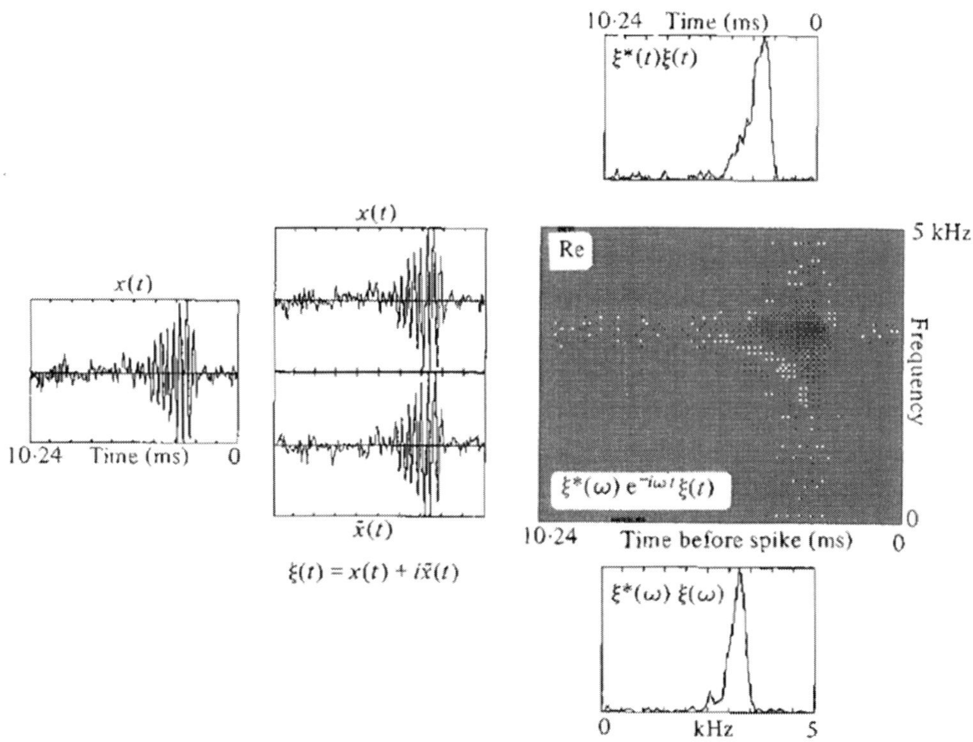

Figure 3. Construction of the 'STRF' on basis of the revcor function for a VCN unit in the cat. From the revcor function x(t), the analytic signal ξ(t) is constructed and its Fourier transform ξ(ω) is obtained. The CoSTID, $\xi^*(\omega)\, e^{-i\omega t}\, \xi(t)$, is calculated. $\xi^*(\omega)$ is the complex conjugate of ξ(ω). The STRF shows a best frequency (BF) of 3.2 kHz and a latency of 2.2 ms. A region of lateral inhibition is visible for frequencies below the BF. From Eggermont et al. (1983c) reprinted with permission from Cambridge University Press.

One can calculate an STRF on basis of the analytic signal of the revcor function, i.e., the average stimulus preceding the spike (Figure 3). However, this CoSTID is based on an averaged signal, whereas the STRF in general is based on averaging RDFs or WDFs of elements of the pre-event stimulus ensemble. The difference between the two representations is a measure of the amount of phase-lock of the neural firings to the stimulus (Eggermont and Smith, 1990).

4.3. The First STRFs for Frog Midbrain Neurons Stimulated with Noise

The CoSTID (Aertsen and Johannesma, 1981b) of the PESE for pseudo-random noise became the basis for calculating the STRF:

> "These results lead to the conclusion that in the context of a formal approach to the investigation of neuron characteristics like the spectro-temporal receptive field and its possible inherent stimulus dependence, an instrument-based (Dynamic Spectrum Analyzer) analysis like the APES shows severe shortcomings, which can only be overcome by using more refined and theoretically more firmly and elegantly based methods of spectro-temporal representation of sound. A possible example of such a method has been described as the complex spectro-temporal intensity density function CoSTID (Rihaczek, 1968; Johannesma and Aertsen, 1979; Johannesma et al., 1981). One of its essential characteristics is that, unlike the sonogram-analysis, it preserves phase-relations which are present in the signal. It has successfully been applied to the characterization of auditory neuron responses to Gaussian wideband noise (Hermes et al., 1981)."

Adopting this approach, Hermes et al. (1981) found that about 30% of the auditory units in the midbrain of the lightly anaesthetized grass frog responded in a sustained way to stationary pseudorandom noise, and computed STRFs. On basis of these STRFs, frequency selectivity, postactivation suppression and lateral inhibition could quantitatively be studied for one and the same stimulus condition. Single units that responded to stationary noise were localized in those parts of the auditory midbrain where axons entered from the olivary nucleus. For these midbrain neurons, excluding spikes from incoming axons, Eggermont et al. (1981) evaluated the STRF against the separate characterizations of frequency-sensitivity and temporal response properties. By factoring the STRF into two marginal density functions $I_1(f)$, and $I_2(t)$, one may reconstruct the joint density by multiplication: $I_1(f)* I_2(t)$ This reconstructed $\hat{I}(f,t)$ was compared to the original $I(f,t)$ for 83 neurons: in 23% of them, the $\hat{I}(f,t)$ appeared to be vastly different from $I(f,t)$. These units were located dominantly in the ventral parts of the auditory midbrain and had a latency exceeding 30 ms. This suggested to us that a spectra-temporal characterization of auditory neurons appears mandatory for investigations in and central from the auditory midbrain.

Epping and Eggermont (1985a) studied neurons in the auditory midbrain of the immobilized grassfrog using the STRF. Stationary Gaussian wide-band noise was presented to 102 units. In 65 units, noise stimulation resulted in an activation pattern clearly discernible from spontaneous activity. In 45 units an STRF could be determined. Several STRF types were observed: monomodal excitatory STRFs comprised about half of the cases (Figure 4a). Bimodal excitatory STRFs, i.e. STRFs with two discrete excitation regions, were observed in about 25% (Figure 4b). Trimodal (Figure 4c) and broadly tuned STRFs comprised about 5%. The remaining 20% of the STRFs were characterized by phenomena such as pure inhihltion (Figure 4d) lateral inhibition (Figure 4e) and post-activation suppression (Figure 4f). The distribution of best frequencies matched the frequency spectrum of the frog's vocalizations. A relative absence of monomodal units was noted in the mid frequency range. The distribution of latencies was bimodal over the range of 7-108 ms. Comparing these results with those from a previous study on lightly anesthetized grassfrogs (Hermes et al., 1981) showed that spontaneous activity, inhibitory phenomena and complex STRFs were common using immobilization, whereas these were rarely observed using anesthesia.

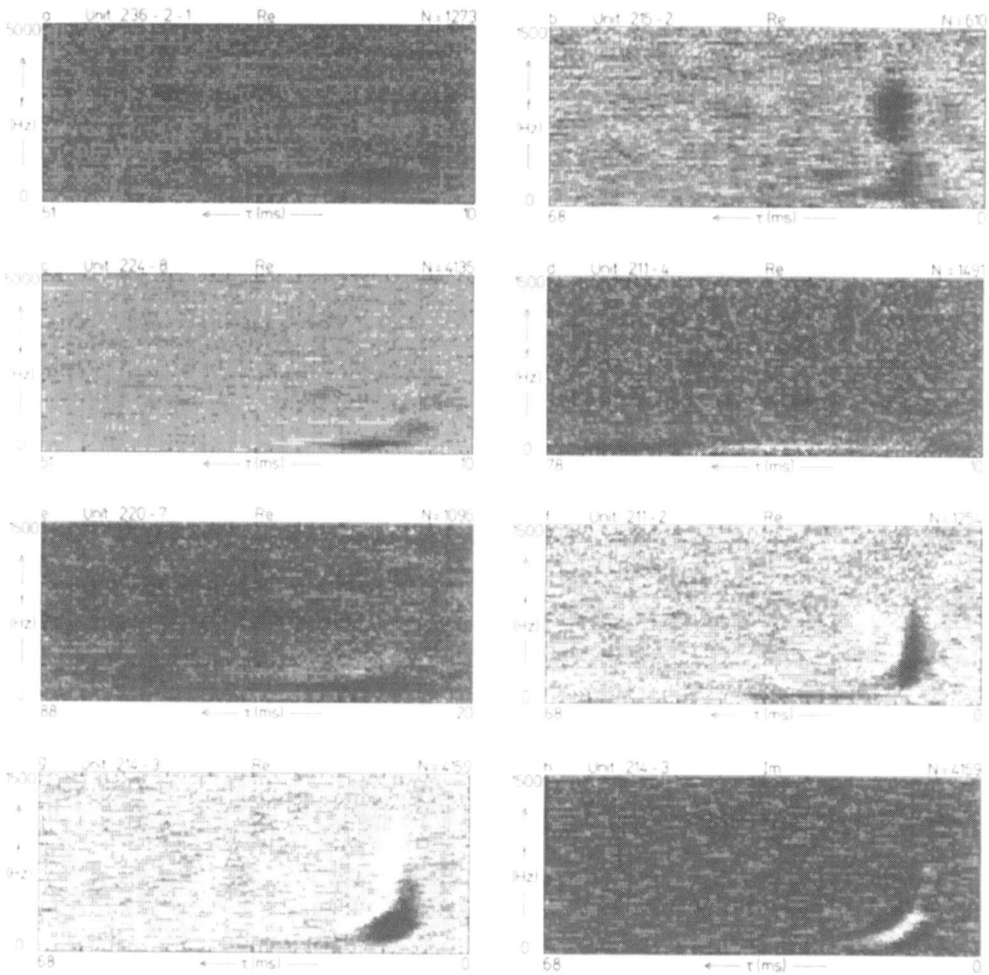

Figure 4. STRF types for continuous noise stimulation. The horizontal axis represents time before an event. The vertical axis represents frequency on a linear scale. Intensity representing activation or inhibition is coded in gray. Only the real (Re) parts of the STRF are shown except for unit 214-3. (a) Monomodal excitatory. (b) Bimodal excitatory. (c) Trimodal excitatory. (d) Inhibitory. (e) sideband Inhibition. (f) post-activation inhibition. (g) STRF indicating a preference for upward sweeping frequencies. (h) Imaginary (Im) part of the STRF for which the real part is shown in g. Reprinted from Hearing Research, Vol 18, W.J.M. Epping, W.J.M. and J.J. Eggermont, Single-unit characteristics in the auditory midbrain of the immobilized grassfrog, Pages 223-243, (1985), with permission from Elsevier.

In a subsequent paper, Epping and Eggermont (1985b) studied the relation between binaural interaction type and spectra-temporal characteristics for single units in the auditory midbrain of the grassfrog. Comparisons of ipsi-, contra- and bilateral spectra-temporal sensitivities, revealed differences in best frequency, latency and temporal discharge pattern. In some units a complex interplay of excitatory and inhibitory monaural influences was demonstrated. A number of units showed multiple activation or suppression areas. The majority of these units exhibited frequency-dependent binaural interaction types (Figure 5).

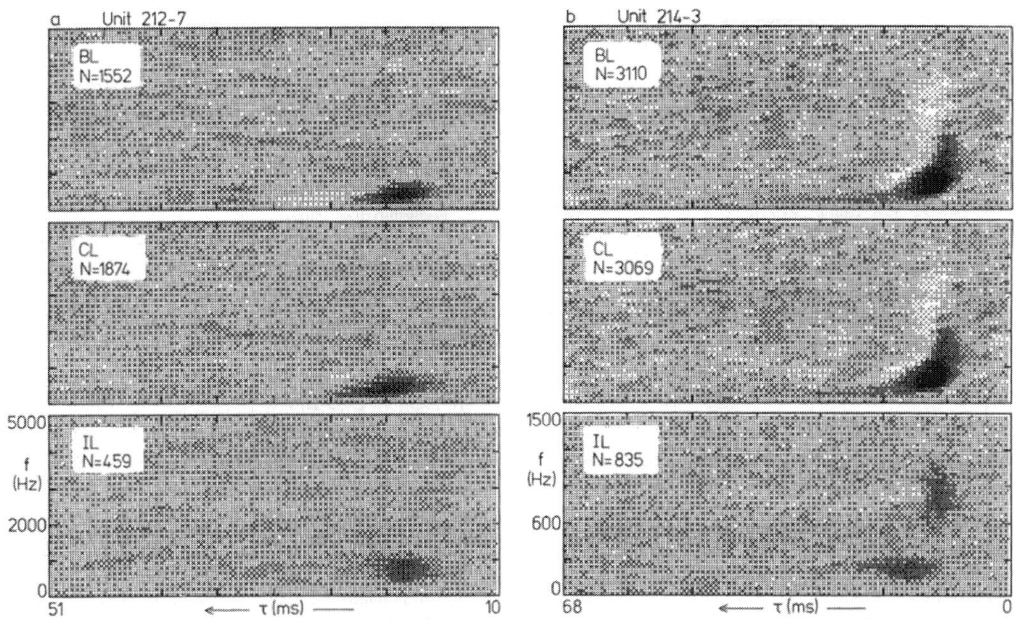

Figure 5. STRFs for continuous wideband noise stimulation presented bi- (BL), contra- (CL) and ipsilaterally (IL) at 90 dB SPL, displayed in the first, second and third rows, respectively. The horizontal axis represents time before a neural event. The vertical axis represents frequency on a linear scale. Intensity representing activation or suppression is coded in grey. Only the real parts of the complex-valued STRFs are shown. Reprinted from Hearing Research, Vol 19, W.J.M. Epping, W.J.M. and J.J. Eggermont, Relation of binaural interaction and spectro-temporal characteristics in the auditory midbrain of the grassfrog. Pages 15-28, (1985), with permission from Elsevier.

5. Crossing the Atlantic: Early Use of the STRF in Mammals

5.1 Auditory Nerve and Cochlear Nucleus

Kim and Young (1984) evaluated the potential use of STRFs and revcors in comparison to frequency-tuning curves of single auditory-nerve fibers (ANFs). Revcors were only useful for ANFs with phase-locking responses, i.e., with CF< 6 kHz, whereas STRFs were able to characterize all units studied (CFs ranging from 0.26-23 kHz). Measures of latency from revcors and STRFs were compatible with those from PSTHs. Frequency tuning curves (FTC) bandwidth derived from revcors exceeded those measured from FTCs at all CFs and increased with sound level. In contrast, STRF bandwidth was invariant to sound level. This likely reflects nonlinear properties of auditory-nerve fiber firing such as two-tone suppression that are absent in the FTC.

For wide-band noise stimulation, low-CF cells in the anteroventral cochlear nucleus (AVCN) are potentially sensitive to changes in the spatiotemporal pattern of discharges across their ANF inputs. To evaluate and characterize this sensitivity, Carney and Friedman (1998) developed a technique whereby the physiological responses of AVCN cells to wide-band noise were analyzed using the simulated response of a population of ANFs to the same noise stimulus. By averaging the simulated two-dimensional spatiotemporal pattern of ANF activity that preceded each AVCN discharge, they derived a two-dimensional reverse-correlation function that characterized the spatiotemporal tuning of each AVCN cell. The derived spatiotemporal tuning pattern represented a feature in the ANF population response that was most likely to precede discharges of the AVCN cell.

Clopton and Backoff (1991) estimated STRFs for neurons in the VCN of the guinea pig. The STRF BF corresponded to the unit's CF estimated by tone pips. The sizes of features in STRFs from the guinea pig VCN appeared significantly smaller in their temporal and spectral extents than those reported in the auditory midbrain of grass frogs and were roughly comparable to the few units reported from cat VCN (cf. Figure 1). Backoff and Clopton (1991) estimated STRFs for chopper and pauser units recorded in guinea pig dorsal cochlear nucleus (DCN) using the same noise stimuli as for the VCN. The STRFs obtained were unique to the DCN, as compared to the VCN (Clopton and Backoff, 1991) in their degree of temporal and spectral complexity. All STRFs had at least one region of elevated energy density (peak region) closely preceding spike occurrence. In addition, some units displayed low-energy regions (likely post-activation suppression) especially for higher stimulus levels.

The STRF obtained with broadband noise could account for some qualitative features of the responses of type IV neurons in cat DCN to broadband noise and spectral notches embedded therein (Nelken et al., 1997). Quantitatively, however, the STRFs failed to predict the responses of type IV units even to simple broadband noise stimuli. For narrowband stimuli, the STRF failed to predict even qualitative features (such as excitatory and inhibitory frequency bands). The responses of DCN type IV units presumably result from interactions of two inhibitory sources, a strong one that is preferentially activated by narrowband stimuli and a weaker one that is preferentially activated by broadband stimuli. These results suggested that the STRF measures effects related to the broadband inhibition, whereas two-tone interactions measure mostly effects related to narrowband inhibition. This explains why models based on two-tone interactions predicted the DCN responses to narrow bands of noise much better then models based on STRFs.

5.2. Midbrain and Cortex

Using random-chord stimuli and STRFs, deCharms et al. (1998) demonstrated that neurons in the primary auditory cortex of the awake monkey have complex spectro-temporal features (Figure 6). The traditional frequency-tuning curve (Figure 6A) was computed by counting the number of spikes elicited from a single auditory cortical neuron by 100-ms pure-tone pips presented at 84 frequencies and eight intensities (scale bar in spikes per stimulus, intensities in decibel SPL). The STRF (Figure 6B) shows the spectro-temporal structure of the same neuron in response to random chords with synchronous onset times for each component in the chord. The STRF in (Figure 6C) was recomputed for the same neuron with a stimulus set for which all individual tone pips were presented at completely random and asynchronous times. The resulting STRF is the same. The neurons shown in (Figure 6D,E) had a receptive field structure with strong sideband inhibition and complex combinations of excitation and inhibition. The neuron shown in (Figure 6F) had an STRF that showed both side-band inhibition and post-activation suppression. Neurons could also show a pattern of response within the STRF is strongly analogous to motion energy detectors (Figure 6G). The red line on the panel illustrates the slope of an FM stimulus that drove the strongest response from this cell. The neurons shown in (Figs. 6B, C, H, and I) had complex multimodal receptive field structures, with multiple excitatory or inhibitory subregions.

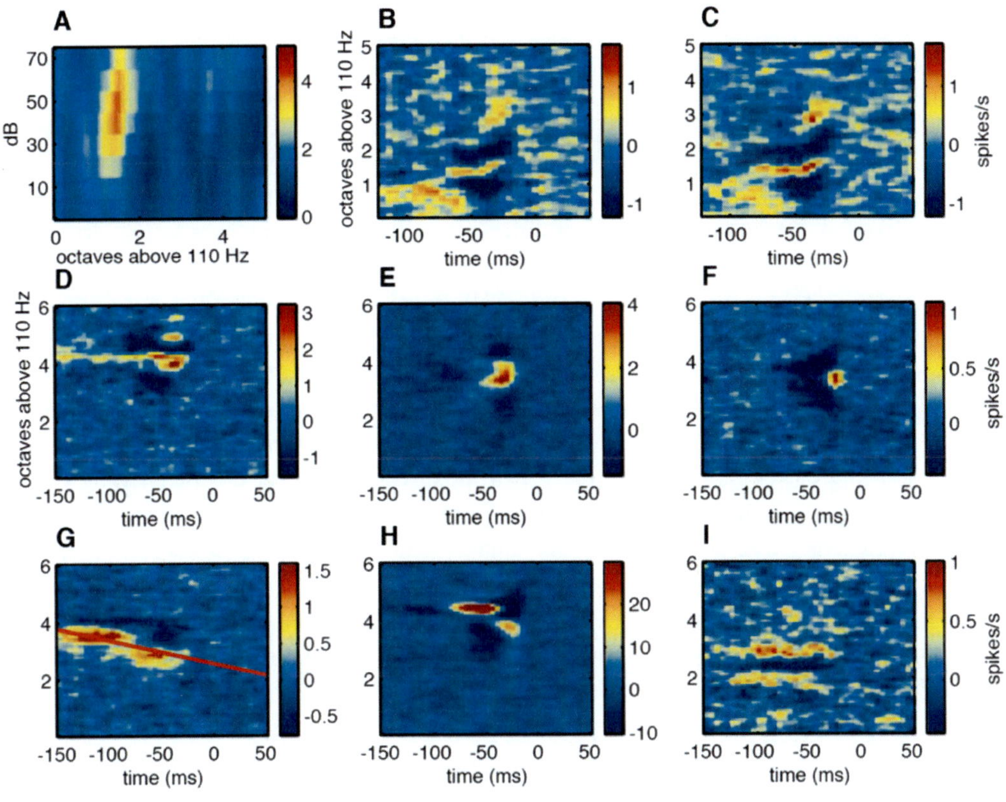

Figure 6. The STRFs (B-I) of neurons in the primary auditory cortex of the awake primate show the pattern of sound features selected for by particular neurons. Part A shows the frequency tuning curve corresponding to the STRF shown in part B. Further description in the text. From deCharms, R.C., Blake, D.T., Merzenich, M.M., 1998. Optimizing sound features for cortical neurons. Science 280, 1439-1443. Reprinted with permission from AAAS.

Rutkowski et al (2002) reported STRFs of single units in the primary (A1) and dorsocaudal (DC) fields, and the ventrorostral belt of the urethane-anaesthetized guinea pig auditory cortex. The STRFs recorded from each cortical area indicated temporal response properties consistent with those shown by traditional peristimulus time histogram analysis. Overall, fields A1 and DC showed no significant differences in the distribution of STRF types. Thus, it appears that both fields display similar spectro-temporal sensitivities to auditory stimuli and therefore, appear to process such stimuli in a parallel fashion. Single units recorded in the ventrorostral belt area showed STRF types similar to those recorded in A1 and DC but with different proportions, suggesting a difference in spectro-temporal processing between the ventrorostral belt and the core areas. Valentine and Eggermont (2004) showed that for random multi-tone stimuli the STRF can, in addition to reverse correlation, also be obtained as the frequency-dependent PSTH (forward correlation), representing the spike times following the onsets of every tone pip over a 100-ms time window. The STRFs obtained with these two methods, reverse and forward correlation, differed in their temporal resolution owing to the smoothing action of the tonepip envelope in the reverse correlation.

It appears that the cortical STRFs in awake animals are more complex than those in anesthetized ones, indicated particularly by the much stronger inhibition visible in awake animals.

6. Experimental and Computational Advances

Despite the appeal of quantitative descriptions of the auditory system using STRF estimates based on GWN stimulation, GWN is a poor stimulus for neurons in higher auditory areas. Stimuli useful for assessing STRFs in higher brain areas included dynamic random chords (Blake and Merzenich, 2002; Rutkowski et al., 2002; Valentine and Eggermont, 2004), and animal vocalizations (Theunissen et al., 2000; Machens et al., 2004). While still broadband, these stimuli have a more specific structure than that of GWN.

Shamma (1996) described the use of a variant of the Gaussian white-noise approach for STRFs based on stimulation with broadband sounds having dynamic spectra. These sounds were named moving ripples. The ripple spectrum has a sinusoidal profile drifting along a logarithmic frequency axis at a constant velocity. The carrier of the profile can be a broadband noise or a series of tones that are equally spaced in frequency.

This stimulus has been used in a series of papers that initially only showed the properties of the responses to such stimuli but did not show STRFs (Schreiner and Calhoun, 1994; Calhoun and Schreiner, 1998; Shamma and Versnel, 1995; Shamma et al., 1995; Versnel et al., 1995), further addressed by Kowalski et al (1996ab) and Versnel and Shamma (1998). Kowalski et al (1996a) used moving ripples to characterize the responses of both single and multiple units in the ferret primary auditory cortex. Neuronal responses to moving ripples were locked to the phase of the ripple, i.e., they exhibit the same periodicity as that of the moving ripple profile. Neural responses were characterized as a function of ripple velocity (temporal property) and ripple frequency (spectral property). STRFs were not shown in this paper, neither in Kowalski et al. (1996b) where they tested the predictive power of the ripple transfer function. They concluded that A1 cells in the ferret may encode the profile of a dynamic spectrum by performing a multiscale spectro-temporal decomposition of the dynamic spectral profile in a largely linear manner. The first STRFs using this method were reported in journal paper form by Klein et al. (2000) and Depireux et al. (2001). An improvement was found in temporally orthogonal ripple combinations (TORCs; Fritz et al., 2003; Elhilali et al., 2004). The spectral ripple stimuli are very effective in eliciting spikes if the frequencies in the spectral peak match the neuron's excitation regions and the neighboring spectral valleys match the neuron's inhibitory side bands. By using stimuli with a large number of peak-valley combinations the spectral tuning of the neuron is estimated. The various ripple stimuli and the random multi-tone stimuli typically have long-term broad flat spectra and random temporal properties that make them useful for reverse correlation procedures.

6.1. A Variety of Ripples

Escabi and Schreiner (2002) compared dynamic moving ripple (DMR) stimuli and ripple noise (RN) to systematically characterize response attributes with the STRF in the central nucleus of the inferior colliculus (ICC). STRFs derived with DMR and RN would be identical for a linear integrating neuron, and ~60% of ICC neurons met this basic requirement. The remaining neurons were distinctly nonlinear; they either responded selectively to DMR or produced no STRFs despite selective activation by spectro-temporal acoustic attributes. Klein et al. (2006) explored the origin of, and relationship between, different ways of measuring and analyzing an STRF. They demonstrated that in the ferret A1 STRFs measured using dynamic ripples, spectro-temporally white noise, and TORCs were very similar, confirming earlier findings that the STRF is a robust linear descriptor of the cell. They also presented a new deterministic analysis framework that allowed estimation of temporal modulation transfer functions, contained in the stimuli and responses.

White noise has power over all possible ripple components. Auditory nerve fibers are able to respond to an extended set of ripple components; however, at the level of A1, the range of densities and modulation rates to which neurons are responsive is quite narrow. Thus, the power of the dynamic spectrum is typically focused over this relevant range of ripple components. The drawback is that the various ripple stimuli are no longer uncorrelated. A partial solution was found in a TORC stimulus. Although uncorrelated, these orthogonal ripples are not independent (Christianson et al., 2008), which can cause nonlinear interactions between them showing up in the STRF. These broadband stimuli likely bias cortical cells in a manner different from that of narrowband or transient stimuli such as tones and clicks. Consequently, predicting details of tone and click responses from the broadband-based STRF has proven to be problematic. Christianson et al. (2008) demonstrated analytically and in simulations that, even when uncorrelated stimuli are used, interactions between simple neuronal nonlinearities and higher-order structure in the stimulus can produce STRFs that show contributions from time–frequency combinations to which the neuron is actually insensitive. Only when spectro-temporally independent stimuli are used, as in the random multitone stimuli, does the STRF reliably indicate features of the underlying receptive field, and even then it provides only a conservative estimate.

6.2. Natural Sounds

Theunissen et al. (2000) found that the STRFs derived using natural sounds were often strikingly different from the STRFs that were obtained using an ensemble of random tone pips. This again emphasizes that the STRF is context dependent and not an invariant characterization of a neuron (Gourévitch et al. 2009). The STRF for natural sounds is still informative and efficient (Theunissen et al. 2004) because it described the basic tuning of the neuron during the processing of complex sounds such as birdsong. Gill et al. (2006) systematically investigated the effects of four factors in the non-linear step in the STRF model: the choice of logarithmic or linear filter frequency spacing, the time-frequency scale, stimulus amplitude compression and adaptive gain control. They quantified the goodness of fit of these different STRF models on data obtained from auditory neurons in the songbird midbrain and forebrain. They found that adaptive gain control and the correct stimulus amplitude compression scheme are crucial to correctly modeling neurons. David et al. (2009) explored ways to account more accurately for responses of neurons in A1 to natural sounds. They compared STRFs for A1 neurons estimated using continuous speech, with STRFs estimated using synthetic ripple noise. For about one-third of the neurons significant differences between these STRFs were found, usually in the temporal dynamics of inhibition and/or overall gain. This shift in tuning resulted primarily from differences in the coarse temporal structure of the speech and noise stimuli. They speculated that synaptic depression may enable efficient encoding of natural auditory stimuli.

6.3. Separability of the STRF

Separability in frequency and time has been investigated in a heuristic way from the very first computation of STRFs from the auditory midbrain (Eggermont et al., 1981). More recently, solid analyses investigated this for ripple-based stimuli and recordings from A1 and IC. Depireux et al. (2001) measured the responses to upward and downward drifting ripples, assuming separability within each direction, to determine if the total bidirectional transfer function is fully separable. In general, the combined transfer function for two directions was not symmetric, and hence units in A1 were not, in general, fully separable. Consequently, many A1 units had complex response properties such as sensitivity to direction of motion, though most inseparable units were not strongly directionally selective. Qiu et al. (2003) reported the properties of monaural STRFs and the relationship between ipsi- and contralateral inputs to neurons of the ICC of cats. First, they used an optimal singular-value decomposition method to approximate auditory STRFs as a sum of time-frequency separable Gabor functions. The STRFs of 60% of collicular neurons are well described by such separable Gabor STRF model, whereas the remaining neurons exhibited obliquely oriented or multiple excitatory/inhibitory subfields that require a non-separable Gabor fitting procedure. Parametric analysis revealed distinct tradeoffs in receptive field size and modulation filtering resolution.

7. Current Use of the STRF

7.1. STRFs Based on Membrane Potentials, Local Field Potentials or Evoked Potentials

Machens et al. (2004) recorded subthreshold membrane potential fluctuations in response to complex sounds, including animal vocalizations, with in vivo whole-cell methods in the rat auditory cortex. Note that this is expected to give different STRFs compared to those based on spikes; typically the STRF frequency-bandwidths are much narrower for spikes. The obtained STRFs had a rich dynamical structure, including excitatory regions positioned in general accord with the prediction of the classical tuning curve. On average, only 11% of the response power to natural stimuli could be predicted by the STRF. This could not be attributed to simple nonlinearities such as adaptation to mean intensity, rectification, or saturation. The highly nonlinear response properties of auditory cortical neurons were attributed to nonlinear interactions between sound frequencies (see also Pienkowski and Eggermont (2010) for spike based STRFs).

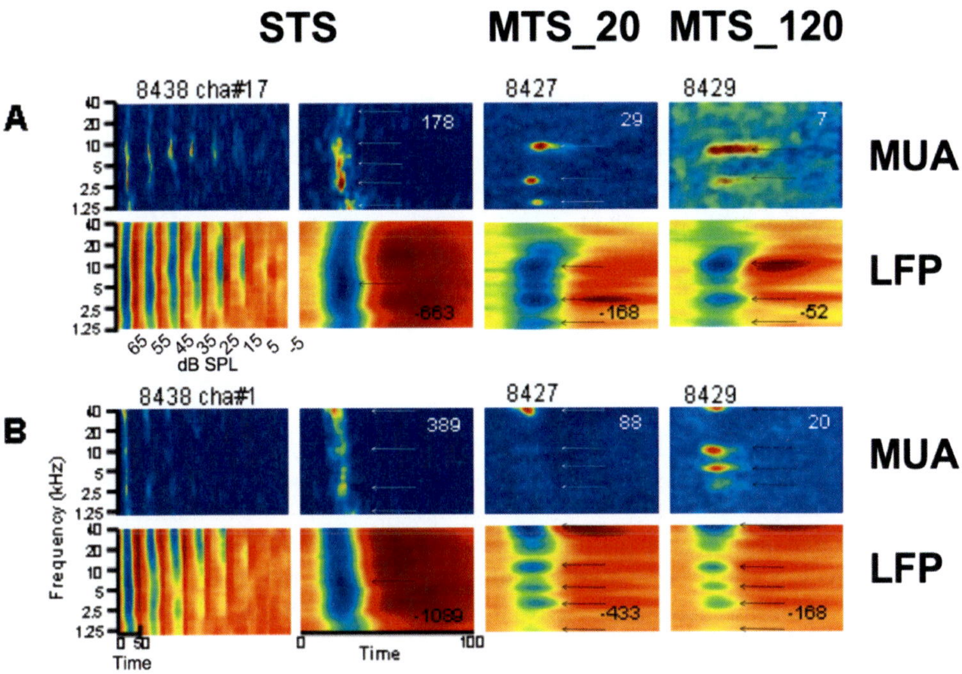

Figure 7. Examples of STRF obtained from LFPs (second and fourth rows) and MUA (first and third rows) from two electrodes (recordings were not simultaneous). The tuning curves are shown in the first column; responses over a 50 ms window (from stimulus onset) obtained with intensity levels between 5 (right) and 65 dB SPL (left) are stacked. The second column shows the STRF derived from the STS condition at the same level (65 dB SPL) used for deriving STRF from the two MTS stimuli. The third and fourth columns show the STRFs derived from MTS_20 (stimulus rate 20/s) and MTS_120 (stimulus rate 120/s), respectively. Numbers within each panel (columns 2-4) indicate the maximum firing rate (for MUA, first and third rows) and the negative peak amplitude (for LFPs, second and fourth rows). For MUA (first and third rows), the color scale indicates the firing rate, from dark blue (minimal responses, corresponding to spontaneous firing rate) to dark red (maximal responses). For LFPs (second and fourth rows), the color indicates the amplitude of the potentials, from dark blue (negative potentials, which correspond to excitatory synaptic potentials; see Results, Individual examples) to dark red (positive potentials). From Noreña et al. (2008). Reprinted with permission from the Society for Neuroscience.

Noreña et al. (2008) obtained STRFs from responses to random multi-frequency stimuli differing in their average spectro-temporal density (i.e., number of tone pips per second). STRFs for different stimulus densities were derived from multi -unit activity (MUA) and local field potentials (LFPs), simultaneously recorded in primary auditory cortex of cats (Figure 7). Consistent with earlier studies, they found that the spectral bandwidth was narrower for MUA than for LFPs. Both neural firing rate and LFP amplitude were reduced when the density of the stimulus ensemble increased. Surprisingly, increasing the spectro-temporal sound density revealed an over-representation of response peaks at frequencies of 3, 5, 10, and 20 kHz, in both MUA- and LFP-derived STRFs. Although the decrease in spectral bandwidth and neural activity with increasing stimulus density can likely be accounted for by forward suppression, the mechanisms underlying the over-representation of the octave-spaced response peaks are unclear.

Ding and Simon (2012) obtained magnetoencephalography (MEG) recordings from human subjects actively listening to spoken narratives, in both simple and cocktail party-like auditory scenes. Note that the MEG represents compound synaptic potentials. By modeling how acoustic features of speech are encoded in ongoing MEG activity as a spectro-temporal response function, they demonstrated that the slow temporal modulations of speech in a broad spectral region were represented bilaterally in auditory cortex by a phase-locked temporal code, i.e., an STRF. For speech presented monaurally to either ear, this phase-locked response was always more faithful in the right hemisphere, but with a shorter latency in the hemisphere contralateral to the stimulated ear. The early sensory response to the attended speech was considerably stronger than that to the unattended speech, demonstrating top-down attentional gain control.

7.2. STRFs for FM Sounds

Single unit responses at the auditory midbrain of the anesthetized rat were characterized by STRFs for random frequency modulated (FM) tones (Poon and Yu, 2000). Roughly half of the neurons showed clearly preferred stimulus time profiles that formed single, double or multiple bands. Neurons with a single-band STRF appeared to be sorted into positive or negative directional sensitivity for FM modulation on the basis of their CF either below or above 10 kHz. STRFs obtained from the same unit at different frequency regions generated a composite receptive field covering a wider frequency range of 2 to 3 octaves. Multiple-bands in a given composite map were often oriented in the same direction (representing upward or downward FM ramps) separated at rather regular frequency intervals. Results showed that the subcortical auditory pathways are capable of detecting multiple FM features and such sensitivity could be useful in detecting multiple-harmonic FM bands present in the vocalization sounds. (Chiu and Poon, 2007).

Andoni et al. (2007) investigated how neurons in the inferior colliculus (IC) of Mexican free-tailed bats responded to the frequency-modulated (FM) direction and velocity of complex signals by extracting their STRFs using upward- and downward-moving ripple stimuli. STRFs were obtained in more than half of the cells sampled. Responses to tones were in close agreement with the STRF and the responses predicted by convolutions compared favorably with responses evoked by those calls. Most neurons were selective for the direction and velocity of spectral motion with a majority favoring the downward FM direction, and most had spectrum–time inseparability that correlated with their direction selectivity.

Using an implanted array of microelectrodes in the primary auditory cortex of two awake owl monkeys Atencio et al. (2007) quantitatively characterized neuronal responses to FM sweeps and to random tonepip stimuli. Tone-pip responses were used to construct STRFs. Classification of FM sweep responses revealed few neurons with high direction and speed selectivity. Most neurons responded to sweeps in both directions and over a broad range of sweep speeds. Characteristic frequency estimates from FM responses were highly correlated with estimates from STRFs, although spectral receptive field bandwidth was consistently underestimated by FM stimuli. Predictions of FM direction selectivity and best speed from STRFs were significantly correlated with observed FM responses, although some systematic discrepancies existed.

7.3. Partitioning the Auditory Bird Brain on Basis of STRFs

Sen et al. (2001) recorded from several regions of the songbird auditory forebrain to a large ensemble of bird songs and used these data to calculate the STRFs. These neurons responded to a wide variety of features in songs ranging from simple tonal components to more complex spectral-temporal structures such as frequency sweeps and multi-peaked frequency stacks. These results reveal successively more complex functional stages of song analysis by neurons in the auditory forebrain, suggestive of hierarchical processing. The most obvious differences were found in the temporal domain, i.e., in increased latencies and response durations. Kim and Doupe (2011) investigated the spatial organization of field L in multiple anatomical planes, using multielectrode array recordings and a stimulus that captures aspects of spectro-temporal modulations of song. The data demonstrated two separate axes along which spectro-temporal aspects of sound were mapped: width of spectral tuning changed systematically from narrow to broad mediolaterally, whereas width of temporal tuning changed markedly, from narrow to broad, from the input to the output layers. These spatial patterns, which were evident in STRFs computed from both multiple and single units, resulted in a mapping of basic STRF types to subregions of field L. This highly organized representation of spectro-temporal features of sound contrasts with current views of mammalian auditory cortex.

In songbirds, vocalizations drive auditory neurons particularly well. Woolley et al. (2006) used STRFs to study the neural encoding of song versus the encoding of a generic sound, modulation-limited noise, by single neurons and the neuronal population in the zebra finch auditory midbrain. The noise was designed to match song in frequency, spectro-temporal modulation boundaries, and power. STRF calculations were balanced between the two stimulus types by forcing a common stimulus subspace. They found that 91% of midbrain neurons showed significant differences in spectral and temporal tuning properties when birds heard song and when birds heard modulation-limited noise. During the processing of noise, spectro-temporal tuning was highly variable across cells. During song processing, the tuning of individual cells became more similar; frequency tuning bandwidth increased, best temporal modulation frequency increased, and spike timing became more precise. The outcome was a population response to song that encoded rapidly changing sounds with power and precision, resulting in a faithful neural representation of the temporal pattern of a song. Woolley et al. (2009) suggested that auditory neurons could be classified into functional groups, each of which plays a specific role in extracting distinct complex sound features. They measured the STRFs of single auditory neurons in the songbird midbrain and forebrain to conspecific song. Based on STRF shape, cells were clustered into functional groups that represented cues for the fundamental acoustic percepts of pitch, timbre, and rhythm. Four major groups were found in the midbrain, and five major groups were found in the forebrain.

7.4. STRFs are Context Dependent

In the best realization of a random chord stimulus (Blake and Merzenich 2002; Tomita and Eggermont 2005; Noreña et al. 2008), the temporal sequence of tone pips of a given frequency is drawn from a Poisson distribution, and different frequencies have temporal sequences independent of each other. As a result, the overall temporal sequence of the stimulus is also a realization of a Poisson process. The density is basically the average overlap in frequency and time of the tone pips. As density increased (column 2-4 in Figure 7), cortical excitatory receptive fields became narrower in the frequency domain and had slightly longer latencies in anesthetized cat AI. The largest changes occurred between the STS (single-tone stimulation) condition and the MTS_20 (multi-tone stimulation at 20/s). Further changes by increasing the tone pip rate to 120/s could have dramatic changes on the spike-based STRF but not for LFP-based STRF (Figure 7B) suggesting changes in AI concurrent to those in the output from the MGBv (the LFPs). Receptive field sensitivity, expressed as the expected change in firing rate after a tone pip onset, decreased by an order of magnitude with increasing density. However, spectral selectivity more than doubled.

Frequency-tuning curves obtained for single tone stimuli typically show a level-dependent bandwidth, suggesting level dependence of STRFs. Valentine and Eggermont (2004), using random chord stimuli, found that in 35% of recordings the excitatory STRF regions in cat AI were very similar for single tone and multi-frequency stimuli across a 60 dB intensity range. In the remaining 65% the common finding was the emergence of an intensity independent STRF shape for the multi-frequency stimuli over an intensity range of 5-65 dB SPL. As a consequence, these cortical neurons tended to show narrower tuning and level invariance for multi-frequency stimuli compared to the V-shaped tuning curves resulting from single frequency stimuli. At lower stimulus levels the spectral bandwidths became very similar for the different densities.

Using broadband sounds to estimate STRFs imperfectly reflects the way neurons process complex stimuli like conspecific vocalizations insofar as natural sounds often show limited bandwidth (see also Nelken et al., 1997; Section 5.1). Using recordings in the primary auditory cortex of anesthetized cats, Gourévitch et al. (2009) showed that presentation of narrowband stimuli not including the best frequency of neurons resulted in the appearance of residual peaks and increased firing rate at some specific spectral edges of stimuli compared with classical STRFs obtained from broadband stimuli (Figure 8). A comparison between columns 2 and 3 shows this very clearly, column 2 represents the STRFs obtained for broadband multi-tone stimulation, and column 3 the averaged result for 6 one-octave-band multi-tone stimuli (individual bands shown in columns 4/5). Potential mechanisms likely involve release from inhibition. This emphasized an important aspect of context dependency of STRFs, namely how the balance of inhibitory and excitatory inputs is able to shape the neural response from the spectral content of stimuli.

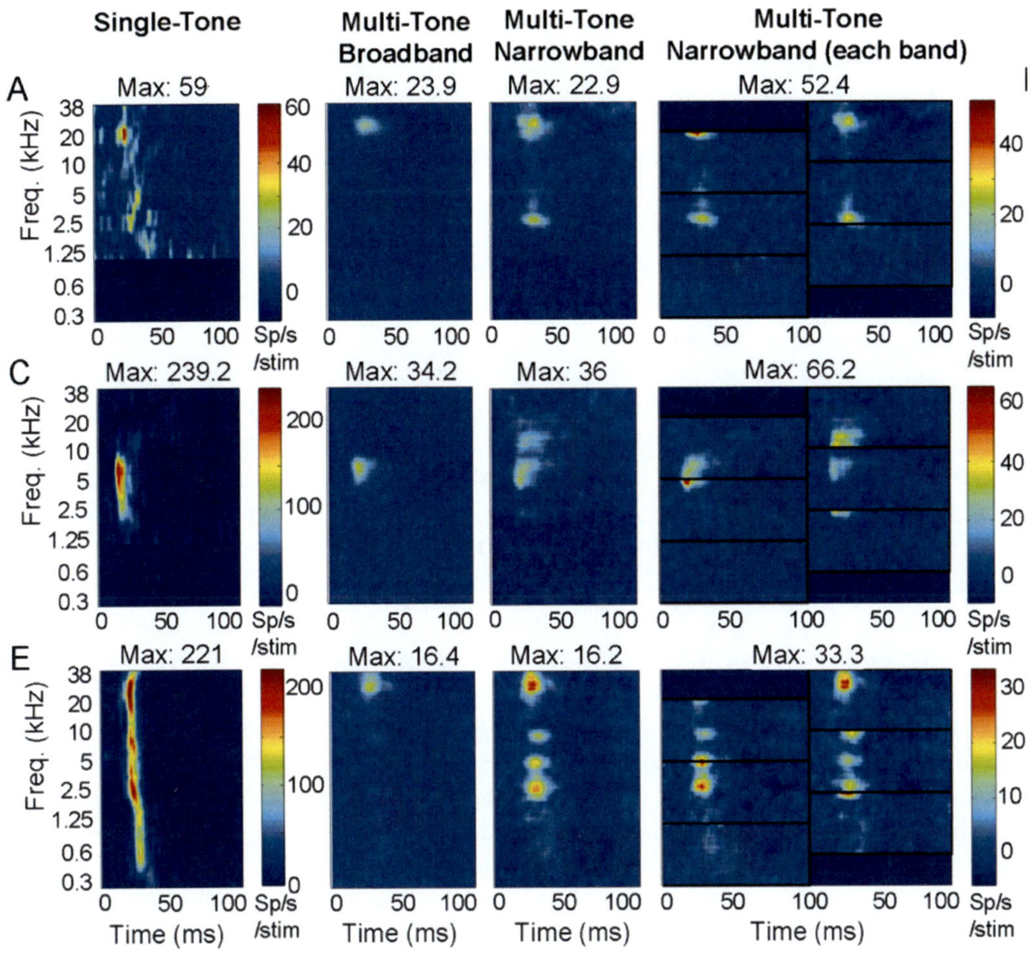

Figure 8. Individual examples illustrating the modifications in the STRFs induced by the presentation of narrowband sounds. (A, C, E) Single unit--based STRFs obtained from the presentation of (left to right) (column 1) single tones separated of 250 ms, (column 2) multiple tones at 24 pips per octave per s over 7 octaves (broadband stimulus), (columns 4 and 5) the same multiple tones organized in 15-s-long bands of 2-octaves wide (narrowband stimulus). Each band shows a 1-octave overlap with the previous and the following bands. Column 3 the sum of the results in columns 4 and 5. Same scales (spikes per stimulus per s) have been used for multiple tones broadband- and narrowband-evoked STRFs in each case (see color bars). From Gourévitch, B., Noreña, A., Shaw, G., Eggermont, J.J., Spectro-temporal receptive fields in anesthetized cat primary auditory cortex are context dependent. Cereb. Cortex, 2009, 19, 1448-1461, by permission of Oxford University Press.

The distribution of neuronal characteristic frequencies over the area of AI roughly reflects the tonotopic organization of the cochlea. However, because the area of AI activated by any given sound frequency increases erratically with sound level (Phillips et al., 1994), it has generally been proposed that frequency is represented in AI not with a rate-place code but with some more complex, distributed code. On the basis of both spike and LFP recordings in cat, Pienkowski and Eggermont (2011) showed that the tonotopic representation in AI is much more level tolerant when mapped with spectro-temporally dense tone pip ensembles than with individually presented tone pips. That is, the tuning properties of individual unit and LFP STRF responses are less variable with sound level under dense compared with sparse stimulation, and the spatial frequency resolution achieved by the AI neural population at moderate stimulus levels (65 dB SPL) is better with densely than with sparsely presented sounds. This implies that nonlinear processing in the central auditory system can compensate (in part) for the level-dependent coding of sound frequency in the cochlea, and suggests that there may be a functional role for the cortical tonotopic map in the representation of complex sounds.

7.5. STRFs Probe Neural Plasticity

Fritz et al. (2003) found that cortical neurons' responses may change their properties to reflect changing behavioral salience of certain sensory features. Attention to salient acoustic features in auditory tasks can influence receptive field properties of cortical neurons (Fritz et al., 2005a). Ferrets were trained on spectral tasks, including tone detection and two-tone discrimination, and on temporal tasks, including gap detection and click-rate discrimination. STRF recorded in A1 changed within minutes of task onset. During spectral tasks, there were specific spectral changes, whereas in the temporal tasks the STRF was changed by sharpening temporal dynamics. In ferrets trained on multiple tasks, distinctive and task-specific STRF changes could be observed in the same cortical neurons in successive behavioral sessions. Fritz et al. (2005b) recorded from A1 in ferrets also trained on a frequency discrimination task. A distinct pattern of STRF change was found, which was characterized by a selective enhancement at the target tone frequency but also by an equally selective depression at the reference tone frequency. When single-tone detection and frequency discrimination tasks were performed sequentially, neurons responded differentially to identical tones, reflecting distinct predictive values of stimuli in the two behavioral contexts. Thus, rapid task-related plasticity is an ongoing process that dynamically adapts cortical STRFs in response to changing acoustic demands. To explore receptive field changes to more complex spectral patterns, Fritz et al. (2007) trained ferrets to detect variable, multi-tone targets in the context of background, rippled noise. Recordings from A1 of behaving ferrets showed a consistent pattern of plasticity with enhancement for each component tone frequency and suppression for inter-tone frequencies. Plasticity was strongest near neuronal best frequency, with fast onset and long persistence. Attention was not needed for the persistence of the receptive field changes. Atiani et al. (2009) subsequently explored the neural correlates of attention effects by measuring rapid changes of STRFs in primary auditory cortex during detection of a target tone embedded in noise. STRF shape changes were excitatory and specific and strongest in cells with best frequencies near the target tone. Cells with best frequencies remote from the target tone were generally suppressed. This enhanced the representation of the target tone relative to the noise. These adaptive STRF changes were largest when the animals performed their task well and suggest that STRF's shape and strength strongly correlate with behavior.

7.6. STRFs and Auditory System Non-Linearity

The transformation of auditory information from the cochlea to the cortex is highly nonlinear, e.g., changing stimulus level can cause a shift in a neuron's preferred frequency. Lesica and Grothe (2008) used STRFs to characterize the effects of stimulus level in the mammalian IC. At low levels, they found that STRFs were relatively simple, typically consisting of a single excitatory region, indicating that the neural response is simply a reflection of the stimulus amplitude at the preferred frequency. In contrast, at high intensities STRFs typically showed a combination of an excitatory region and one or more inhibitory regions, often in a spectro-temporally inseparable arrangement. Versnel et al. (2009) characterized STRFs of single units in alert monkey IC by using a variety of broadband sounds. A variety of dynamic STRFs, with a strong preference for low ripple densities, and weak direction selectivity was found. Most cells preferred dynamic rippled stimuli above pure amplitude modulated noise. The data of Versnel et al (2009), together with those of Andoni et al. (2007) and Lesica and Grothe (2008), indicate that responses can be predicted on the basis of STRFs similarly well in IC as in A1.

While the STRF can predict the overall course of the response to a novel stimulus, it is unable to account for aspects of the neural output, which are inherently nonlinear. Shechter and Depireux (2010) measured the STRFs of neurons in A1 of the awake ferret using ripple stimuli. They quantified the degree of nonlinearity of these neurons by comparing their responses to those predicted from their respective STRFs. The responses of most cells in A1 showed a second-order relation to the stimuli used to evoke them. Thus, the nonlinearity of these cells was not solely the result of spike rate rectification or saturation. By using a static polynomial nonlinearity, the predictive power of the STRF could significantly be improved (cf Eggermont et al., 1983 ab).

The effects of nonlinear interactions between different sound frequencies on the responses of neurons in cat AI were investigated by Pienkowski and Eggermont (2010). They stimulated with relatively dense, Poisson-distributed trains of tone pips (with frequency ranges spanning five octaves, 16 frequencies/octave, and mean rates of 20 or 120 pips /s; MTS_20 and MTS_120 in Figure 7), and examined within-frequency (or auto-frequency) and cross-frequency interactions We used the Wiener–Volterra approach to analyze nonlinear cross-frequency interactions in STRFs exhibiting two distinct excitatory peaks ("dual-peaked"), a single excitatory peak ("single-peaked"), and a single excitatory peak flanked by one or more inhibitory valleys ("peak-valley"). We found evidence of combination-sensitivity for the two peaks in only a minority (<25%) of dual-peak interactions, although never a supralinear facilitation of the isolated-pip response. Second-order kernels invariably demonstrated a depression of (first-order) excitation, but in combination-sensitive units, that depression was reduced during cross-frequency compared to auto-frequency interactions. That is, combination-sensitive units responded more strongly to a pair of pips drawn from different excitatory-frequency bands compared to those from the same-frequency bands, though in both cases the average response to a pip was sublinear. In recordings with single-peaked and peak-valley STRFs, responses to excitatory frequencies by nonexcitatory (single-peaked) and inhibitory (peak-valley) frequencies were also depressed at short (<50 ms) interstimulus lags, but facilitated at longer lags of <50–200 ms. This favors detection of onset responses to e.g., consonants, with potential enhancement for longer lasting stimulus components such as vowels. This facilitation was stronger and more prevalent in peak-valley compared to single-peaked units. Finally, facilitative-type interactions in all three STRF types decreased with increasing spectro-temporal stimulus density.

7.7. STRFs Used to Assess Neural Connectivity

Miller et al. (2001) focused on the transformation of sensory representations in the lemniscal auditory thalamocortical network (MGBv-AI) in the cat. While stimulating with a complex sound, they recorded simultaneously from functionally connected cell pairs in the ventral medial geniculate body and AI. Thalamic action potentials that immediately preceded or potentially caused a cortical spike were more selective than the average thalamic spike for spectro-temporal stimulus features. Thus, for some thalamic cells, spikes are not propagated through cortex independently but interact with other inputs onto the same target cell. The spectro-temporal nature of these interactions was found to be cooperative or antagonistic to the average receptive field of the thalamic cell. Therefore some thalamic spikes carry more receptive field information than average and cooperate to constrain the information communicated through a cortical cell. Spectral integration, as measured by excitatory bandwidth and spectral modulation preference, was similar for MGBv and AI (Miller et al., 2002). Temporal modulation rates derived from the STRFs were higher in MGBv (best modulation frequency = 32.4 Hz, limiting rate = 62.9 Hz) compared to cortex (best modulation frequency = 16.6 Hz, limiting rate = 37.4 Hz). No correlation between spectral and temporal integration properties was found, suggesting that the excitatory-inhibitory interactions underlying preference in each domain are largely independent.

Excitatory pyramidal neurons and inhibitory interneurons constitute the main elements of cortical circuitry and have distinctive morphologic and electrophysiological properties. Pyramidal neurons have longer duration APs and discharge as regular-spiking units (RSUs), whereas basket and chandelier cells, which are inhibitory interneurons, have shorter APs and are fast-spiking units (FSUs). To compare these neuronal classes, Atencio and Schreiner (2008) stimulated cat AI neurons with a dynamic moving ripple stimulus and constructed single-unit STRFs. FSUs had shorter latencies, broader spectral tuning, greater stimulus specificity, and higher temporal precision than RSUs. The STRF structure of FSUs was more separable, suggesting more independence between spectral and temporal processing regimens. The nonlinearities associated with the two cell classes were indicative of higher feature selectivity for FSUs. Atencio and Schreiner (2010a) then studied the relationships between functional connectivity and receptive field properties in a columnar microcircuit by simultaneously recording from single neurons in cat AI in response to broadband dynamic moving ripple stimuli. STRFs were used to estimate the relationship between receptive field parameters and the functional connectivity between pairs of neurons. Cross-correlation between units in different layers was consistent with information flow from thalamic input layers to cortical output layers. Correlation strength and STRF similarity were greatest for intralaminar neuron pairs and in supragranular layers and weaker for interlaminar projections. Interlaminar correlation co-varied with several STRF parameters. Correlation properties and receptive field relationships differed for vertical and horizontal connections. Thus, the mode of local processing in supragranular layers differs from that in infragranular layers. To further examine the layer-specific processing of acoustic modulation information, Attencio and Schreiner (2010b) simultaneously recorded from multiple AI laminae in the anesthetized cat. STRFs were obtained for dynamic moving ripple stimuli. Temporal and spectral modulation transfer functions (tMTFs, sMTFs) were calculated and compared across layers. On average, neural responses followed higher temporal modulations in layer IV compared to layer II/III and VI. tMTFs were mainly band-pass in granular layer IV and became more low-pass in infragranular layers. Compared with layer IV, sMTFs were broader and their upper cutoff frequencies higher in layers V and VI. In about 70% of individual penetrations, temporal modulation preference was similar across layers. By contrast, only about 30% of penetrations showed consistent spectral modulation preferences across layers.

Along the iso-frequency domain in cat AI, regions with predominantly narrowly tuned (NT) neurons are segregated from regions with more broadly tuned (BT). Attencio and Schreiner (2012) identified these NT and BT regions with STRFs to broad-band ripple stimuli. The durations of STRF excitatory and inhibitory subfields were shorter and the best temporal modulation frequencies were higher for BT neurons than for NT neurons, following the 'standard' frequency-time resolution trade off. For NT neurons, the bandwidth of excitatory and inhibitory subfields was matched, whereas for BT neurons it was not. However, spectrotemporal interactions and nonlinear input/output behavior appeared similar for both neuronal subgroups. They suggested that spectral integration modules (BT vs. NT) in AI differ in what specific stimulus aspects are processed, but they are similar in the manner in which stimulus information is processed.

8. Outlook

The average STRF is a robust linear descriptor of a neuron's or population response to complex stimuli. Within this STRF, non-linear aspects of the transformation from stimulus to response are buried; they can be extracted by computing STRFs based on stimulus functionals. In simple form this computation is based on polynomial correlation with the higher order orthogonal Hermite polynomials, which for normalized power are x^2-1, x^3-3x, x^4-6x^2+3, etc., i.e., one correlates spike times with the transformed stimulus x. This only evaluates the main diagonals of the stimulus-response non-linearity matrix but gives at least an indication of the presence of non-linearities (Eggermont et al., 1983c, Eggermont 1993). In reverse correlation techniques, the requirement of vast numbers of spikes is likely prohibitive to go beyond third order. Using more rapidly converging basis functions to decompose the neural non-linearity may alleviate these practical problems. Volterra kernels can be estimated far more accurately (and from shorter data-records) by use of the Laguerre expansion technique adapted to point-process inputs. This technique employs the orthonormal basis of Laguerre functions to expand the system kernels, and then uses least-squares fitting to estimate the requisite expansion coefficients (Marmarelis and Berger, 2005). A more basic problem will, however, remain: a Gausian noise stimulus, continuous or spectrally filtered, will linearize the neurons stimulus-response relation (Spekreijse and Oosting, 1970), so that the non-linearities that manifest themselves for 'simple' stimuli cannot be predicted. Use of linear-nonlinear methods are ad-hoc correction/estimation procedures that aim to deal with this problem. The remainder of this book is specifically aimed at providing the background of these techniques.

Acknowledgments

I like to thank Ad Aertsen for confirming my memories of the conception years of the STRF and commenting on an earlier version of the manuscript. This work was supported by the Campbell McLaurin Chair for Hearing Deficiencies and Alberta Innovates-Health Solutions.

References

Aertsen, A.M.H.J., Johannesma, P.I.M., 1980. Spectro-temporal receptive fields of auditory neurons in the grassfrog. I. Characterization of tonal and natural stimuli. *Biol. Cybern.* 38, 223-234.

Aertsen AM, Johannesma PI. (1981a) The spectro-temporal receptive field. A functional characteristic of auditory neurons. *Biol Cybern*. 42(2):133-43.

Aertsen AM, Johannesma PI. (1981b) A comparison of the spectro-temporal sensitivity of auditory neurons to tonal and natural stimuli. *Biol Cybern*. 42(2):145-56.

Aertsen, A.M.H.J., Olders, J.H.J., Johannesma, P.I.M., 1981. Spectrotemporal receptive fields of auditory neurons in the grassfrog. III. Analysis of the stimulus-event relation for natural stimuli. *Biol. Cybern*. 39, 195-209.

Aertsen AMHJ, Johannesma PIM, Bruijns J, Koopmans PWM (1984) Second-order representation of signals. In: *Localization and orientation in biology and engineering*, pp 38-41; Varju D, Schnitzler H-U (eds). Berlin Heidelberg Springer.

Andoni S, Li N, Pollak G D. 2007. Spectrotemporal Receptive Fields in the Inferior Colliculus Revealing Selectivity for Spectral Motion in Conspecific Vocalizations. *The Journal of Neuroscience* 27(18): 4882– 4893

Atencio CA, Blake DT, Strata F, Cheung SW, Merzenich MM, Schreiner CE. 2007. Frequency-modulation encoding in the primary auditory cortex of the awake owl monkey. *J Neurophysiol*. 98(4):2182-95.

Atencio CA, Schreiner CE. 2008. Spectrotemporal processing differences between auditory cortical fast-spiking and regular-spiking neurons. *J Neurosci*. 28(15):3897-910.

Atencio CA, Schreiner CE. 2010a. Laminar diversity of dynamic sound processing in cat primary auditory cortex. *J Neurophysiol*. 103(1):192-205.

Atencio CA, Schreiner CE. 2010b. Columnar connectivity and laminar processing in cat primary auditory cortex. *PLoS ONE* 5(3): e9521.

Atencio CA, Schreiner CE. 2012. Spectrotemporal Processing in Spectral Tuning Modules of Cat Primary Auditory Cortex. *PLoS ONE* 7(2): e31537

Atiani S, Elhilali M, David, SV, Fritz JB, Shamma SA. 2009. Task Difficulty and Performance Induce Diverse Adaptive Patterns in Gain and Shape of Primary Auditory Cortical Receptive Fields. *Neuron* 61, 467–480.

Backoff, P.M., Clopton, B.M., 1991. A spectrotemporal analysis of DCN single unit responses to wideband noise in guinea pig. *Hear. Res*. 53, 28-40.

Blake, D.T., Merzenich, M.M., 2002. Changes of AI receptive fields with sound density. *J. Neurophysiol.* 88, 3409-3420.

Calhoun BM, Schreiner CE. 1998. Spectral envelope coding in cat primary auditory cortex: linear and non-linear effects of stimulus characteristics. *Eur J Neurosci* 10: 926-940.

Carney LH, Friedman M. 1998. Spatiotemporal Tuning of Low-Frequency Cells in the Anteroventral Cochlear Nucleus. *The Journal of Neuroscience* 18(3): 1096–1104.

Chiu TW, Poon PWF. 2007. Multiple-Band Trigger Features of Midbrain Auditory Neurons Revealed in Composite Spectro-Temporal Receptive Fields *Chinese Journal of Physiology* 50(3): 105-112.

Christianson, G.B., Sahani, M., Linden, J.F., 2008. The consequences of response nonlinearities for interpretation of spectrotemporal receptive fields. *J. Neuroscie*. 28, 446-455.

Clopton, B.M., Backoff, P.M., 1991. Spectrotemporal receptive fields of neurons in cochlear nucleus of guinea pig. *Hear. Res*. 52, 329-344

David, S.V., Mesgarani, N., Fritz, J.B., Shamma, S.A., 2009. Rapid synaptic depression explains nonlinear modulation of spectro-temporal tuning in primary auditory cortex by natural stimuli. *J. Neurosci*. 29, 3374-3386

de Boer, E. (1967) Correlation studies applied to the frequency resolution of the cochlea. *J. Audit. Res*. 7, 209-217.

de Boer, E. (1968) Reverse correlation I. *Proc. K. Ned. Acad. Wet*. C71, 472-486.

de Boer, E. (1969) Reverse correlation II. *Proc. K. Ned. Acad. Wet*. C72, 129-151.

de Boer, E. (1973) On the principle of specific coding. *J. Dynamical Systems, Measurement and Control* 95G 265-273.

de Boer, E. and de Jongh, H.R. (1978) On cochlear encoding: potentialities and limitations of the reverse correlation technique. *J. Acoust. Sot. Am*. 63, 115-135.

De Boer E, Jongkees LBW. 1968. On cochlear sharpening and cross-correlation methods. *Acta oto-laryngologica* 65, 97-104

de Boer, E. and Kuijper, P. (1968) Triggered correlation. *IEEE Trans. BME* 15, 169-179.

deCharms, R.C., Blake, D.T., Merzenich, M.M., 1998. Optimizing sound features for cortical neurons. *Science* 280, 1439-1443.

Depireux, D.A., Simon, J.Z., Klein, D.J., Shamma, S.A., 2001. Spectro-temporal response field characterization with dynamic ripples in ferret primary auditory cortex. *J. Neurophysiol*. 85, 1220-1234.

Ding N, Simon JZ. 2012. Neural coding of continuous speech in auditory cortex during monaural and dichotic listening. *J Neurophysiol* 107: 78–89.

Eggermont, J.J., 1993. Wiener and Volterra analyses applied to the auditory system. *Hear. Res*. 66, 177-201.

Eggermont JJ. (2011) Context Dependence of Spectrotemporal Receptive Fields with Implications for Neural Coding. *Hearing Research* 271: 123-132.

Eggermont, J.J., Aertsen, A.M.H.J., Hermes, D.J. and Johannesma, P.I.M. (1981): Spectro-temporal characterization of auditory neurons: redundant or necessary? *Hearing Research* 5: 109-121.

Eggermont, J.J., Aertsen, A.M.H.J., Johannesma, P.I.M., 1983a. Quantitative characterization procedure for auditory neurons based on the spectra-temporal receptive field. *Hear. Res*. 10, 167-190.

Eggermont, J.J., Aertsen, A.M.H.J., Johannesma, P.I.M., 1983b. Prediction of the responses of auditory neurons in the midbrain of the grass frog based on the spectro-temporal receptive field. *Hear. Res*. 10, 191-202

Eggermont, J.J., Johannesma, P.I.M., Aertsen, A.M.H.J., 1983c. Reverse-correlation methods in auditory research. *Q. Rev. Biophys.* 16, 341-414.

Eggermont, J.J., Smith, G.M.,1990. Characterizing auditory neurons using the Wigner and Rihacek distributions: a comparison. *J. Acoust. Soc. Am.* 87, 246-259.

Elhilali, M., Fritz, J.B., Klein DJ, Simon JZ, Shamma, S.A., 2004. Dynamics of Precise Spike Timing in Primary Auditory Cortex. *The Journal of Neuroscience*, 24(5): 1159 –1172

Epping, W.J.M., Eggermont, J.J., 1985a. Single-unit characteristics in the auditory midbrain of the immobilized grassfrog. *Hear. Res.* 18, 223-243.

Epping, W.J.M. and Eggermont, J.J. (1985b): Relation of binaural interaction and spectro-temporal characteristics in the auditory midbrain of the grassfrog. *Hearing Research* 19: 15-28

Escabí ME, Christoph E. Schreiner CE. 2002. Nonlinear Spectrotemporal Sound Analysis by Neurons in the Auditory Midbrain.*The Journal of Neuroscience* 22(10): 4114–4131

Fritz, J., Shamma, S., Elhilali, M., Klein, D., 2003. Rapid task-related plasticity of spectrotemporal receptive fields in primary auditory cortex. *Nat. Neurosci.* 6, 1216-1223.

Fritz, J., Elhilali, M., Shamma, S., 2005a. Active listening: task-dependent plasticity of spectrotemporal receptive fields in primary auditory cortex. *Hear. Res.* 206, 159-176.

Fritz, J.B., Elhilali, M., Shamma, S.A., 2005b. Differential dynamic plasticity of A1 receptive fields during multiple spectral tasks. *J. Neurosci.* 25, 7623–7635.

Fritz, J.B., Elhilali, M., Shamma, S.A., 2007. Adaptive changes in cortical receptive fields induced by attention to complex sounds. *J. Neurophysiol.* 98, 2337-2346.

Gill P, Zhang J, Woolley SMN, Fremouw T, Theunissen FE. 2006. Sound representation methods for spectro-temporal receptive field Estimation. *J Comput Neurosci* 21(1):5-20.

Gourévitch, B., Noreña, A., Shaw, G., Eggermont, J.J., 2009. Spectro-temporal receptive fields in anesthetized cat primary auditory cortex are context dependent. *Cereb. Cortex* 19, 1448-1461.

Hermes, D.J., Aertsen, A.M., Johannesma, P.I., Eggermont, J.J., 1981. Spectro-temporal characteristics of single units in the auditory midbrain of the lightly anaesthetized grass frog (Rana temporaria L) investigated with noise stimuli. *Hear. Res.* 5, 147-178.

Johannesma, P.I.M. (1972) The pre-response stimulus ensemble of neurons in the cochlear nucleus. In: B.L. Cardozo (Ed.), *Proceedings of the IPO symposium on Hearing Theory.* Eindhoven: IPO. pp. 58-69.

Johannesma, P.I.M., Aertsen, A.M.H.J. 1979. Neural image of sound in the grassfrog. In: Hearing mechanisms and speech, Creutzfeld, O., Scheich, H., Schreiner, Chr. (eds.). Exp. *Brain Res.* [Suppl. II]: 79-86.

Johannesma P, Aertsen A. 1982. *Statistical and Dimensional Analysis of the Neural Representation of the Acoustic Biotope of the Frog Journal of Medical Systems*, 6 (4): 399-421.

Johannesma, P., Aertsen, A., Cranen, B., van Erning, L., 1981. The phonochrome: a coherent spectra-temporal representation of sound. *Hear. Res.* 5, 123-145.

Kim G, Doupe A. 2011. Organized Representation of Spectrotemporal Features in Songbird Auditory Forebrain. *The Journal of Neuroscience* 31(47):16977–16990

Kim, P.J., Young, E.D., 1994. Comparative analysis of spectro-temporal receptive fields, reverse correlation functions, and frequency tuning curves of auditorynerve fibers. *J. Acoust. Soc. Am.* 95, 410-422.

Klein, D.J., Depireux, D.A., Simon, J.Z., Shamma, S.A., 2000. Robust spectrotemporal reverse correlation for the auditory system: optimizing stimulus design. *J. Comput. Neurosci.* 9, 85-111.

Klein, D.J., Simon, J.Z., Depireux, D.A., Shamma, S.A., 2006. Stimulus-invariant processing and spectrotemporal reverse correlation in primary auditory cortex. *J. Comput. Neurosci.* 20, 111-136.

Kowalski, N., Depireux, D.A., Shamma, S.A., 1996a. Analysis of dynamic spectra in ferret primary auditory cortex. I. Characteristics of single-unit responses to moving ripple spectra. *J. Neurophysiol.* 76, 3503-3523.

Kowalski N, Depireaux DA, Shamma SA. 1996b. Analysis of dynamic spectra in ferret primary auditory cortex. II. Prediction of unit responses to arbitrary dynamic spectra. *J Neurophysiol* 76: 3524–3534.

Lesica, N.A., Grothe, B., 2008. Dynamic spectrotemporal feature selectivity in the auditory midbrain. *J. Neurosci.* 28, 5412-5421.

Machens, C.K., Wehr, M.S., Zador, A.M., 2004. Linearity of cortical receptive fields measured with natural sounds. *J. Neurosci.* 24, 1089-1100.

Marmarelis VZ, Berger TW. 2005. General methodology for nonlinear modeling of neural systems with Poisson point-process inputs. *Mathematical Biosciences* 196: 1–13.

Marmarelis, P.Z. and Marmarelis, V.Z. (1978) *Analysis of physiological systems: the white noise approach.* Plenum Press, New York.

Miller LM, Escabí MA, Read HL, Schreiner CE. 2001. Functional Convergence of Response Properties in the Auditory Thalamocortical System.*Neuron* 32, 151–160.

Miller LM, Escabí MA, Read HL, Schreiner CE. 2002. Spectrotemporal receptive fields in the lemniscal auditory thalamus and cortex. *J Neurophysiol* 87: 516–527.

Nelken, I., Kim, P.J., Young, E.D., 1997. Linear and nonlinear spectral integration in type IV neurons of the dorsal cochlear nucleus. II. Predicting responses with the use of nonlinear models. *J. Neurophysiol.* 78, 800-811.

Noreña, A.J., Gourévitch, B., Pienkowski, M., Shaw, G., Eggermont, J.J., 2008. Increasing spectrotemporal sound density reveals an octave-based organization in cat primary auditory cortex. *J. Neurosci.* 28, 8885-8896.

Palm, G. and Pöpel, B. (1985) Volterra representation and Wiener-like identification of non-linear systems: scope and limitations. *Quart. Rev. Biophysics* 18, 135-164.

Pienkowski M, Eggermont JJ. (2010) Nonlinear Cross-Frequency Interactions in Primary Auditory Cortex Spectrotemporal Receptive Fields: A Wiener-Volterra Analysis. *J Comput Neurosci* 28: 285-303.

Pienkowski, M. and Eggermont, J.J. (2011) Sound frequency representation in primary auditory cortex is level tolerant for moderately loud, complex sounds. *J. Neurophysiol,* 106: 1016-1027.

Phillips DP, Semple MN, Calford MB, Kitzes LM. (1994) Level-dependent representation of stimulus frequency in cat primary auditory cortex. *Exp Brain Res* 102: 210–226.

Poon PWF, Yu PP. 2000. Spectro-temporal receptive ®elds of midbrain auditory neurons in the rat obtained with frequency modulated stimulation *Neuroscience Letters* 289: 9-12

Qiu A, Schreiner CE, Escabí MA. 2003. Gabor analysis of auditory midbrain receptive fields: spectro-temporal and binaural composition. *J Neurophysiol* 90: 456-476.

Rihaczek AW. 1968. Signal Energy Distribution in Time and Frequency *IEEE Trans on Information Theory IT*-14: 369-374

Rutkowski, R.G., Shackleton, T.M., Schnupp, J.W., Wallace, M.N., Palmer, A.R., 2002. Spectrotemporal receptive field properties of single units in the primary, dorsocaudal and ventrorostral auditory cortex of the guinea pig. *Audiol. Neurootol.* 7, 214-227.

Schnupp J, Nelken I, King A. 2010. *Auditory Neuroscience: Making Sense of Sound.* MIT Press.

Schreiner CE, Calhoun BM. 1994. Spectral envelope coding in cat primary auditory cortex. Properties of ripple transfer functions. *Auditory Neuroscience* 1: 39-61.

Sen, K., Theunissen, F.E., Doupe, A.J., 2001. Feature analysis of natural sounds in the songbird auditory forebrain. *J. Neurophysiol.* 86, 1445-1458.

Shamma SA. 1996. Auditory cortical representation of complex acoustic spectra as inferred from the ripple analysis method. *Network: computation in neural systems* 7: 439-476.

Shamma S, Versnel H, Kowalski N. 1995. Ripple analysis in the ferret primary auditory cortex. I. Response characteristics of single units to sinusoidally rippled spectra *J. Audit. Neurosci.* 1: 233–54

Shamma S, Versnel H. 1995. Ripple analysis in the ferret primary auditory cortex. II. Prediction of unit responses to arbitrary spectral profiles *J. Audit. Neurosci.* 1: 255–70

Shechter B, Depireux DA. 2010. Nonlinearity of coding in primary auditory cortex of the awake ferret. *Neuroscience* 165: 612-620.

Spekreijse H, Oosting J. 1970. Linearizing: A method for analysing and synthesizing nonlinear systems. *Kybernetik* 7: 23-31.

Theunissen, F.E., Sen, K., Doupe, A.J., 2000. Spectral-temporal receptive fields of nonlinear auditory neurons obtained using natural sounds. *J. Neurosci.* 20, 2315-2331.

Theunissen FE, Woolley SMN, Hsu A, Fremouw T. 2004. Methods for the analysis of auditory processing in the brain. *Ann. N.Y. Acad. Sci.* 1016: 187–207

Tomita, M., Eggermont, J.J., 2005. Cross-correlation and joint spectro-temporal receptive field properties in auditory cortex. *J. Neurophysiol.* 93, 378-392.

Valentine, P.A., Eggermont, J.J., 2004. Stimulus dependence of spectro-temporal receptive fields in cat primary auditory cortex. *Hear. Res.* 196, 119-133.

van Gisbergen JAM, Grashuis JL, Johannesma PIM, Vendrik AJH. 1975. Neurons in the cochlear nucleus Investigated with tone and noise stimuli. *Exp. Brain Res.* 23, 387—406.

Versnel H, Kowalski N, Shamma SA. 1995. Ripple analysis in ferret primary auditory cortex: III. Topographic distribution of ripple response parameters. *Aud Neurosci* 1:271–285.

Versnel H, Shamma SA. 1998. Spectral-ripple representation of steady-state vowels in primary auditory cortex. *J Acoust Soc Am* 103(5): 2502-2514

Versnel, H., Zwiers, M.P., van Opstal, A.J., 2009. Spectrotemporal response properties of inferior colliculus neurons in alert monkey. *J. Neurosci.* 29, 9725-9739.

Wallace MN, Rutkowski RG, Shackleton TM, Palmer AR. 2000. Phase-locked responses to pure tones in guinea pig auditory cortex. *Neuroreport* 11, 3989-3993

Wallace MN, Coomber B, Sumner CJ, Grimsley JMS, Shackleton TM, Palmer AR. 2011. Location of cells giving phase-locked responses to pure tones in the primary auditory cortex. *Hearing Research* 274: 142-151.

Woolley SMN, Gill PR, Fremouw T, Theunissen FE. 2009. Functional Groups in the Avian Auditory System. *The Journal of Neuroscience* 29(9): 2780 –2793

Woolley, S.M., Gill, P.R., Theunissen, F.E., 2006. Stimulus-dependent auditory tuning results in synchronous population coding of vocalizations in the songbird midbrain. *J. Neurosci.* 26, 2499-2512.

In: Handbook of Modern Techniques in Auditory Cortex ISBN: 978-1-62808-894-6
Editors: Didier A. Depireux and Mounya Elhilali

Chapter 2

A Linear System's View to the Concept of STRFs

***Mounya Elhilali*[1], *Shihab Shamma*[2,3], *Jonathan Z. Simon*[2,3,4] *and Jonathan B. Fritz*[3]**
[1]Department of Electrical & Computer Engineering, Johns Hopkins University, Baltimore, Maryland, US
[2]Department of Electrical & Computer Engineering, University of Maryland, College Park, Maryland, US
[3]Institute for Systems Research, University of Maryland, College Park
[4]Department of Biology, University of Maryland, College Park, Maryland, US

1. Introduction

A key requirement in the study of sensory nervous systems is the ability to effectively characterize neuronal response selectivity. In the visual system, striving for this objective yielded remarkable progress in understanding the functional organization of the visual cortex and its implications to perception. For instance, the discovery of ordered feature representations of retinal space, color, ocular dominance, orientation, and motion direction in various cortical fields has catalyzed extensive studies into the anatomical bases of this organization, its developmental course, and the changes it undergoes during learning or following injury. In the primary auditory cortex (A1), response selectivity of the neurons (also called their *receptive fields*) is ordered topographically according to the frequency they are most tuned to, an organization inherited from the cochlea. Beyond their tuning, however, A1 responses and receptive fields exhibit a bewildering variety of dynamics, frequency bandwidths, response thresholds, and patterns of excitatory and inhibitory regions. All this has been learned over decades of testing with a large variety of acoustic stimuli (tones, clicks, noise, and natural sounds) and response measures (tuning curves, rate-level functions, and binaural maps).

A response measure that has proven particularly useful beyond the feature-specific measures enumerated earlier is the notion of a generalized *spatiotemporal*, or equivalently for the auditory system, the *spectro-temporal receptive field* (STRF). It is distinguished from other measures by its broader descriptive power (encompassing both dynamics and spectral selectivity) and its relatively noncommittal nature (not requiring too much prior knowledge such as frequency tuning or threshold). In the last two decades, the STRF has become widely employed in all sensory systems (Aertsen & Johannesma, 1981; De Valois & De Valois, 1988; DeAngelis, Ohzawa, & Freeman, 1995; Gosselin & Schyns, 2002; Hochstein & Shapley, 1976; Sripati, Yoshioka, Denchev, Hsiao, & Johnson, 2006), and especially in the auditory system where it had found its original promise, development, and examination of its value and liability (Aertsen & Johannesma, 1981; De Boer, 1967; de Boer & de Jongh, 1978; Sripati et al., 2006). The STRF has primarily been viewed as a linear characterization of the complex stimulus-response transformations seen in sensory neurons. However, there are well-understood limitations of the STRF ability to capture all the essential details of a sensory neuron's response. These stem from the existence of a host of known nonlinearities such as spiking threshold, rate saturation, synaptic-depression that can complicate the interpretation of the STRF and render its representation stimulus dependent or meaningless. Nevertheless, the utility of the STRF has inspired deeper and broader examination of its constraints and pitfalls, of ways to circumvent them (Atencio, Sharpee, & Schreiner, 2008; Christianson, Sahani, & Linden, 2008; David, Hayden, & Gallant, 2006; Nagel & Doupe, 2008) or even exploit them to learn more about the nonlinearities in the system (Ahrens, Linden, & Sahani, 2008; Klein, Simon, Depireux, & Shamma, 2006; Theunissen, Sen, & Doupe, 2000). In the following sections, we explore the mathematical bases of the STRF, its richness and limitations, and ways to estimate it reliably. We then briefly review its utility in a wide range of investigations, including the cortical encoding of sound and the exploration of learning and rapid plasticity during behavior.

2. Systems Approach to Characterizing Cortical Neurons

Approaches to understanding sound processing in the auditory system, particularly at the level of auditory cortex, have often treated neurons as "black-box" devices; i.e. systems whose internal workings are opaque, but that can be mathematically described solely in terms of their input-output relationship. Each neuron is then understood as a transducer that is driven via sensory stimulation by external sounds to evoke a neural response. In absence of any stimulation, the neuron is in its spontaneous (or quiet) state. When presented with a sensory input, the neuron is driven to spike either actively above its spontaneous state; or in a suppressive manner below its spontaneous state. The pattern of neural firing depends on the characteristics of the sensory stimulation and its match to the neuron's own tuning properties.

By understanding how a stimulus can drive a neuron to fire in an excitatory or inhibitory fashion, one gains better insight into the functional role of this neuron in sensory information processing, its tuning characteristics, and predictive knowledge of the neuron's behavior under any stimulation conditions.

Clearly, the ability to fully describe the workings and behavior of neurons (even if treated as black boxes) is often impossible. The transducer view of neurons is only possible when the neuron's output is controlled *solely* by its sensory input. Most sub-cortical stages can be reduced –somewhat- to this transducer view. Such is not the case for sensory cortex, where many neurons appear to play a role not only in sensory encoding, but also in memory, decision and behavior; therefore integrating information across a neural network spanning one or many neural loci. As the circuitry becomes more intricate, it is often impossible to understand the role of a single neuron in abstraction of the complex dynamics of the network in which it exists.

With this caveat in mind, on can still employ a number of tools to gain elementary insight into the sensory information encoding of cortical neurons, the topic of interest in this issue. Systems theory provides the mathematical language to characterize the behavior of neurons (or systems in general), and provide a better understanding of their function (Bender, 2000). For many complex systems, such as the nervous system, this characterization often focuses on investigating the dependencies of the output function (neural response) on the input function (input stimulation). This approach adopts the viewpoint of *functionals*, in which the signal as a whole is considered, rather than its values at given points in time. In other words, the neuron is viewed as a transducer of an input signal $s(t)$ to a neural response $r(t)$ via a mapping F:

$$r(t) = F[s(t)] \tag{1}$$

$F[.]$ is a functional (function of a function) of the input signal $s(t)$. By treating the neuron as a black-box and limiting its characterization to its input-output function, we are deriving a good understanding of its behavior without incorporating any knowledge of its internal mechanisms (e.g. ionic channels), its biophysical principles or anatomical structure. Such simplification is neither uncommon (Isermann & Munchhof, 2011; Rugh, 1981; Sastry, 1999), nor unwarranted when dealing with a complex structure such as cortical neurons.

The simplest form of systems is linear and time-invariant (LTI). A linear system obeys two keys rules: homogeneity and superposition. The former means that the response to stimuls s that is scaled by a factor α is also scaled by the same amount. The later means that a cell driven by the sum of two stimuli s_1+s_2 responds to the sum of the responses to the individual stimuli. A time-invariant system is one whose behavior depends on its state, independent of time; so that the system's response to a given stimulation does not depend on the time it is applied.

LTI systems that are single-input, single-output can be represented by the familiar convolution integral:

$$r(t) = \int_{-\infty}^{\infty} h(\tau)s(t-\tau)d\tau \tag{2}$$

where $s(t)$ is the input and $r(t)$ the output of the system. The kernel $h(t)$ is called the impulse response of the system, which is the limit of the sequence of responses when the system is excited with input that tends towards an impulse $\delta(t)$.

Intuitively, the convolution represents the correlation between the system's impulse response $h(\tau)$ and the time-reversed input around a given instant $s(t-\tau)$ to produce the output at time t. This operation is repeated for all time t, as the input signal continues to evolve. Thus, the system produces the strongest response when the input matches the system function $h(t)$. In this regard, $h(t)$ is sometimes thought of as a filter that selectively operates on the input signal in order to enhance or suppress certain components. Alternatively, one can think of *h(t)* as a set of weights which defines the output at time *t* as the weighted sum over the values of the input. If the system is not causal, this dependency would extend to the past, present and future values of *s(t)*; while for a causal system, this dependency is limited to only past and present values of *s(t)*. The ease of working with linear, time-invariant systems stems from the fact that *h(t)* gives a *full* description of the black box model. It provides the mapping between *any* input signal and its corresponding output signal. If we know *h(t)*, we know everything there is to know about the system and can fully predict its behavior.

An equivalent representation of the convolution equation (Eq. 2) operates in Frequency domain. Denote the Fourier transform of *s(t)* as *S(f)*, defined as

$$S(f) = \int_{-\infty}^{\infty} s(t)e^{-j2\pi ft}dt \tag{3}$$

where $j = \sqrt{-1}$. Taking the Fourier transform of both sides of Eq. 2 yields

$$R(f) = H(f)S(f) \tag{4}$$

H(f) is called the transfer function of the system. It is related in a one-to-one mapping to the system impulse response *h(t)* (via the Fourier transform); and just like *h(t)*, knowing *H(f)* means knowing everything there is to know about the behavior of the LTI system under study. The Fourier-domain equation reinforces the notion that linear systems only output frequencies that are uniquely determined by the same frequencies in the input; in other words, the output $R(f_0)$ depends solely on $S(f_0)$ and no other components of *S(f)*. The output $R(f_0)$ is simply an amplification of $S(f_0)$ by an amount dictated by $H(f_0)$. Therefore, the output of a linear system to a pure tone is also a pure tone of the same frequency; possibly amplified or dampened, and likely shifted in phase.

Such linearity cannot be expected or realistic in a system so plagued with nonlinearities such as the auditory system. A pure tone typically induces responses at the harmonics of the input frequency. The output to two pure tones is generally composed of the sum and differences of the harmonics of the input frequencies. This and a plethora of other nonlinear phenomena have been demonstrated throughout the auditory pathway, including two-tone suppression, dynamic intensity compression, lateral inhibition, masking and masking release phenomena as well as unpredictable responses to natural stimuli (Goldstein, 1967; Nelken, 2004; Pickles, 2008).

When dealing with nonlinear systems, the convolution equation can be generalized to a more universal class of systems using Volterra series (Volterra, 1959):

$$r(t) = \vartheta_0 + \int_{-\infty}^{\infty} \vartheta_1(\tau)s(t-\tau)d\tau + \int_{-\infty}^{\infty}\int_{-\infty}^{\infty} \vartheta_2(\tau_1,\tau_2)s(t-\tau_1)s(t-\tau_2)d\tau_1 d\tau_2 + \int_{-\infty}^{\infty}\int_{-\infty}^{\infty}\int_{-\infty}^{\infty} \vartheta_3(\tau_1,\tau_2,\tau_3)s(t-\tau_1)s(t-\tau_2)s(t-\tau_3)d\tau_1 d\tau_2 d\tau_3 + \cdots \tag{5}$$

$\vartheta_n(\tau_1, \tau_2, \ldots, \tau_n)$ is called the nth order Volterra kernel with independent variables $\tau_1, \tau_2, \ldots, \tau_n$. It describes the nth order nonlinearity of the system (Mathews & Sicuranza, 2000; Rugh, 1981). *n* is called the order of the system, and can in theory be infinite. Note that Volterra series still assume that the system is time-invariant. It is clear that the convolution integral (Eq. 2) is a special case of the Volterra series equation (Eq. 5) by setting $\vartheta_n(\tau_1, \tau_2, \ldots, \tau_n) = 0 \text{ for } n > 1$.

Now, if we take the Fourier transform of both sides of Eq. 5, we get:

$$Y(f) = V_0\delta(f) + V_1(f)X(f) + \int_{-\infty}^{\infty} V_2(f_1, f - f_1)X(f_1)X(f - f_1)df_1 +$$

$$\int_{-\infty}^{\infty}\int_{-\infty}^{\infty} V_3(f_1, f_2, f - f_1 - f_2)X(f_1)X(f_2)X(f - f_1 - f_2)df_1df_2 + \cdots \quad (6)$$

where is the n-dimensional Fourier transform of $\vartheta_n(\tau_1, \tau_2, \ldots, \tau_n)$. Just like LTI systems, knowledge of the Volterra kernels (in either the time-domain or frequency-domain) allows one to quantify the strength of the system nonlinearity and to quantify the nonlinear energy transfer.

Generally, Eq. 5 or Eq. 6 can be difficult to handle and practically challenging to determine especially for a system with unknown order *n*. The number of terms in the operators does grow both with degree of nonlinearity in the system as well as input dimensionality. This greatly limits their applicability to low-dimensional systems with mild nonlinearities; and even then, the computation tends to be quite tedious and involved.

A simpler formulation of the same functional has been proposed by Wiener, which reformulated the Volterra series representation into sums of multidimensional convolutions that are *mutually uncorrelated*; i.e. orthogonal with respect to zero-mean Gaussian white noise –GWN– (Wiener, 1958). By construction, the Wiener functional of order *n* can be obtained from the original Volterra kernels by a procedure similar to Gram-Schmidt orthogonalization; and is nothing but linear combinations of Volterra kernels up to order *n* (Ogunfunmi, 2007; Rugh, 1981). Their orthogonal nature also allows the Wiener series to be truncated after *n* functionals, giving the best n^{th} order polynomial approximation to the system (given GWN input). Higher order Wiener functionals are independent and can be added without affecting the estimate of the lower order ones already computed. On the other hand, the relationship between the Wiener kernels and the system properties is more blurred. For instance, the first-order Wiener functional is not the only term containing the linear convolution; all odd order functionals contain a linear term; so truncating the Wiener series would misrepresent the contribution of the linear and other nonlinear components to the system's behavior.

The use of GWN stimulation and Wiener-series has proven quite successful in modeling neural processing in a number of sensory systems; particularly at the peripheral level (Eggermont, 1993; Johnson, 1980; Marmarelis & Marmarelis, 1978; Wickesberg, Dickson, Gibson, & Geisler, 1984). While somewhat successful, such white-noise technique has proven quite inadequate and inapplicable to central auditory loci, particularly auditory cortex for a number of reasons. The most obvious one being that white noise stimulation is quite stationary and fails to elicit responses from cortical neurons.

The Spectro-Temporal Receptive Field (STRF)

Cortical neurons are more responsive to rich sounds with non-static spectro-temporal structures. As sounds journey up the auditory system to sensory cortex, they come readily represented into their dynamic spectra. The cortical input is mapped onto a spectro-temporal representation; as tonotopically-organized temporal neural activity. It is therefore important to tie the spectro-temporal space with the functional definition presented above.

To take the structure of the input to cortical neurons into account and also begin to gauge the role of the spectro-temporal structure of sound, we can revisit the formulation of the Volterra series model of a system; particularly its bilinear or quadratic term. From Eq. 5, the second order term of the Volterra series can be written as:

$$\begin{aligned} V_2[s(t)] &= \int_{-\infty}^{\infty}\int_{-\infty}^{\infty} \vartheta_2(\tau_1,\tau_2)s(t-\tau_1)s(t-\tau_2)d\tau_1 d\tau_2 \\ &= \int_{-\infty}^{\infty}\int_{-\infty}^{\infty} \hat{\vartheta}_2(\tau,\theta)s\left(t-\tau-\frac{\theta}{2}\right)s(t-\tau+\frac{\theta}{2})d\tau d\theta \quad ,\tau=\frac{\tau_1+\tau_2}{2},\theta=\tau_2-\tau_1 \\ &= \int_{-\infty}^{\infty}\int_{-\infty}^{\infty} STRF_{V_2}(\tau,f)W(t-\tau,f)d\tau d\theta \end{aligned} \tag{7}$$

where we recognize the quadratic term as the Wigner-Ville distribution[1] of the input signal $s(t)$; $W_s(t,f)=\int s\left(t-\frac{\theta}{2}\right)s(t+\frac{\theta}{2})e^{-j2\pi f\theta}d\tau$; i.e. the Fourier transform of the signal's autocorrelation function. Here, $STRF_{V_2}$ is defined as:

$$STRF_{V_2}(\tau,f) \equiv \int_{-\infty}^{\infty} \hat{\vartheta}_2(\tau,\theta)e^{-j2\pi f\theta}d\theta \tag{8}$$

and can be thought of as Fourier transform of the second-order Volterra kernel. Eq. 7 gives a derivation of an STRF based on the Wigner-Ville distribution; and can be shown to be easily related to STRFs derived from other time-frequency representations of the signal via a filtering operation (Theunissen et al., 2000). The class of bilinear time-frequency representations of signals is inter-convertible with respect to one another, as smoothed or convolved versions of each other. Whether the Wigner-Ville, Choi-Williams distribution, the

[1] The presence of complex conjugation of *s(t)* in the equations is ignored since all stimuli are real-valued.

Gabor transform or the spectrogram representation, they can all be written in general form as (Cohen, 1995; Grochenig, 2001; Sang-Won Nam & Powers, 2003):

$$C_s(t,f) = \iiint_{-\infty}^{\infty} \Psi(\xi,\theta) e^{-j2\pi\xi(t-\tau)} \underbrace{s(\tau+\tfrac{\theta}{2})s^*(\tau-\tfrac{\theta}{2})e^{-j2\pi f\theta}}_{\sim\text{Wigner-Ville distribution}} \, d\theta d\tau d\xi \qquad (9)$$

where $\Psi(\xi,\theta)$ is a kernel that determines the influence of cross-terms on the time-frequency function. Note that for the Wigner-Ville distribution. The choice of time-frequency representation to use depends on ease of interpretation and applicability to the sound class of interest (Eggermont & Smith, 1990; Kim & Young, 1994; Theunissen et al., 2000). It is also important to consider representations with proper support to enable mapping back and forth between $STRF_{V_2}$ (i.e. the Fourier transform of the second-order Volterra kernel) and any other equivalent STRF representation of the neuron (see (Klein, Depireux, Simon, & Shamma, 2000) for a discussion).

Regardless of the choice of spectro-temporal representation of the stimulus *s(t)*, Eq. 7 shows that the second-order Volterra functional can be thought of as a linear system that processes the Wigner-Ville distribution of the stimulus (or other equivalent representations).

3. Construction of Spectro-Temporal Receptive Fields

Reverse Correlation

The most common way of constructing STRFs uses the classic *reverse correlation* method (De Boer & Kuyper, 1968). This technique amounts to computing the cross-correlation between an input stimulus $S(t,f)$ and neural response $r(t)$; i.e. $C(t,f)=<S(\tau-t,f)r(\tau)>$, where <.> corresponds to averaging over time. If the input signal is a spectro-temporal GWN, its autocorrelation function is a pure two-dimensional impulse, i.e, $\Phi(\tau,x)=\delta(\tau,x)$, since the only nonzero correlations are those between each time-frequency channel and itself; hence corresponding to an impulse function. One can in fact show that when driven with white noise, this cross-correlation $C(t,f)$ corresponds to the *impulse response* of the neuron (Bracewell, 1999); therefore fully determining the system function (of course, assuming the system obeys principles of linearity and time-invariance).

Computing the cross-correlation $C(t,f)$ can be technically done in a number of ways. The term "reverse-correlation" emphasizes the notion that one centers this computation around the response $r(t)$, and looks back at the stimulus that precedes it (Fig. 1). As the neuron produces a spike, reverse-correlation postulates that the neuron must have "heard" a sensory input that it "likes", therefore driving it to fire. So one looks back at the immediate past of the input just preceding the spike and saves it. As more spikes are generated, the inputs $S(t,f)$ preceding spikes are averaged out. Features that are consistently driving the neuron to fire will add up while features that are irrelevant will "wash-out", leaving a crisp representation of the neuron's preference of time-frequency features. Anchoring the computation around the system output makes reverse-correlation very adequate for spiking systems, such as neurons, whose outputs translate to a binary code of 0's and 1's; hence limiting the computation to only few instances when the neuron fires a spike. All instances during which the neuron is operating sub-threshold are irrelevant for this computation; since they contribute only zero to the summation. The time averaging operation reduces to a computation that grows linearly with the number of spikes generated by the neuron. One can in fact follow the evolution of this computation in real-time. As sound progresses over time, a sequence of stimulus patterns can be averaged in an online fashion each time the neuron spikes, until a pattern emerges; or some measure of estimation convergence is satisfied. This method has been applied widely throughout the neuroscience literature in studying behavior of sensory neurons (De Boer & Kuyper, 1968; Johnson, 1980; Jones & Palmer, 1987; Ringach, Sapiro, & Shapley, 1997).

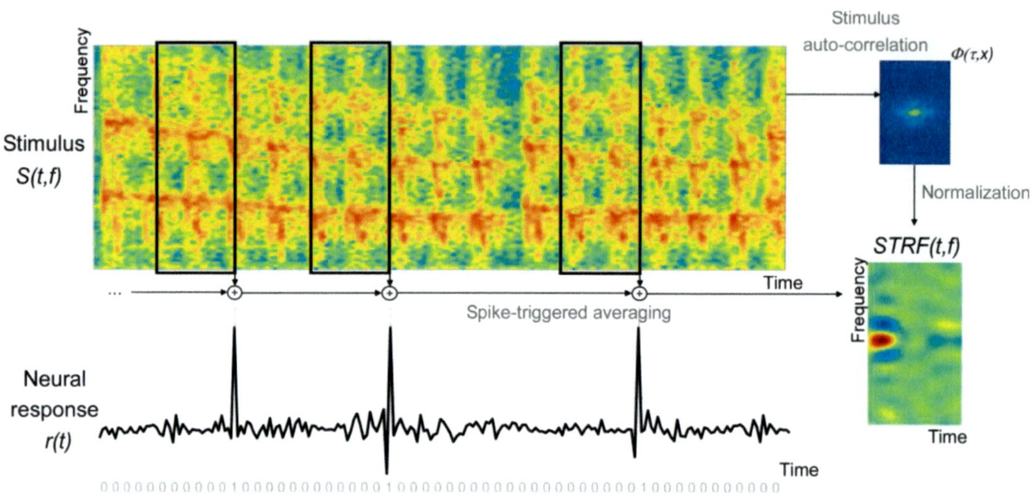

Figure 1. Spike-triggered averaging for estimating the spectro-temporal receptive field. Instances from the stimulus spectrogram that precede a spike are averaged together (and can be normalized by the stimulus auto-correlation) to derive an estimate of the tuning properties of the neuron; what spectral and temporal features in the input stimulus triggered the neuron to fire an action potential.

It is important to note here that the reverse-correlation method yields the second order Wiener kernel; which is in principle not equivalent to the second order Volterra kernel or the STRF as derived in Eq. 7. However, the distinction between the two is often ignored as neurophysiologists often assume that the system's order does not extend to higher orders n; hence making the two metrics equivalent.

Aside from the mathematical foundation of the reverse correlation technique, it is important to appreciate the intuition that if the time-frequency space is sampled randomly and uniformly, and assuming the system is LTI, knowing how each time-frequency bin drives a neuron gives us a complete description of the neuron's behavior (De Boer & Kuyper, 1968). Aside from the absurdity of trying to reduce complex neurons to simple LTI systems (as discussed throughout this book), the spike-triggered method is further limited by its reliance on a uniform sampling of time-frequency space. Nevertheless, the limitations of GWN have been circumvented by using more interesting stimuli that share a lot of the characteristics of GWN such as moving ripples, TORCs or other modulated broadband sounds (Escabi & Read, 2003; Klein et al., 2000; Kowalski, Depireux, & Shamma, 1996; Miller, Escabi, Read, &

Schreiner, 2002). The spike-triggered averaging methodology has also been extended to more general sound classes such as animal vocalizations, natural sounds and human speech. Though it yields a biased representation of the STRF, compensation can be applied by normalizing the representation using second-order statistics of the input (Aertsen & Johannesma, 1981; David, Mesgarani, Fritz, & Shamma, 2009; Eggermont, Aertsen, & Johannesma, 1983; Ringach et al., 1997; Theunissen et al., 2000).

Estimation Errors

It is clear that the receptive field is not an invariant characterization of the spectro-temporal properties of auditory neurons. It is an approach that is riddled with problems. It varies with stimulus type including bandwidth, temporal dynamics, intensity, richness of spectro-temporal properties or any other properties that determine the effectiveness of a stimulus in driving a neuron; an issue considered in chapter 3. It also changes with different levels of analysis (see chapter 4), and poses great challenges for validation as a true transfer function of neurons (see chapter 7). Nevertheless, it remains one of the great tools available to neurophysiologists to provide a window (albeit narrow) into complex processing taking place throughout the sensory system, particularly at the level of auditory cortex.

A number of issues should however be carefully considered when working with the concept of STRF: (i) Sensory stimulation is a crucial component to the procedure of deriving receptive fields. It is a critical factor in determining whether a neuron is driven to its full dynamic range or under-stimulated. In addition, as has been shown in a number of studies, different stimulus ensembles with different spectro-temporal characteristics appear to thrust neurons into different operating states; yielding STRFs that are *different* linearizations of the true behavior of a neuron around different points (Machens, Wehr, & Zador, 2004). (ii) What form of time-frequency representation is appropriate to use when dealing with cortical neurons? This issue has to be carefully considered; especially at the level of auditory cortex where numerous investigation have demonstrated a lack of phase locking to rapidly changing stimuli (>30Hz). Stimuli such as ripples and broadband noises are usually designed with that knowledge in mind. Even natural sounds, animal vocalizations and speech exhibit similar slow dynamics. Such phenomenon has often justified the use of smooth envelope profiles of the stimulus spectrogram (or other forms of time-frequency representations); rather than the spectrogram itself. In doing so, the emergent STRF captures *only* the slow spectro-temporal characteristics of the sound that usually modulates a richer structure composed of the signal carrier and its fine-structure interaction terms as the sound travels through the auditory pathway. Carefully considering the appropriate space for representing the signal can unravel more about processing by cortical neurons; particularly their seeming multiplexing ability at eliciting responses to the sound envelope, which itself gates phase-locked responses to the sound fine structure (Elhilali, Fritz, Klein, Simon, & Shamma, 2004). (iii) In most studies employing STRFs as neural measure, the linearity assumptions impose inclusion of only steady-state portions of the neural response. In doing so, one bypasses the use of the phasic behavior of neurons at onset; which is believed to drive the neurons around a different operating point, hence heightening the nonlinear behavior (Shechter, Dobbins, Marvit, & Depireux, 2009). What constitute *steady-space* responses is not well understood; and this issue is further compounded by processes of neural adaptation that changes the neuron's behavior as the sensory input is extended over time. (iv) All derivations of receptive fields (including the general Volterra series approach) have an underlying assumption that the system is time-invariant. Such assumption is challenged by compelling experimental evidence for receptive field plasticity, both during development (de Villers-Sidani, Chang, Bao, & Merzenich, 2007; Hubel & Wiesel, 1963) and the adult brain (for review, see (J. Fritz, Elhilali, & Shamma, 2005; Weinberger, 2007)) or induced by arousal, attention, and stimulus and behavioral context. (v) The STRF is ultimately an average measure; how much data is needed to derive a 'good' estimate of a neuron's STRF; depends on a number of ill-understood issues including the neuron's variability, degree of nonlinearity (or alternatively the plausibility of the linearity assumption for that particular neuron) as well as other sources of noise or variability (e.g. inherent system variability, experimental noise). (vi) It is important to keep in mind is that STRF derivations presented earlier, based on Volterra series, Wiener series or reverse correlation are approximating a functional that maps a deterministic input $s(t)$ onto a stochastic output: a sequence of spike trains. When applying the methods above to the nervous system, it is customary to average the output process to measure the underlying spiking rate of the neuron. Such approximation does not come without its perils. It causes great variations in the estimates of the STRF function. One has to carefully consider the long-term variations of the spiking rate and whether time-averaging is valid for the specific experimental settings investigated.

Interpretation of the Spectro-Temporal Receptive Field

One of the chief impacts of the STRF technique was generalizing the concept of a classic response field (RF) to the spectro-temporal domain (Depireux, Simon, Klein, & Shamma, 2001; Escabi & Schreiner, 2002; Klein et al., 2000; Miller et al., 2002; Nelken & Young, 1997; Theunissen et al., 2000; Yeshurun, Wollberg, Dyn, & Allon, 1985). It is greatly related to frequency tuning curves – a classic descriptor used to probe the spectral properties of a neuron; or indirectly to measure the matrix of synaptic weights to the neuron from tonotopically-organized inputs. The correspondence between a frequency tuning curve and the spectral axis of a neuron's STRF is not exactly one-to-one. Each is derived using different sets of stimuli with different dynamics and is likely probing the system under different states. Nevertheless, there is great agreement between the two. The STRF undoubtedly overcomes a number of limitations that beset the classic tuning curve.

The STRF procedure operates under the assumption that the system under investigation integrates information linearly; but makes no assumptions about the relationship or independence of the spectral and temporal attributes of the response. As such, it is indeed more informative than the classic tuning curve. The x-axis represents time or delay between sensory stimulation and neural response. The y-axis represents the frequency tuning; ideally spanning the entire range of hearing of the animal. It is important to note that the STRF reflects the effect of the dynamic spectrum of sound on the sensory neuron. It is the conjunction of its time and frequency characteristics, rather than just the individual contributions of each of them. Because of its two-dimensional construction, it can be interpreted in two complementary ways: rows vs. columns. The former views the STRF an array of frequency-dependent dynamical filters; while the later interprets the STRF as time-dependent spectral weighting function.

The STRF reveals numerous characteristics about the underlying sensory neuron investigated, all in one function:

- Spectral characteristics (features shared to some extent with the classic tuning curve): its spectral tuning, its frequency-response bandwidth, presence of excitatory peaks or inhibitory sidebands,
- Temporal characteristics: the response latency, refractoriness, modulation rate tuning;
- Spectro-temporal characteristics: frequency-modulation direction selectivity (for FM sweeps moving upwards or downwards).

4. The Rosetta Stone of STRFs

In this section, we consider the interpretation of the STRF form, and in particular how its temporal and spectral dimensions might be interdependent, how one can infer from the STRF form its sensitivity to spectral and temporal features such as directional and spectral bandwidth sensitivity.

Rank and Separability

The *rank* of a two dimensional function, such as an STRF, captures one aspect of how simple the function is. When a two dimensional function is the simple product of two one-dimensional functions, i.e. $h(t,x)=f(t)g(x)$, this captures an important notion of simplicity. When this occurs, the function is of rank 1. When the sum of two products is required, e.g. $h(t,x)=f_A(t)g_A(x)+f_B(t)g_B(x)$, the function is of rank 2. (In cases of rank 2 and higher, we demand that each temporal function $f_i(t)$ be linearly independent of every other temporal function $f(t)$, and the same for the spectral functions $g(x)$; otherwise we could have used a smaller number of terms.) A rank 2 function is clearly not as simple as a rank 1 function, but nevertheless can be expressed rather concisely. In general, the *rank* of any two dimensional function is the minimum number of simple products needed to describe the function (When the functions are approximated as discrete, the definition of rank is identical to the definition of the algebraic rank of a matrix).

An STRF of rank 1, also called *fully separable,* can be written:

$$h^{FS}(t,x) = f(t)g(x) \tag{10}$$

which has this simple interpretation: the temporal processing of the STRF is performed independently of the spectral processing (and of course vice versa). A simple model of a neuron with this property is that its spectral processing is due purely to inputs from presynaptic neurons with a range of center frequencies, while the temporal processing is due to integration in the soma of all inputs arriving from all dendrites. For many peripheral neurons, this model is a good one. An STRF of rank 1 is also called fully separable because its processing separates cleanly into independent spectral and temporal processing stages. The example STRF in Figure 2a is fully separable, and this can be verified by noting that all spectral (vertical) cross- sections have the same shape (the shape of the spectral function $g(x)$), differing only in amplitude (and possible sign). Similarly, all temporal (horizontal) cross-sections have the same shape (the shape of the temporal function $f(t)$), differing only in amplitude (and possibly sign).

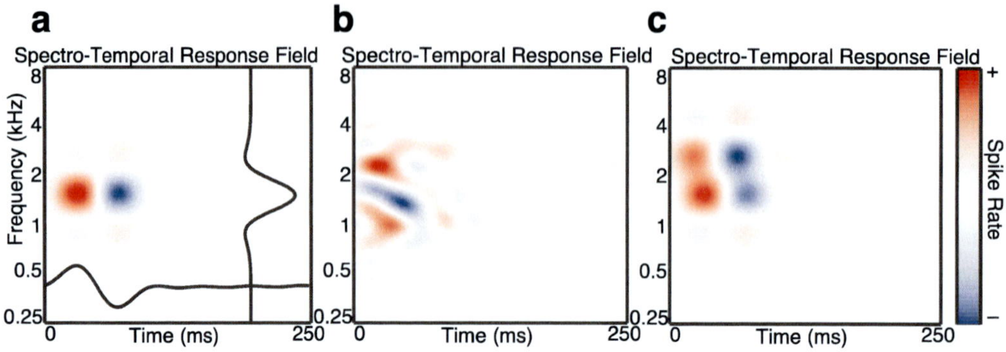

Figure 2. a. A simulated fully separable STRF, with spectral and temporal one-dimensional cross-sections as inserts (all horizontal slices have the same profile, as do vertical slices). b. A simulated high rank STRF with no particular symmetries. c. A simulated temporally symmetric and quadrant separable STRF of rank 2. This STRF's symmetry is not obviously visible. This STRF was created by adding to the STRF in a the same STRF except with the spatial cross-section shifted upward by 3/4 octave and the temporal cross- section Hilbert-rotated (see below) by 30°.

An STRF of rank 2 is somewhat less simple and is somewhat less straightforward to interpret.

$$h^{R2}(t,x) = f_A(t)g_A(x) + f_B(t)g_B(x) \tag{11}$$

One interpretation comes from noting that this can be written as the sum of two fully separable STRFs, $f_A(t)g_A(x)$ and $f_B(t)g_B(x)$. This implies a possible, but less than satisfying, interpretation: the neuron has exactly two neural inputs, each of which has a fully separable STRF, and then simply adds them. Below we will present more realistic interpretations, consistent with known physiology. An STRF described by a generic two-dimensional function would not necessarily have the same physiologically motivated interpretations or models.

An STRF of general rank *N* can be written as the sum of N terms:

$$h^{RN}(t,x) = f_A(t)g_A(x) + f_B(t)g_B(x) + \cdots f_z(t)g_z(x) \tag{12}$$

As the rank of an STRF increases, more and more complexity is permitted. Figure 2b demonstrates a simulated STRF of high rank (though still well localized in time and spectrum). STRFs of this complexity are not seen in A1 (Klein et al., 2006). In general, *higher rank* implies more STRF complexity. On the other hand, *lower rank* suggests there is a specific property (constraint) that causes this simplicity.

Singular Value Decomposition Analysis of the STRF

Singular Value Decomposition (SVD) is a method that can be applied to any finite dimensional matrix (e.g. a discretized version of the STRF) to establish both its rank and a unique re-expression of the matrix as the sum of terms whose number is the rank of the matrix (Hansen, 1997; Press, Flannery, Teukolsky, & Vetterling, 1992). The SVD decomposition of a matrix M takes the form of the sum of N terms:

$$M_{ij} = \Lambda_A u_{Ai} v^T{}_{Aj} + \Lambda_B u_{Bi} v^T{}_{Bj} + \cdots + \Lambda_Z u_{Zi} v^T{}_{Zj} \tag{13}$$

where N is the rank of the matrix, u and v are vectors normalized to have unit power, and each Λ is the term's RMS power. If we discretize the STRF into a finite number of frequencies and time steps, $x=\{x_i\}=\{x_1,x_2,...x_M\}$ and $t=t_j=(t_1,...,t_N)$, so that $h(t_i,t_j)=\{h_{ij}\}=h(t_1,...t_N;x_1,...x_M)$, we see the N terms,

$$h_{ij} = \Lambda_A u_A(x_i) v_A(t_j) + \Lambda_B u_B(x_i) v_B(t_j) + \cdots + \Lambda_z u_z(x_i) v_Z(t_j) \tag{14}$$

where N is the rank of the STRF, the u and v vectors are normalized to have unit power, and each Λ is the RMS power of its term. This is the same as Eq. 12, except that time and frequency have been discretized, and thus the STRF has been discretized also.

What makes SVD unique among decompositions is that (i) it automatically orders the terms by decreasing power: $\Lambda_A > \Lambda_B > ... > \Lambda_Z$; (ii) each column $u_A, u_B, ..., u_Z$ is orthogonal to all the others; 3) each row v_A^T , v_B^T ,..., v_Z^T is orthogonal to all the others. The mathematical specifics are described well in textbooks (see, e.g., (Press et al., 1992) and will not be covered here. Mathematically, SVD is intimately related to Principle Component Analysis (PCA), and both are used for a variety of analytic purposes, including noise reduction (Hansen, 1997). Physiologically, however, (as with PCA) there is in general no universal physiological interpretation to specific components, since distinct physiological contributions to the singular value expansion are, in general, not constrained to be orthogonal to each other.

Since measured STRFs are made with noisy measurements (the noise arising from both neural variability and instrument noise), the true rank of the STRF must be estimated. There are a variety of methods to do this (Stewart, 1993) but they all use the same conceptual framework: once the power of the noise is estimated, then all SVD components with power greater than the noise can be considered signal, and the number of components satisfying this criterion is the estimate of the rank. This estimate of rank is biased (more noise results in a lower rank estimate), but it has been shown that noise is not an impediment to measuring high rank (Klein et al., 2006).

SVD also motivates us to recast Eq. 12 into its N terms in continuous form

$$h^{RN}(t,x) = \Lambda_A u_A(x) v_A(t) + \Lambda_B u_B(x) v_B(t) + \cdots + \Lambda_z u_z(x) v_Z(t) \tag{15}$$

where the u and v functions have unit power and each Λ is the RMS power of its term. Compared to Eq. 12, it more complex, but it is less arbitrary: decompositions of the form of Eqs. 10, 11, and 12 are not unique since amplitude can be arbitrarily shifted between the temporal and spectral components. In Eq. 14, all amplitude information is explicitly shared within each term by each Λ_i coefficient. When the technique of SVD, which is designed for discrete matrices, is applied to continuous two-dimensional functions, as in the case of Eq. 14, it is called the Singular Value Expansion (Hansen, 1997). We will go back and forth between the continuous and discretized versions of the STRF without loss of generality (so long as N is finite), depending on which formalism is more beneficial.

There are a few important exceptions, however, to the statement above that there are typically no physiological interpretation to the specific components in the Singular Value Expansion. This occurs when one of the temporal (or spectral) component functions is the Hilbert Transform of another. In this case, as will be shown below, the two functions have identical spectral characteristics, and are orthogonal only because they differ in phase.

Hilbert Transform and Partial Hilbert Transforms/Rotations

We now discuss the Hilbert transform, a standard tool in signal processing, and necessary for the phenomenon of temporal symmetry. The Hilbert transform of a function produces the same function but with all its phase components shifted by 90°. This can be seen in the Fourier domain. For a function $f(t)$ with Fourier transform $F(\omega)$, i.e.

$$F(\omega) = \mathcal{F}_\omega[f(t)] = \int dt f(t) \mathrm{e}^{-j\omega t}$$
$$f(t) = \mathcal{F}_t^{-1}[F(\omega)] = (2\pi)^{-1} \int d\omega F(\omega) \mathrm{e}^{j\omega t} \quad , \tag{16}$$

where the Hilbert transform, designated by $H[.]$ or $\wedge$, is defined by

$$\hat{f}(t) = \mathcal{H}[f(t)] = \mathcal{F}_t^{-1}\left[\mathrm{sgn}(\omega) e^{j\pi/2} F(\omega)\right], \tag{17}$$

where is a rotation by 90° in the complex plane (the role of sgn(ω) guarantees that the Hilbert transform of a real function is itself a real function). This rotation of phase by 90° means that the Hilbert transform of any sine wave is a cosine wave, and the Hilbert transform of any cosine wave is the negative sine wave, but unlike differentiation, the amplitude is unchanged by the operation.

An important property of the Hilbert transform is that it is orthogonal to the original function, and yet it still has the same frequency content (aside from the DC component, i.e. its mean, which is zeroed out). $\hat{f}(t)$ is said to be "in quadrature" with $f(t)$; a demonstration is illustrated in Figure 3. For the remainder of this section, we assume that any function $f(t)$ which will be Hilbert transformed has mean zero (or has had its mean subtracted manually).

The double application of a Hilbert transform, since applying two successive 90° rotations is equivalent to one 180° rotation, is just a sign inversion.

$$\mathcal{H}[\mathcal{H}[f(t)]] = \hat{\hat{f}}(t) = -f(t) \tag{18}$$

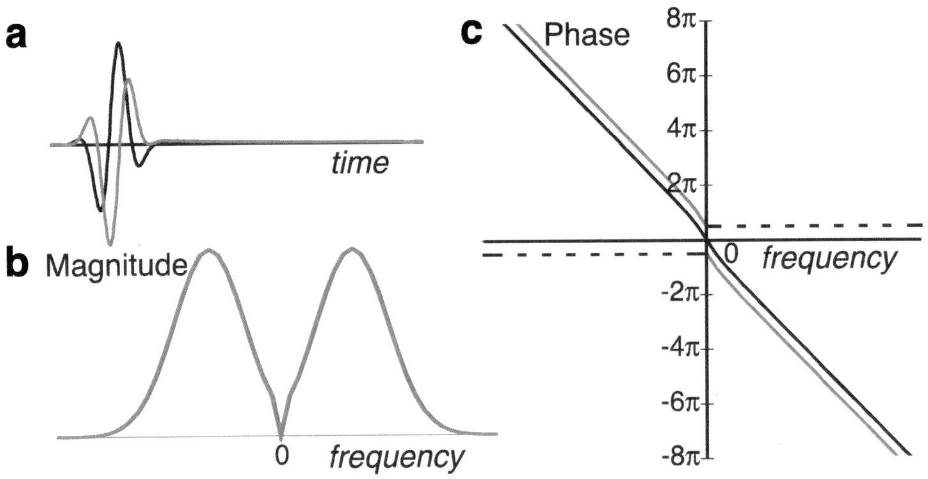

Figure 3. An example of a function and its Hilbert transform. a. A function (in black) overlaid with its Hilbert transform (in gray); the two are orthogonal. b. The magnitude of the Fourier transform of the function (in black) overlaid with the magnitude of the Fourier transform of its Hilbert transform (in gray); they overlap exactly. c. The phase of the Fourier transform of the function (in black) overlaid with the phase of the Fourier transform of its Hilbert transform (in gray); the difference is exactly ±90°(dashed line).

It is also useful to define a partial Hilbert transform. As pointed out above, a Hilbert transform of a function can be viewed as a 90° rotation in a mixing angle plane, so one can define a partial version of the transform

$$f^{\theta}(t) = \sin\theta\,\hat{f}(t) + \cos\theta\,f(t) \tag{19}$$

In this convention, note that

$$\hat{f}(t) = f^{\pi/2}(t),\; f(t) = f^{0}(t), \text{ and } \hat{\hat{f}}(t) = f^{\pi}(t) = -f(t).$$

Thus a partial Hilbert transform still has the same frequency content as the original function, but its phase "rotation" is not restricted to 90° and can be any angle on the complex plane.

Physiological examples of the Hilbert transform have been demonstrated in the visual system, and have been named "lagged" cells (De Valois, Cottaris, Elfar, Mahon, & Wilson, 2000; Humphrey & Weller, 1988; Mastronarde, 1987a; Mastronarde, 1987b). These lagged cells are located in the Lateral Geniculate Nucleus (LGN), one of the visual thalamic nuclei. We will continue this nomenclature and call any neuron whose impulse response is the Hilbert transform of another the lagged version of the latter. We will further generalize, and call any neuron whose impulse response is the partial Hilbert transform (Hilbert rotation) of another, the "partially lagged" version of the latter. Note that the lag is a phase lag, not a time lag.

The full and partial Hilbert transform/rotation is not restricted to the time domain and is equally applicable to the spectral domain (Simon, Depireux, Klein, Fritz, & Shamma, 2007).

Temporal Symmetry

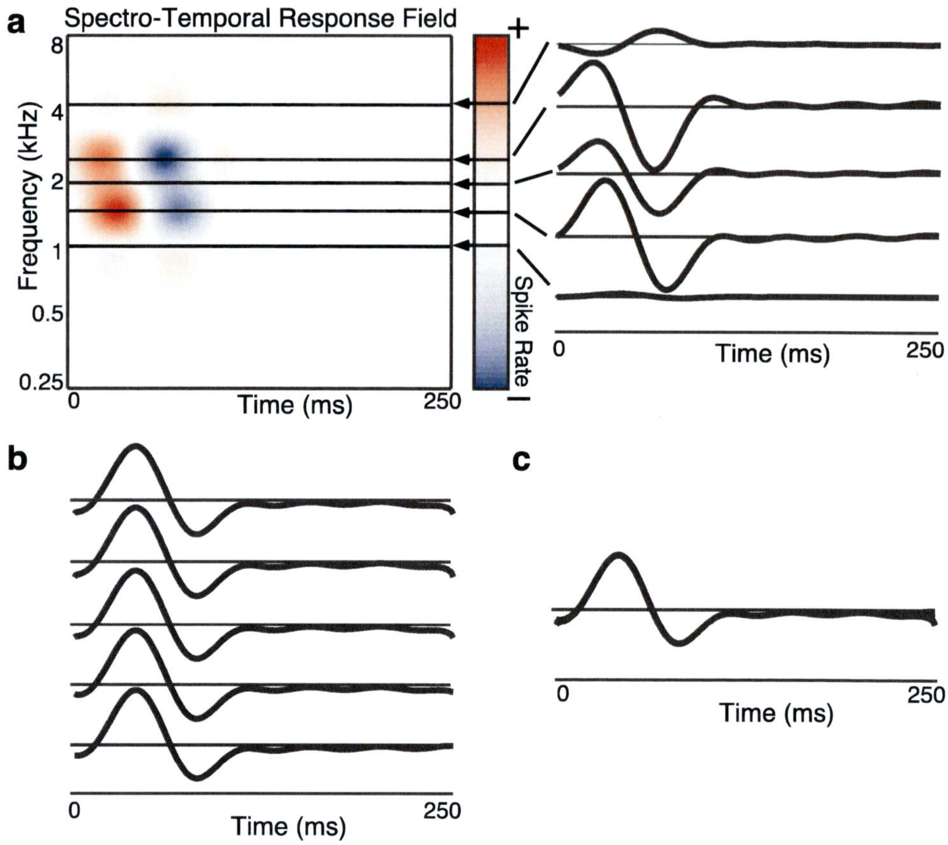

Figure 4. a. The simulated temporally symmetric and quadrant separable STRF from Figure 1c, and five fixed-frequency cross-sections, corresponding to five temporal impulse responses. b. The same five impulse responses but individually Hilbert-rotated and rescaled. c. The same Hilbert-rotated and rescaled impulse responses superimposed. The Hilbert-rotation phases were calculated by taking the negative phase of the complex correlation coefficient between the analytic signal of each temporal cross-section and the analytic signal of the 4th temporal cross-section.

An important class of STRFs consists of those for which all temporal cross-sections (i.e. each cross section at a constant spectral index *xc*), of the given STRF are related to each other by a simple scaling, *g*, and rotation, θ, of the same time function:

$$h(t,x_c) = g_{x_c} f^{\theta_{x_c}}(t), \tag{20}$$

where each scaling and rotation can depend on x_c. Since this is then true for all spectral indices *x*, we call the system Temporally Symmetric and write it in the functional form:

$$h^{TS}(t,x) = g(x) f^{\theta(x)}(t) \tag{21}$$

The meaning is still the same: all temporal cross-sections are related to each other by a simple scaling and rotation of the same time function. There is only one function of *t*, i.e. *f(t)*, and Hilbert rotations of it (demonstrated in Figure 4).

Using the definition of the Hilbert rotation Eq. 19, we can re-express Eq. 21 to explicitly show that a temporally symmetric STRF is rank 2 (i.e. is the sum of two linearly independent product terms):

$$\begin{aligned} h^{TS}(t,x) &= g(x) f^{\theta(x)}(t) \\ &= g(x)\cos\theta(x) f(t) + g(x)\sin\theta(x)\hat{f}(t) \\ &= f(t) g_A(x) + \hat{f}(t) g_B(x) \end{aligned} \tag{22}$$

where

$$\begin{aligned} g_A(x) &= g(x)\cos\theta(x) \\ g_B(x) &= g(x)\sin\theta(x) \\ \tan\theta(x) &= \frac{g_B(x)}{g_A(x)} \\ g^2(x) &= g_A^2(x) + g_B^2(x). \end{aligned}$$

We will often use the form of Eq. 22, which is completely equivalent to Eq. 21. In Eq. 22 it is explicit that a temporally symmetric STRF has rank 2 and cannot have higher rank.

Temporally symmetric STRFs, because of the symmetry relating the two temporal functions, fall into a very special subcategory of rank 2 STRFs. For these STRFs, it turns out there *are* physiological interpretations for the individual components. The neural benefit of temporally symmetric STRFs is to allow modulation spectral selectivity without also being hampered by modulation phase selectivity (Simon et al., 2007). Not also that not all rank 2 STRFs are temporally symmetric: there are a wide variety of simple counter-examples (Simon et al., 2007).

For systems, which are not exactly temporally symmetric but are of rank 2, or for systems, which have been truncated by SVD to rank 2, we can define an index of temporal symmetry, η_t. This index ranges from 0 to 1, where $\eta_t = 1$ for the temporally symmetric case and $\eta_t = 0$ when the two time functions are temporally unrelated. First we put Eq. 22, which is explicitly rank 2, into the form of Eq. 14:

$$h^{R2}(t,x) = \Lambda_A u_A(x) v_A(t) + \Lambda_B u_B(x) v_B(t) \tag{23}$$

Since the u and v functions have unit power, we define the index of temporal symmetry to be the magnitude of the normalized complex inner product between the two temporal analytic signals (Cohen, 1995)

$$\eta_t = \left| \int \tfrac{1}{2} \left(v_A(t) + j\hat{v}_A(t) \right)^* \left(v_B(t) + j\hat{v}_B(t) \right) dt \right|, \tag{24}$$

where * is the complex conjugate operator. The rank 1 case, since it is automatically temporally symmetric, is also given the value $\eta_t = 1$. Temporal symmetry's cousin, spectral symmetry, is described in (Klein et al., 2006).

Temporal Symmetry and Quadrant Separability

When the STRF is separable, the Spectro-Temporal Modulation Transfer Function (MTF_{ST}), the two-dimensional Fourier Transform of the STRF, is also separable, because the Fourier transform of the STRF is given by the simple products of the Fourier transforms of $f(t)$ and $g(x)$. It was noticed that even when the STRF is not separable, the quadrants of the MTF_{ST} are still individually separable (Depireux et al., 2001; Klein et al., 2006; Kowalski et al., 1996), but neither the significance nor the origin of this property was well understood. It was demonstrated in (Simon et al., 2007) that when the STRF is of rank 2, quadrant separability and temporal symmetry are intimately related mathematically properties, manifesting differently as temporal symmetry in the STRF and quadrant separability in the MTF_{ST}. Mathematically, quadrant separability in the MTF_{ST} can manifest in two other ways in a rank 2 STRF: spectral symmetry (the spectral analog of temporal symmetry) or total directional selectivity. To our knowledge, spectral symmetry has not been observed physiologically. Total directional selectivity, in contrast, has been much discussed in the vision literature when STRF is interpreted as the visual Spatio-Temporal Response Field: both temporal and spectral functions are added in quadrature (Adelson & Bergen, 1985; Barlow & Levick, 1965; Borst & Egelhaaf, 1989; Chance, Nelson, & Abbott, 1998; De Valois et al., 2000; Emerson & Gerstein, 1977; Heeger, 1993; Maex & Orban, 1996; McLean & Palmer, 1994; Smith, Snowden, & Milne, 1994; Suarez, Koch, & Douglas, 1995; Watson & Ahumada, 1985). Mathematically, quadrant separable STRF of rank 4 are also possible, but we are not aware of their presence in any physiological system.

5. STRFs and Cortical Processing

The STRF concept has proven valuable in the understanding of auditory cortical processing and its applications in audio systems ranging from speech and speaker recognition, to enhancements of speech signals and cochlear implants. Their first valuable contribution has been to provide an effective summary of the representation of sound features in the primary auditory cortex (Atencio et al., 2008; Theunissen et al., 2000; Versnel, Kowalski, & Shamma, 1995). A key finding has been the realization that the huge variety of auditory cortical responses in frequency tuning, dynamics, and other features can be integrated in models of auditory processing that view the cortex as a 'multiscale' spectro-temporal analyzer that decomposes the signal into a rich representation that can be effectively harnessed for a variety of applications (Chi, Ru, & Shamma, 2005). For example, complex signals such as speech and music can be analyzed in this cortical model to understand how phonetic information is represented (Mesgarani, David, Fritz, & Shamma, 2008), or how timbres of different musical instruments are encoded (Patil, Pressnitzer, Shamma, & Elhilali, 2012). The uniqueness of the representation of the different types of signals allows us further to separate speech from interfering noise, to detect the presence of speech compared to non-speech (Mesgarani, Slaney, & Shamma, 2006), and to separate multiple speakers (Elhilali & Shamma, 2008).

STRFs have proven valuable in plasticity and development studies as a summary of a neuron's response properties *even if incomplete.* The reason is that in many cases, it is not the completeness of the representation that is of interest, but rather *how* the (admittedly incomplete) representation changes during behavior or learning. In this role, the STRF has demonstrated a robustness and versatility that was not initially appreciated. For instance, auditory cortical STRFs often provide an estimate of the *relative* sensitivity of a neuron to different frequencies and temporal dynamics. Therefore, when examining the effects of attention and learning, changes in neuronal responsiveness are often unpredictable in their dynamics or spectral configurations, or are very small and augment already very noisy responses. The STRF counters both of these challenges. Thus, by virtue of its generalized nature (not being specific to a particular feature or response dimension), changes in the neuronal sensitivity in one of multiple dimensions can readily be spotted and characterized (J. Fritz, Elhilali, Klein, & Shamma, 2003). Furthermore, these response changes are often very difficult to discern or interpret (as spectral or temporal changes) in the firing rates themselves. STRFS by their nature are simultaneous *relative* measures of a neuron's responsiveness to many frequencies and dynamics. Consequently, the effect of attention and learning (and behavior in general) is often seen as changes in the STRF shape that can be readily interpreted as changes in the relative sensitivity of the neuron to different frequencies (J. B. Fritz, Elhilali, & Shamma, 2005), or in the temporal parameters of the STRF such as its latency (J. Fritz et al., 2005).

Another interesting use of the STRFs is in characterizing global response properties of a large population of cells or cortical areas for the purpose of summarizing its representational properties, and how that may change due to learning and plasticity. Specifically, in many situations, cortical neurons encode considerable details about the underlying sensory stimuli, and the encoded information is likely to change with stimulus context and behavioral conditions in a manner that is difficult to discern across large sets of single neuron data because of the complexity of cortical receptive fields. STRFs help overcome this problem because they facilitate methods of stimulus *reconstruction* to study how complex sounds are encoded in A1. In such a method, measured STRFs are used to *invert* the responses and hence map population responses to an estimate of the stimulus spectrogram (Mesgarani, David, Fritz, & Shamma, 2009). This enables one to perform a direct comparison between an original stimulus spectrogram and its reconstruction following learning or from responses during attention to particular cues in a behavioral paradigm. In fact, by estimating the fidelity of such reconstructions using generalized spectrally and temporally modulated noise stimuli, one can determine the range over which A1 neurons can faithfully encode such spectro-temporal features. Finally, contrasting stimulus reconstructions under different behavioral states can reveal a novel view of the rapid changes in spectro-temporal response properties induced by different attentional and motivational states.

There is much ongoing research to develop new STRF measurement procedures and structures, and to combine them with new methodologies that go beyond the simple methods discussed here. For instance, generalizing the STRFs to include nonlinear phenomena (Atencio et al., 2008; Christianson et al., 2008; Nagel & Doupe, 2008), inhibitory interactions (Schinkel-Bielefeld, David, Shamma, & Butts, 2012), and more flexible structures are among the goals being pursued. Also, STRFs are now being regularly estimated with a variety of specialized complex sounds such as bird vocalizations and speech (David, Mesgarani, & Shamma, 2007; Theunissen et al., 2000), measurements that yield STRFs that are tailored to describe more faithfully cortical responses to these sounds. Furthermore, STRFs have now transcended their initial use in single unit recordings and are currently being widely used as a tool to summarize responses in human subjects recorded with fMRI (Zatorre & Belin, 2001), MEG (Ding & Simon, 2012), EEG (Power, Reilly, & Lalor, 2011), and ECoG (Mesgarani & Chang, 2012).

Conclusion

As the divergent impressions of the seven blind men touching the elephant suggests, there are many ways to characterize the receptive field properties of auditory neurons, ranging from classical frequency response areas with responses to tone bursts covering a wide range of frequencies and amplitudes, to click rate tuning for temporal MTF, to pure amplitude tuning at CF, to STRFs derived from artificial stimuli (white noise, dynamic ripples, TORCs) or natural sounds.

As this chapter shows, the STRF is a useful and powerful measure to characterize steady state response properties of auditory neurons, combining a broad description of both temporal dynamics and spectral selectivity. However, although the STRF provides an excellent linear characterization of complex stimulus-response transformations observed in neurons throughout the auditory pathway, there is considerable range in the degree to which neural responses can be described or approximated by a linear model.

The STRF description is a very appealing approach to taming the cortical zoo of diverse neuronal receptive fields. The richness and variety of STRFs makes it possible to encode arbitrary sounds and responses can be used for stimulus reconstruction (Mesgarani & Chang, 2012; Mesgarani et al., 2009). Even within A1 there is considerable diversity between modules of narrow and broadly tuned neurons, and also laminar diversity - neurons in granular layers are “more linear” i.e. they are better describe by a model with one relevant stimulus feature (Sharpee, Atencio, & Schreiner, 2011). Input neurons in layer IV have stimulus feature preferences that are more separable in frequency/time space than those in supra or infra-granular levels. In contrast, output layers in A1 show STRFs with more complex shapes, such as elongated subfields or repeating bands of excitation or suppression (Atencio & Schreiner, 2010).

But, not all neurons in A1 have sufficient linearity in their spiking response to inputs that they can be well described by STRFs – nevertheless, these highly non-linear or “Jackson Pollock” cells may play a very important role in auditory processing. The trade-off of the

STRF approach is that you lose the ability to characterize a fairly large percentage of auditory responsive cells in A1. What percentage of cells in A1 have STRFs? Estimates of the percentage varies from ~30% to 70%, and this percentage goes down considerably as you move to higher cortical areas. However, there are still beautiful STRFs even several synapses higher up – as shown in the example neuron recorded from macaque monkey rostral STG (Figure 5) (see (Hackett, 2011) for neuroanatomical location of rSTG).

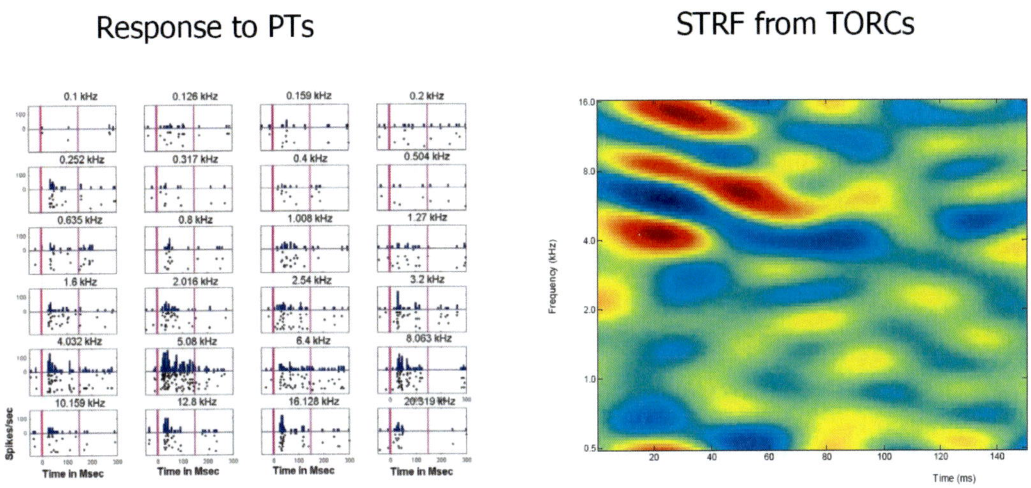

Figure 5. Example of recording in the rostral STG of the monkey, showing an STRF at least 2-3 synapses beyond A1. Most neurons in rSTG (34/53 or 64%) had receptive fields made up of several narrow frequency bands.

Concern about the lack of general applicability to all cortical cells combines with wariness of the STRF that arises from its limited predictive power (Laudanski, Edeline, & Huetz, 2012), and also because of the presence of nonlinearities (spiking threshold, rate saturation, rectification, synaptic depression, modulation of responses by stimulus context, attentional effects and other state-dependent effects) that cast doubt on the linear assumptions underlying the STRF. Various approaches have been taken to go beyond the STRF by new analysis techniques that add input or output nonlinearities, simplified second order interaction terms, feedback kernels, spectro-temporal contrast kernels or multiple feature dimensions (Ahrens et al., 2008; Atencio et al., 2008; Calabrese, Schumacher, Schneider, Paninski, & Wooley, 2011; Rabinowitz, Willmore, Schnupp, & King, 2012). These STRF-nonlinearity models represent exciting new approaches to describing neural function in A1, and generally also have greater predictive success.

The shape of STRFs depends on the choice of stimulus and properties of the stimulus ensemble (Aertsen & Johannesma, 1981; Blake & Merzenich, 2002; David et al., 2009; Laudanski et al., 2012; Machens et al., 2004; Theunissen et al., 2000; Valentine & Eggermont, 2004; Woolley, Gill, & Theunissen, 2006), and STRFs generated from the prevailing ripple stimuli generally lack predictive power for communication calls and other natural sounds. This realization has lead to the use of different stimulus classes (conspecific vocalizations, such as birdcalls or speech) to generate STRFs that have enhanced predictive power for the sounds in these classes (David et al., 2007; Laudanski et al., 2012; Nagel & Doupe, 2008).

One valuable use of the STRF has been to explore the effects of selective attention on cortical filters (Atiani, Elhilali, David, Fritz, & Shamma, 2009; David, Fritz, & Shamma, 2012; J. Fritz et al., 2003; J. B. Fritz et al., 2005; J. B. Fritz, Elhilali, & Shamma, 2007). In addition to its effect on gain control, attention also appears to be able to independently re-shape receptive fields by rapidly changing synaptic input weightings to enhance processing of relevant stimulus features. These dynamic task-driven changes are captured and observed in ~60% of STRFs and have lead to the insight that this reshaping can be described as the convolution of the STRF with a contrast filter emphasizing foreground over background stimuli (J. B. Fritz et al., 2007; Mesgarani, Fritz, & Shamma, 2010).

These results in the awake, behaving animal suggests that the STRF is highly adaptive and reflects top-down influences such as attention, as well as bottom-up influences such as statistics of the ongoing stimulus ensemble or soundscape. So, to make it more complicated, and interesting, the elephant in the story of the seven blind men is a dynamic elephant that changes shape in response to cognitive and stimulus context.

References

Adelson, E. H., & Bergen, J. R. (1985). Spatiotemporal energy models for the perception of motion. *Journal of the Optical Society of America.A, Optics & Image Science, 2*, 284-299.

Aertsen, A. M. H. J., & Johannesma, P. I. M. (1981). The spectro-temporal receptive field. *Biological Cybernetics, 42*, 133-143.

Ahrens, M. B., Linden, J. F., & Sahani, M. (2008). Nonlinearities and contextual influences in auditory cortical responses modeled with multilinear spectrotemporal methods. *The Journal of Neuroscience, 28*(8), 1929-1942. doi:10.1523/JNEUROSCI.3377-07.2008

Atencio, C. A., & Schreiner, C. E. (2010). Laminar diversity of dynamic sound processing in cat primary auditory cortex. *Journal of Neurophysiology, 103*(1), 192-205.

Atencio, C. A., Sharpee, T. O., & Schreiner, C. E. (2008). Cooperative nonlinearities in auditory cortical neurons. *Neuron, 58*(6), 956-966. doi:10.1016/j.neuron.2008.04.026

Atiani, S., Elhilali, M., David, S. V., Fritz, J. B., & Shamma, S. A. (2009). Task difficulty and performance induce diverse adaptive patterns in gain and shape of primary auditory cortical receptive fields. *Neuron, 61*(3), 467-480. doi:10.1016/j.neuron.2008.12.027

Barlow, H. B., & Levick, W. R. (1965). The mechanism of directionally selective units in rabbit's retina. *The Journal of Physiology, 178*(3), 477-504.

Bender, E. (2000). *An introduction to mathematical modeling*. New York: Dover.

Blake, D. T., & Merzenich, M. M. (2002). Changes of AI receptive fields with sound density. *Journal of Neurophysiology, 88*(6), 3409-3420. doi:10.1152/jn.00233.2002

Borst, A., & Egelhaaf, M. (1989). Principles of visual motion detection. *Trends in Neurosciences, 12*(8), 297-306.

Bracewell, R. (1999). *The fourier transform and its applications* , McGraw-Hill.

Calabrese, A., Schumacher, J. W., Schneider, D. M., Paninski, L., & Wooley, S. M. N. (2011). A generalized linear model for estimating spectrotemporal receptive fields from responses to natural sounds. *PLoS ONE, 6*(1), e16104.

Chance, F. S., Nelson, S. B., & Abbott, L. F. (1998). Synaptic depression and the temporal response characteristics of V1 cells. *The Journal of Neuroscience, 18*(12), 4785-4799.

Chi, T., Ru, P., & Shamma, S. A. (2005). Multiresolution spectrotemporal analysis of complex sounds. *The Journal of the Acoustical Society of America, 118*(2), 887-906.

Christianson, G. B., Sahani, M., & Linden, J. F. (2008). The consequences of response nonlinearities for interpretation of spectrotemporal receptive fields. *The Journal of Neuroscience, 28*(2), 446-455.

Cohen, L. (1995). *Time-frequency signal analysis*. Englewood Cliffs, NJ: Prentice-Hall.

David, S. V., Fritz, J. B., & Shamma, S. A. (2012). Task reward structure shapes rapid receptive field plasticity in auditory cortex. *Proceedings of the National Academy of Sciences of the United States of America, 109*(6), 2144-2149. doi:10.1073/pnas.1117717109; 10.1073/pnas.1117717109

David, S. V., Mesgarani, N., Fritz, J. B., & Shamma, S. A. (2009). Rapid synaptic depression explains nonlinear modulation of spectro-temporal tuning in primary auditory cortex by natural stimuli. *Journal of Neuroscience, 29*(11), 3374-3386.

David, S. V., Hayden, B. Y., & Gallant, J. L. (2006). Spectral receptive field properties explain shape selectivity in area V4. *Journal of Neurophysiology, 96*(6), 3492-3505. doi:10.1152/jn.00575.2006

David, S. V., Mesgarani, N., & Shamma, S. A. (2007). Estimating sparse spectro-temporal receptive fields with natural stimuli. *Network: Computation in Neural Systems, 18*(3), 191-212. doi:10.1080/09548980701609235

De Boer,E. (1967). Correlation studies applied to the frequency resolution of the cochlea. *Journal of Auditory Research, 7*(2), 209-217.

de Boer, E., & de Jongh, H. R. (1978). On cochlear encoding: Potentialities and limitations of the reverse-correlation technique. *The Journal of the Acoustical Society of America, 63*(1), 115-135.

De Boer, E., & Kuyper, P. (1968). Triggered correlation. *Biomedical Engineering, IEEE Transactions On, BME-15*(3), 169-179.

De Valois, R. L., & De Valois, K. K. (1988). *Spatial vision*. New York, Oxford: University Press.

De Valois, R. L., Cottaris, N. P., Elfar, S. D., Mahon, L. E., & Wilson, J. A. (2000). Some transformations of color information from lateral geniculate nucleus to striate cortex. *Proceedings of the National Academy of Sciences of the United States of America, 97*(9), 4997-5002.

de Villers-Sidani, E., Chang, E. F., Bao, S., & Merzenich, M. M. (2007). Critical period window for spectral tuning defined in the primary auditory cortex (A1) in the rat. *The Journal of Neuroscience, 27*(1), 180-189. doi:10.1523/JNEUROSCI.3227-06.2007

DeAngelis, G. C., Ohzawa, I., & Freeman, R. D. (1995). Receptive-field dynamics in the central visual pathways. *Trends in Neurosciences, 18*(10), 451-458.

Depireux, D. A., Simon, J. Z., Klein, D. J., & Shamma, S. A. (2001). Spectro-temporal response field characterization with dynamic ripples in ferret primary auditory cortex. *Journal of Neurophysiology, 85*(3), 1220-1234.

Ding, N., & Simon, J. Z. (2012). Emergence of neural encoding of auditory objects while listening to competing speakers. *Proceedings of the National Academy of Sciences of the United States of America, 109*(29), 11854-11859. doi:10.1073/pnas.1205381109

Eggermont, J. J. (1993). Wiener and volterra analyses applied to the auditory system. *Hearing Research, 66*(2), 177-201.
Eggermont, J. J., Aertsen, A. M., & Johannesma, P. I. (1983). Quantitative characterisation procedure for auditory neurons based on the spectro-temporal receptive field. *Hearing Research, 10*(2), 167-190.
Eggermont, J. J., & Smith, G. M. (1990). Characterizing auditory neurons using the wigner and rihacek distributions: A comparison. *The Journal of the Acoustical Society of America, 87*(1), 246-259.
Elhilali, M., Fritz, J. B., Klein, D. J., Simon, J. Z., & Shamma, S. A. (2004). Dynamics of precise spike timing in primary auditory cortex. *Journal of Neuroscience, 24*(5), 1159-1172. doi:10.1523/JNEUROSCI.3825-03.2004
Elhilali, M., & Shamma, S. A. (2008). A cocktail party with a cortical twist: How cortical mechanisms contribute to sound segregation. *Journal of the Acoustical Society of America, 124*(6), 3751-3771. doi:10.1121/1.3001672
Emerson, R. C., & Gerstein, G. L. (1977). Simple striate neurons in the cat. II. mechanisms underlying directional asymmetry and directional selectivity. *Journal of Neurophysiology, 40*(1), 136-155.
Escabi, M. A., & Read, H. L. (2003). Representation of spectrotemporal sound information in the ascending auditory pathway. *Biological Cybernetics, 89*(5), 350-362.
Escabi, M. A., & Schreiner, C. E. (2002). Nonlinear spectrotemporal sound analysis by neurons in the auditory midbrain. *Journal of Neuroscience, 22*(10), 4114-4131.
Fritz, J., Elhilali, M., Klein, D. J., & Shamma, S. A. (2003). Dynamic adaptive plasticity of spectro-temporal receptive fields in the primary auditory cortex of the behaving ferret [Abstract]. *Society for Neuroscience Meeting, New Orleans, LA,*
Fritz, J., Elhilali, M., & Shamma, S. (2005). Active listening: Task-dependent plasticity of spectrotemporal receptive fields in primary auditory cortex. *Hearing Research, 206*(1-2), 159-176. doi:10.1016/j.heares.2005.01.015
Fritz, J. B., Elhilali, M., & Shamma, S. A. (2005). Differential dynamic plasticity of A1 receptive fields during multiple spectral tasks. *Journal of Neuroscience, 25*(33), 7623-7635. doi:10.1523/JNEUROSCI.1318-05.2005
Fritz, J. B., Elhilali, M., & Shamma, S. A. (2007). Adaptive changes in cortical receptive fields induced by attention to complex sounds. *Journal of Neurophysiology, 98*(4), 2337-2346. doi:10.1152/jn.00552.2007
Goldstein, J. L. (1967). Auditory nonlinearity. *The Journal of the Acoustical Society of America, 41*(3), 676-689.
Gosselin, F., & Schyns, P. (2002). A new framework for visual categorization. *Trends in Cognitive Sciences,* (6), 70-76.
Grochenig, K. (2001). *Foundations of time-frequency analysis*. Boston, MA: Birkhauser.
Hackett, T. A. (2011). Information flow in the auditory cortical network. *Hearing Research, 271*(1-2), 133-146. doi:10.1016/j.heares.2010.01.011; 10.1016/j.heares.2010.01.011
Hansen, P. C. (1997). *Rank-deficient and discrete ill-posed problems: Numerical aspects of linear inversion*. Philadelphia: SIAM.
Heeger, D. J. (1993). Modeling simple-cell direction selectivity with normalized, half-squared, linear operators. *Journal of Neurophysiology, 70*(5), 1885-1898.
Hochstein, S., & Shapley, R. M. (1976). Linear and nonlinear spatial subunits in Y cat retinal ganglion cells. *The Journal of Physiology, 262*(2), 265-284.

Hubel, D. H., & Wiesel, T. N. (1963). Receptive fields of cells in striate cortex of very young, visually inexperienced kittens. *Journal of Neurophysiology, 26*, 994-1002.

Humphrey, A. L., & Weller, R. E. (1988). Functionally distinct groups of X-cells in the lateral geniculate nucleus of the cat. *The Journal of Comparative Neurology, 268*(3), 429-447.

Isermann, R., & Munchhof, M. (2011). *Identification of dynamic systems: An introduction with applications* Springer.

Johnson, D. H. (1980). Applicability of white-noise nonlinear system analysis to the peripheral auditory system. *The Journal of the Acoustical Society of America, 68*(3), 876-884.

Jones, J. P., & Palmer, L. A. (1987). An evaluation of the two-dimensional gabor filter model of simple receptive fields in cat striate cortex. *Journal of Neurophysiology, 58*(6), 1233-1258.

Kim, P. J., & Young, E. D. (1994). Comparative analysis of spectro-temporal receptive fields, reverse correlation functions, and frequency tuning curves of auditory-nerve fibers. *The Journal of the Acoustical Society of America, 95*(1), 410-422.

Klein, D. J., Depireux, D. A., Simon, J. Z., & Shamma, S. A. (2000). Robust spectrotemporal reverse correlation for the auditory system: Optimizing stimulus design. *Journal of Computational Neuroscience, 9*(1), 85-111.

Klein, D. J., Simon, J. Z., Depireux, D. A., & Shamma, S. A. (2006). Stimulus-invariant processing and spectrotemporal reverse correlation in primary auditory cortex. *Journal of Computational Neuroscience, 20*(2), 111-136.

Kowalski, N., Depireux, D. A., & Shamma, S. A. (1996). Analysis of dynamic spectra in ferret primary auditory cortex. I. characteristics of single-unit responses to moving ripple spectra. *Journal of Neurophysiology, 76*(5), 3503-3523.

Laudanski, J., Edeline, J. M., & Huetz, C. (2012). Differences between spectro-temporal receptive fields derived from artificial and natural stimuli in the auditory cortex. *PloS One, 7*(11), e50539. doi:10.1371/journal.pone.0050539; 10.1371/journal.pone.0050539

Machens, C. K., Wehr, M. S., & Zador, A. M. (2004). Linearity of cortical receptive fields measured with natural sounds. *The Journal of Neuroscience, 24*(5), 1089-1100. doi:10.1523/JNEUROSCI.4445-03.2004

Maex, R., & Orban, G. A. (1996). Model circuit of spiking neurons generating directional selectivity in simple cells. *Journal of Neurophysiology, 75*(4), 1515-1545.

Marmarelis, P., & Marmarelis, V. (1978). *Analysis of physiological systems: The white noise approach*. New York: Plenum.

Mastronarde, D. N. (1987a). Two classes of single-input X-cells in cat lateral geniculate nucleus. I. receptive-field properties and classification of cells. *Journal of Neurophysiology, 57*(2), 357-380.

Mastronarde, D. N. (1987b). Two classes of single-input X-cells in cat lateral geniculate nucleus. II. retinal inputs and the generation of receptive-field properties. *Journal of Neurophysiology, 57*(2), 381-413.

Mathews, V., & Sicuranza, G. (2000). *Polynomial signal processing*. New York: Wiley.

McLean, J., & Palmer, L. A. (1994). Organization of simple cell responses in the three-dimensional (3-D) frequency domain. *Visual Neuroscience, 11*(2), 295-306.

Mesgarani, N., & Chang, E. F. (2012). Selective cortical representation of attended speaker in multi-talker speech perception. *Nature, 485*(7397), 233-236. doi:10.1038/nature11020

Mesgarani, N., David, S. V., Fritz, J. B., & Shamma, S. A. (2008). Phoneme representation and classification in primary auditory cortex. *The Journal of the Acoustical Society of America, 123*(2), 899-909. doi:10.1121/1.2816572

Mesgarani, N., Fritz, J., & Shamma, S. (2010). A computational model of rapid task-related plasticity of auditory cortical receptive fields. *Journal of Computational Neuroscience, 28*(1), 19-27. doi:10.1007/s10827-009-0181-3; 10.1007/s10827-009-0181-3

Mesgarani, N., Slaney, M., & Shamma, S. A. (2006). Content-based audio classification based on multiscale spectro-temporal features. *IEEE Transaction on Speech and Audio Processing, 14*(3), 920-930.

Mesgarani, N., David, S. V., Fritz, J. B., & Shamma, S. A. (2009). Influence of context and behavior on stimulus reconstruction from neural activity in primary auditory cortex. *Journal of Neuroscience, 102*(6), 3329-3333.

Miller, L. M., Escabi, M. A., Read, H. L., & Schreiner, C. E. (2002). Spectrotemporal receptive fields in the lemniscal auditory thalamus and cortex. *Journal of Neurophysiology, 87*(1), 516-527.

Nagel, K. I., & Doupe, A. J. (2008). Organizing principles of spectro-temporal encoding in the avian primary auditory area field L. *Neuron, 58*(6), 938-955. doi:10.1016/j.neuron.2008.04.028

Nelken, I. (2004). Processing of complex stimuli and natural scenes in the auditory cortex. *Current Opinion in Neurobiology, 14*(4), 474-480.

Nelken, I., & Young, E. D. (1997). Linear and nonlinear spectral integration in type IV neurons of the dorsal cochlear nucleus. I. regions of linear interaction. *Journal of Neurophysiology, 78*(2), 790-799.

Ogunfunmi, T. (2007). *Adaptive nonlinear system identification: The volterra and wiener model approaches (signals and communication technology)* Springer.

Patil, K., Pressnitzer, D., Shamma, S., & Elhilali, M. (2012). Music in our ears: The biological bases of musical timbre perception. *PLoS Computational Biology, 8*(11), e1002759. doi:10.1371/journal.pcbi.1002759

Pickles, J. O. (2008). *An introduction to the physiology of hearing* (Third ed.) Emerald Group Publishing Limited.

Power, A. J., Reilly, R. B., & Lalor, E. C. (2011). Comparing linear and quadratic models of the human auditory system using EEG. *Annual International Conference of the IEEE Engineering in Medicine and Biology Society.IEEE Engineering in Medicine and Biology Society.Conference, 2011*, 4171-4174. doi:10.1109/IEMBS.2011.6091035

Press, W. H., Flannery, B. P., Teukolsky, S. A., & Vetterling, W. T. (1992). *Numerical recipes: The art of scientific computing* Cambridge University Press.

Rabinowitz, N. C., Willmore, B. D., Schnupp, J. W., & King, A. J. (2012). Spectrotemporal contrast kernels for neurons in primary auditory cortex. *The Journal of Neuroscience, 32*(33), 11271-11284. doi:10.1523/JNEUROSCI.1715-12.2012; 10.1523/JNEUROSCI.1715-12.2012

Ringach, D., Sapiro, G., & Shapley, R. (1997). A subspace reverse-correlation technique for the study of visual neurons. *Vision Research, 37*(17), 2455-2464.

Rugh, W. (1981). *Nonlinear system theory: The volterra/wiener approach*. Baltimore, MD: Johns Hopkins Univ. Press.

Sang-Won Nam, & Powers, E. J. (2003). Volterra series representation of time-frequency distributions. *Signal Processing, IEEE Transactions On, 51*(6), 1532-1537.

Sastry, S. (1999). *Nonlinear systems* Springer.
Schinkel-Bielefeld, N., David, S. V., Shamma, S. A., & Butts, D. A. (2012). Inferring the role of inhibition in auditory processing of complex natural stimuli. *Journal of Neurophysiology, 107*(12), 3296-3307. doi:10.1152/jn.01173.2011
Sharpee, T. O., Atencio, C. A., & Schreiner, C. E. (2011). Hierarchical representations in the auditory cortex. *Current Opinion in Neurobiology, 21*(5), 761-767.
Shechter, B., Dobbins, H. D., Marvit, P., & Depireux, D. A. (2009). Dynamics of spectro-temporal tuning in primary auditory cortex of the awake ferret. *Hearing Research, 256*(1-2), 118-130. doi:10.1016/j.heares.2009.07.005; 10.1016/j.heares.2009.07.005
Simon, J. Z., Depireux, D. A., Klein, D. J., Fritz, J. B., & Shamma, S. A. (2007). Temporal symmetry in primary auditory cortex: Implications for cortical connectivity. *Neural Computation, 19*(3), 583-638.
Smith, A. T., Snowden, R. J., & Milne, A. B. (1994). Is global motion really based on spatial integration of local motion signals? *Vision Research, 34*(18), 2425-2430. doi:10.1016/0042-6989(94)90286-0
Sripati, A. P., Yoshioka, T., Denchev, P., Hsiao, S. S., & Johnson, K. O. (2006). Spatiotemporal receptive fields of peripheral afferents and cortical area 3b and 1 neurons in the primate somatosensory system. *The Journal of Neuroscience, 26*(7), 2101-2114. doi:10.1523/JNEUROSCI.3720-05.2006
Stewart, G. W. (1993). Determining rank in the presence of error. In M. S. Moonen, G. H. Golub & B. L. Moor (Eds.), *Linear algebra for large scale and real- time applications* (pp. 1-19). Dordrecht: Kluwer Academic Publishers.
Suarez, H., Koch, C., & Douglas, R. (1995). Modeling direction selectivity of simple cells in striate visual cortex within the framework of the canonical microcircuit. *The Journal of Neuroscience, 15*(10), 6700-6719.
Theunissen, F. E., Sen, K., & Doupe, A. J. (2000). Spectral-temporal receptive fields of nonlinear auditory neurons obtained using natural sounds. *Journal of Neuroscience, 20*(6), 2315-2331.
Valentine, P. A., & Eggermont, J. J. (2004). Stimulus dependence of spectro-temporal receptive fields in cat primary auditory cortex. *Hearing Research, 196*(1-2), 119-133. doi:10.1016/j.heares.2004.05.011
Versnel, H., Kowalski, N., & Shamma, S. A. (1995). Ripple analysis in ferret primary auditory cortex. III. topographic distribution of ripple response parameters. *Journal of Auditory Neuroscience, 1*, 271-286.
Volterra, V. (1959). *Theory of functionals and integral and integro-differential equations*. New York: Dover Publications.
Watson, A. B., & Ahumada, A. J. (1985). Model of human visual-motion sensing. *Journal of the Optical Society of America.A, Optics & Image Science, 2*, 322-341.
Weinberger, N. M. (2007). Auditory associative memory and representational plasticity in the primary auditory cortex. *Hearing Research, 229*(1-2), 54-68. doi:10.1016/j.heares.2007.01.004
Wickesberg, R. E., Dickson, J. W., Gibson, M. M., & Geisler, C. D. (1984). Wiener kernel analysis of responses from anteroventral cochlear nucleus neurons. *Hearing Research, 14*(2), 155-174.
Wiener, N. (1958). *Nonlinear problems in random theory*. New York: Technology Press and Wiley.

Woolley, S. M., Gill, P. R., & Theunissen, F. E. (2006). Stimulus-dependent auditory tuning results in synchronous population coding of vocalizations in the songbird midbrain. *The Journal of Neuroscience, 26*(9), 2499-2512. doi:10.1523/JNEUROSCI.3731-05.2006

Yeshurun, Y., Wollberg, Z., Dyn, N., & Allon, N. (1985). Identification of MGB cells by volterra kernels. I. prediction of responses to species specific vocalizations. *Biological Cybernetics, 51*(6), 383-390.

Zatorre, R. J., & Belin, P. (2001). Spectral and temporal processing in human auditory cortex. *Cerebral Cortex, 11*(10), 946-953.

In: Handbook of Modern Techniques in Auditory Cortex
Editors: Didier A. Depireux and Mounya Elhilali
ISBN: 978-1-62808-894-6

Chapter 3

Stimulus Choices for Spike-Triggered Receptive Field Analyses

Craig A. Atencio and Christoph E. Schreiner
Coleman Memorial Laboratory,
Department of Otolaryngology-Head and Neck Surgery,
and UCSF Center for Integrative Neuroscience
University of California, San Francisco, California, US

I. Principles

Spike-triggered analyses can reveal the spectral and temporal conditions under which a neuron is activated, and can be expressed in the form of the spectrotemporal receptive field (STRF). STRF analysis is at the core of many approaches to study and understand the form and function of the auditory system. However, the outcome of such an analysis may depend on the initial selection of spectrotemporal stimulus parameters. Numerous studies with different stimulus configurations, combined with various, and in certain ways differing, analytical approaches to STRF analysis, seem to make it difficult to navigate between studies and to assess their theoretical rigor and validity.

Indeed, the many available stimuli of interest make it challenging to choose the right approach to estimate STRFs. Additionally, for those wishing to have a rigorous and theoretically sound interpretive framework in which to view STRF results, it may be difficult to discern potential problems or advantages of the approaches and how the stimuli and methods, and the results they supply, can be compared across studies.

To allay these concerns and the perceived challenges of the approach, we will visit here the main types of stimuli that have been used and briefly discuss the analytical approaches that have been applied to estimate STRFs. These two aspects must be treated together, since the applied stimulus will influence the type of analysis that may be employed. When unsuitable or incomplete stimulus sets are mixed with an inappropriate analysis the results may be challenging to interpret or, at least, promote misleading or even false interpretations with questionable conclusions.

Thus, to make progress, we need to be cognizant of the underlying neural model and the assumptions that accompany the model. We must assess the class of systems to which the neural model belongs and what it can accomplish. After classifying the neural model, we may consider the appropriate stimuli for the experiments.

For the analyses we will discuss in this chapter, the system to be modeled is the single neuron, and the model of the system describes the relationship between the stimulus and the spiking response. In the auditory system, as in other sensory modalities, neurons are considered to belong to the Volterra class of nonlinear signal processing systems. The Volterra class of systems have finite memory, are time-invariant, non-chaotic, and non-oscillatory (Marmarelis, 2004). The STRF approach is only appropriate for systems with these characteristics. In auditory regions that have been examined extensively, neurons satisfy these requirements reasonably: they have finite memory, are non-chaotic and are non-oscillatory. They are also time-invariant, since under the conditions typically used to measure STRFs, the stimulus statistics remain constant and there is only limited adaptation and plasticity (Elhilali et al., 2007).

We can probe Volterra systems with appropriately chosen stimuli. One requirement for stimulating Volterra systems is essential and pre-eminent: "A key requirement for nonlinear system modeling is that the ensemble of input waveforms contains most, if not all, frequencies and amplitudes of interest (i.e. cover the entire bandwidth and dynamic range of the system under study)."(Marmarelis, 2004).

This implies that "the system must be tested exhaustively over its entire bandwidth and dynamic range in order to observe all possible nonlinear interactions." (Marmarelis, 2004). The STRF that is estimated will approximate the correct receptive field to the extent that the stimulus satisfies these requirements.

This leads to the two fundamental principles of STRF stimulation:

1) Stimuli must cover the bandwidth/stimulus preferences of the neuron; and
2) The technique that is used must be able to correct for any correlations in the stimulus ensemble.

Therefore, the stimulus must have sufficient bandwidth, in terms of frequency extent and spectrotemporal features, to excite the neuron, and the receptive field estimate must be unbiased. The STRF estimation technique must be capable of correcting for any correlations that are present in the stimulus ensemble. If the technique cannot correct for correlations in the stimulus, then the estimated STRF will only be a biased estimate of the neuron's receptive field.

When the core principles of STRF stimulation are violated the meaning and significance of the resulting function may be difficult or impossible to understand. For example, if the full bandwidth of the neuron is not covered, then important nonlinear interactions may not be elicited. If the stimulus is not appropriate for the STRF method, e.g., by containing specific types of correlations, then the results may again be difficult to interpret, since the technique cannot remove the effects of the correlations and thus it cannot deliver unbiased STRF estimates. The degree of deviation of the STRF - due to inappropriate stimulus choice - from the 'true' STRF is difficult to assess and may vary from minor magnitude changes to major shape alterations and component omissions.

In the following, we discuss different aspects of stimuli for spike-triggered analyses. We first discuss the most widely used, the most powerful, or the most theoretically tractable techniques for spike-triggered analyses. We next discuss the major classes of stimuli that have been used to stimulate auditory neurons. After that we consider the manner in which the stimuli may be represented. We then survey previous studies and discuss the various analytical approaches and the stimuli that were employed. We conclude by providing a synthesis of stimuli and approaches to enable researchers to make appropriate decisions for their experimental conditions.

II. Analysis

Overview

The ideal spectrotemporal receptive field (STRF) is a complete description of the time and frequency stimulus preferences of a neuron. The STRF describes the spectrotemporal stimulus features that, when presented to a neuron, will cause a neuron to fire. The term STRF normally implies a single linear filter that describes the stimulus processing of the neuron. In this context, the STRF is often approximated as the spike-triggered average (STA). The STA is the average stimulus that precedes a spike.

However, the full STRF description may encompass more than a single linear filter. If the STRF is comprised of multiple components, or linear filters, then the STA approach may not be sufficient to appropriately approximate the STRF. Studies in the auditory midbrain and cortex have shown that some neurons have STRFs with multiple components (Atencio et al., 2008, 2009; Andoni and Pollak, 2011). Atencio and colleagues have shown that neurons in cat primary auditory cortex (AI) are often best described by an STRF with at least two components (Atencio et al., 2008, 2009). The number and/or strength of these components varied systematically with the laminar anatomy of cortex. Also, STRFs with multiple components have been discovered in central stations of bats and song birds (Andoni and Pollak, 2011; Sharpee et al., 2011b). Therefore, the term "STRF" must be used with caution, since the appropriate neural model must be determined for results to be interpreted in the correct framework. Only when the STRF is confirmed to have only one component is it appropriate to think of it as a single linear filter.

Since the STRF may have multiple components, it may be modeled as a set of linear filters. Since each filter represents a stimulus feature that, in conjunction with all other filters, models the neuron's stimulus selectivity, the set of filters can be viewed as a subspace of stimulus dimensions. The STRF can be approximated as a set of linear filters because neurons in the auditory system reasonably satisfy the requirements of Volterra systems: they have fading memory, they are time-invariant, they are non-chaotic, and they are non-oscillatory (Boyd and Chua, 1985; Westwick and Kearney, 1998).

The STRF approach is built upon the Volterra kernel expansion method, which describes a nonlinear system in terms of a series of functionals. The series of functionals is analogous to a Taylor series, where a function is approximated by a series of polynomials. In a Volterra series, a nonlinear dynamic system is approximated as a series of functionals that contain the information necessary to characterize the nonlinear processing of the system. Thus, many functionals may be needed for a moderately nonlinear system. However, the Volterra expansion can be equivalently represented as a two part model: a set of filters in a filter bank (part 1) whose outputs are processed by a static nonlinearity (part 2). The dimensionality of the nonlinearity depends on the number of filters in the filter bank. Thus, the key innovation in reformulating the Volterra series was that the dynamics and nonlinearities could be separated and are available for individual scrutiny and interpretation.

As Marmarelis noted, "... a general model of the Volterra class of systems can take a block-structured form wherein the basis functions constitute the impulse responses of a filter bank whose outputs are feeding into a multi-input static nonlinearity $f(v1, \ldots, vj, \ldots)$. For a selected basis ... the modeling problem reduces to estimating the multivariate function $f(.)$. Of course, the latter will be different for different bases." (Marmarelis et al., 1999).

Therefore, a neural system can be represented by one or several linear filters followed by static nonlinearities (Palm, 1979). This model is called a Linear-Nonlinear model in the neuroscience literature, though in engineering reports it is termed a Wiener-Bose system (Figure 1). There are relatively few requirements for this description to be appropriate:

"Note that the formal decomposition of a nonlinear dynamic system into a linear filter bank (representing the dynamics) and a multi-input static nonlinearity is valid for all systems that have square-integrable kernels (5). In discrete-time representations, this condition becomes one of square summability, which is satisfied by the condition of absolute summability defining the Volterra class of systems." (Marmarelis, 1997).

Therefore, the LN model is neither ad-hoc nor inappropriate (Pienkowski et al., 2009). In fact, it follows from a straightforward application of the theoretically sound Volterra systems identification approach.

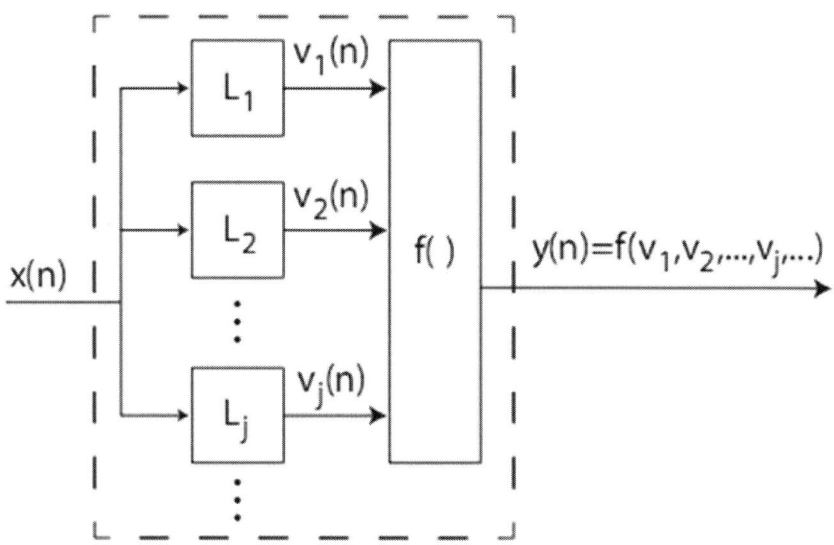

Figure 1. Schematic of the Linear-Nonlinear (LN) model. The model structure is also known as a Wiener-Bose system. The stimulus x(n) is processed by a bank of linear filters, whose output is sent to a nonlinear gain function, or nonlinearity, f(). The response of the system, y(n), is the output of the nonlinear gain. Model schematic adapted from (Marmarelis, 1989, 1997).

Since the LN model can be used to represent the processing of a neuron, the problem of identifying a system reduces to estimating the components of the linear filter bank and the associated nonlinear input/output function. While many approaches have been described, there is one prime principle that must be heeded: The choice of stimulus constrains the analysis approach that may be applied.

Analytical Approaches

In the following, we review analytical approaches that are highly used, very powerful, and have undergone extensive theoretical testing (Figure 2). We begin by discussing the spike-triggered average technique, which recovers a single linear filter. We then discuss techniques that allow multiple STRF components to be estimated.

A. Spike-triggered average (STA)

The STRF is most commonly represented as the spike-triggered average (STA). The STA is calculated by averaging the stimuli that directly precede a spike (Figure 2). This procedure is known as reverse correlation (de Boer and Kuyper, 1968). The STA may also be obtained through linear regression of the stimulus/response relationship (DiCarlo et al., 1998; Paninski, 2003). In the following discussion, by STA we mean all approaches that utilize an average of stimuli that precede a spike, whether this average is normalized or not. The STA may be interpreted in several ways: as the average stimulus feature that precedes a spike, a relevant stimulus dimension, the optimal stimulus, a linear filter, or a spectrotemporal feature to which the neuron is tuned (deCharms et al., 1998; Bialek and de Ruyter van Steveninck, 2005).

To gain insight into the methodology, we need to understand how the stimulus affects the STA. Each stimulus is assumed to be represented as a function of time and frequency. The set of all stimuli that are presented to the neuron is termed the stimulus ensemble. The set of stimuli that precede a spike is termed the spike-triggered stimulus ensemble. For a simple case, where the stimulus has two frequencies and two time bins, we represent an individual time-frequency stimulus as:

$$S(f,t_k) = \begin{bmatrix} s(f_1,t_{k-1}) & s(f_1,t_k) \\ s(f_2,t_{k-1}) & s(f_2,t_k) \end{bmatrix} = \begin{bmatrix} s_1 & s_3 \\ s_2 & s_4 \end{bmatrix}$$

t_k is the kth time bin in the stimulus. The time interval between stimulus samples, $t_k - t_{k-1}$, is determined by the user and is based on the temporal modulation processing capacity of the system under study. In the auditory midbrain a time interval of 1 ms is usually sufficient, in the thalamus it may be 1-5 ms, and in the cortex it is usually 5 ms (Joris et al., 2004). The number of pre-spike time points must also be specified, and in practice this is determined by the memory of the neuron.

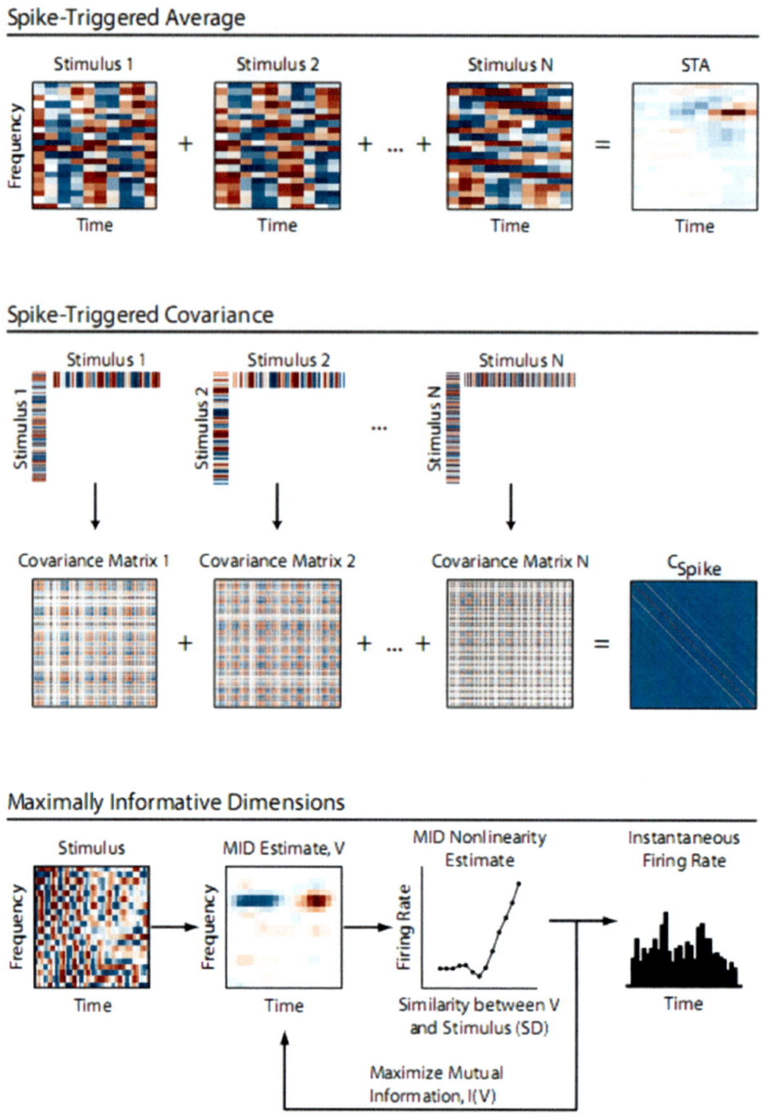

Figure 2. Analytical approaches for estimated STRFs. *Top*: to estimate the spike-triggered average (STA), the stimuli preceding a spike are obtained, and then summed. After a sufficient number of spikes, the excitatory (red) and inhibitory (blue) subfields emerge within the STA. *Middle*: in Spike-Triggered Covariance (STC), the stimuli that precede a spike are obtained. Each single stimulus is reshaped into a column and a row vector. The outer product of the vectors produces a covariance matrix for stimulus that preceded a spike. The sum of the stimulus covariance matrices is the spike-conditional covariance matrix, C_{Spike}. To obtain STRF filter components, the eigenvectors and eigenvalues of C_{Spike} are estimated. For each significant eigenvalue, the corresponding eigenvector is an STRF component, or linear filter. In most applications, the STA is removed from each stimulus covariance matrix estimate, though this step has been omitted here for simplicity. *Bottom*: in Maximally Informative Dimensions (MID) analysis, an iterative search is made for a filter V that captures the most mutual information between the stimulus and the response. At each iteration, the algorithm estimates the filter V and nonlinear gain function (nonlinearity). The algorithm first adjusts the filter's excitatory and inhibitory subregions. Then, the algorithm estimates the information by calculating the nonlinearity. The nonlinearity relates the output of the filter to the response of the neuron. Upon convergence the final filter estimate V is the first MID.

In the midbrain the memory is usually less than ~50 ms, in the thalamus it is less than ~100 ms, and in cortex it is less than ~200 ms (these roughly correspond to the time constant of forward masking in each station).

We can formulate the estimation problem as a linear model. First, the stimuli that were presented are collected into a matrix. Each row of the matrix represents one of the presented stimuli. The columns in each row represent the time and frequency components of the stimulus. As above, we assume that the receptive field has two time components and two frequency components. For the case of *N* stimuli, the linear model may now be written as (DiCarlo et al., 1998; Blake and Merzenich, 2002):

$$r_{predicted} = \begin{bmatrix} s_{1,1} & s_{1,2} & s_{1,3} & s_{1,4} \\ \vdots & \vdots & \vdots & \vdots \\ s_{N,1} & s_{N,2} & s_{N,3} & s_{N,4} \end{bmatrix} \begin{bmatrix} b_1 \\ b_2 \\ b_3 \\ b_4 \end{bmatrix}$$

$$= Xb$$

Here the STA is denoted as the vector *b*, and the stimulus is contained in the matrix X. The subscripts of the stimuli differ from those of the STA because for the stimulus the absolute time does not have significance. On the other hand, the time bins in the STA have a physiological interpretation: they represent the time before a spike occurred. *b*, the STA, is in column vector form, though for display purposes it is reshaped into the standard time-frequency matrix representation. Since the response and stimulus are known, the problem reduces to estimating *b*, the STA. We note that the filter can be recovered without taking the nonlinearity into account (de Boer and Kuyper, 1968; Chichilnisky, 2001). Therefore, to obtain *b* using least squares, we need to solve the normal equations for the linear model. To do this, the predicted firing rate of the model is replaced by the observed firing rate. For a linear model, the normal equations show how the filter may be obtained:

$$\left(X^T X\right) b = X^T r_{observed}$$

The matrix to the left of *b* represents the autocorrelations in the stimulus, while the terms to the right of the equal sign represent the correlation between the stimulus and the observed response (i.e., reverse correlation). We solve for *b* by inverting the stimulus autocorrelation matrix. The resulting filter is:

$$b = \left(X^T X\right)^{-1} X^T r_{observed}$$

After the filter is determined, the nonlinearity may be estimated from the data and incorporated into the Linear-Nonlinear model (Schwartz et al., 2006).

In this framework, the issues which ensue from this approach become evident. Three main approaches have been used to estimate *b*. In the first, the autocorrelation matrix of the stimulus is directly inverted in the time-frequency domain and is used to obtain the STA.

When the response is a spike train, with M spikes, and when second order correlations are non-existent or minimal, the STA is estimated as:

$$
\begin{aligned}
b &= \left(X^T X\right)^{-1} X^T r_{observed} \\
&= (I)^{-1} X^T r_{observed} \\
&= X^T r_{observed} \\
&= X^T \begin{bmatrix} 1 \\ 0 \\ \vdots \\ 1 \end{bmatrix} \\
&= \sum_{i=1}^{M} \begin{bmatrix} s_{i,1} \\ s_{i,2} \\ s_{i,3} \\ s_{i,4} \end{bmatrix} \\
&= \sum_{i=1}^{M} S_i(f,t)
\end{aligned}
$$

Since the second order correlations in the stimulus were minimal, the autocorrelation matrix was replaced by the identity matrix. Since the spike train contained 1's and 0's (spike or no spike, respectively), only the 1's contribute to the solution. The stimuli that correspond to the spikes are the spike-triggered stimulus ensemble. Therefore, the STA is the sum of the stimuli that preceded a spike. If desired, b may also be scaled according to the number of spikes and the units of the stimulus.

Though this procedure is efficient and simple, problems may arise (Paninski, 2003). Specifically, applied stimuli can have at most second order correlations. Many noise-type sounds satisfy this condition; natural sounds, however, do not. If there are higher order correlations, then the inversion of the stimulus autocorrelation matrix, $\left(X^T X\right)^{-1}$, cannot correct for the correlations, and the STA will be biased.

If the stimulus ensemble has only second order correlations, then in practice the main difficulty is inverting the autocorrelation matrix. If stimuli that contribute to neural firing have not been adequately sampled, then the inversion will amplify noise.

Two main methods have been used to invert ill-conditioned autocorrelation matrices. The first approach, subspace regression, uses singular value decomposition to obtain the pseudoinverse (Theunissen et al., 2000; Kim and Doupe, 2011). The pseudoinverse is used to represent the inverse of the autocorrelation matrix as $\left(X^T X\right)^{-1} = \sum_i \frac{v_i u_i^T}{\sigma_i}$. Therefore, the pseudoinverse is a weighted sum of outer products of the singular vectors v_i and u_i. The number of singular values and corresponding outer products can be limited by removing those that reduce the predictive power of the model or if they amplify noise (i.e. when is small).

The second approach is to use Ridge Regression to introduce a stabilizing factor which will make the matrix inversion better conditioned (Draper and Smith, 1981; Machens et al., 2004; Lesica and Grothe, 2008). In Ridge Regression, the solution to the normal equations is modified as:

$$b = \left(X^T X + \lambda I\right)^{-1} X^T r_{observed}$$

λ stabilizes the inverse by adding a constant to the diagonal of the stimulus autocorrelation matrix. This allows a decorrelated STA to be calculated when the inverse of the correlation matrix is ill-conditioned. Note, however, that this does not obviate the problem of natural sounds: these sounds have higher than second order stimulus correlations, and thus using them to estimate the STA may result in unsound estimates (Voss and Clarke, 1975; Sharpee et al., 2004). Further, a heuristic method is needed to choose the optimal value for λ. λ is often chosen to minimize the error between the observed and predicted responses, though this procedure is not guaranteed to lead to the correct receptive field estimate.

The second part of the Linear-Nonlinear model is the nonlinearity. After the STA has been estimated, the nonlinearity may be computed (Atencio and Schreiner, 2012). The nonlinearity describes the probability of spike generation for each stimulus. This nonlinear, memory-less input/output function describes how the correlation between the stimulus and the linear filter is translated to the response of the neuron. The following steps are used to calculate the nonlinearity. First, each stimulus segment, $S_i(f,t)$, that elicited a spike, is correlated with the STA by projecting it onto the STA via the inner product $z = S_i \cdot STA$. These projections represent the similarity between the stimulus and the filter, and they characterize the probability distribution $P(z \mid spike)$. Next, all stimuli that were presented, without regard to a spike, are projected onto the STA, forming the prior distribution, $P(z)$. The mean and standard deviation of $P(z)$, μ and σ, are then calculated, and and are transformed to units of standard deviation by using to obtain the distributions and $P(x)$. This transforms the values of x to units of standard deviation (SD). The nonlinearity for the STA is then computed as , where is the average firing rate of the neuron. Thus, the nonlinearity describes the likelihood of a spike given the similarity between the STA and the stimulus.

In summary, the STA is an efficient estimate of a single linear filter that does not require much computational cost. The most appropriate stimulus for STA analyses is a broad-band, noise-like stimulus that may be characterized by second-order correlations. The stimulus is not required to be Gaussian, though it must not have higher than second-order correlations. As the stimulus deviates from this requirement the estimated STA becomes more biased (Sharpee et al., 2004). Therefore, if natural sounds are to be used with this approach, the statistics of each natural sound stimulus ensemble need to be assessed.

B. Spike-Triggered Covariance

A second approach to estimating receptive fields is Spike-triggered Covariance (STC; Figure 2). The details of each application of STC may vary, though the goal is the same: to compute the covariance of the stimuli that preceded a spike (Marmarelis, 1997; Lewis et al.,

2002b; Touryan et al., 2002; Rust et al., 2005; Pillow and Simoncelli, 2006). Since the STA is a linear sum of stimuli, it represents the mean of the spike-triggered stimulus ensemble, and how it differs from the complete stimulus ensemble.

Alternatively, the STC metric quantifies changes in the variance of the spike-triggered stimulus ensemble relative to the complete stimulus ensemble. The covariance matrix for spike-triggered stimuli is:

$$C_{spike} = \sum_{i=1}^{M} (S_i - b)(S_i - b)^T$$
$$= \sum_{i=1}^{M} \left(S_i S_i^T - bb^T \right)$$

where

$$S_i S_i^T = \begin{bmatrix} s_{i,1} \\ s_{i,2} \\ s_{i,3} \\ s_{i,4} \end{bmatrix} \begin{bmatrix} s_{i,1} & s_{i,2} & s_{i,3} & s_{i,4} \end{bmatrix}$$
$$= \begin{bmatrix} s_{i,1}s_{i,1} & s_{i,1}s_{i,2} & s_{i,1}s_{i,3} & s_{i,1}s_{i,4} \\ s_{i,2}s_{i,1} & s_{i,2}s_{i,2} & s_{i,2}s_{i,3} & s_{i,2}s_{i,4} \\ s_{i,3}s_{i,1} & s_{i,3}s_{i,2} & s_{i,3}s_{i,3} & s_{i,3}s_{i,4} \\ s_{i,4}s_{i,1} & s_{i,4}s_{i,2} & s_{i,4}s_{i,3} & s_{i,4}s_{i,4} \end{bmatrix}$$

For each stimulus that elicited a spike, the outer product of that stimulus with itself is computed. *M* is the number of spikes, is a column vector of the *i*th stimulus that preceded a spike, *b* is the STA in column vector form, and *T* is the transpose operator. Thus, is the sum of outer products, or covariance matrices, of the stimuli that preceded a spike, and therefore it quantifies the pairwise interactions in the stimulus. If desired, may be scaled according to the number of spikes.

After is obtained it is decomposed to find its eigenvectors and eigenvalues. The statistical significance of each eigenvalue is then determined. For each significant eigenvalue, the corresponding eigenvector represents an STRF component, or linear filter, that describes the stimulus selectivity of the neuron. Since the STA, *b*, is subtracted out from the spike-triggered ensemble, the STA is orthogonal to the eigenvectors from STC. The dimensionality of the STRF is determined by the total number of linear filters, which is the STA and the set of significant eigenvectors.

Since STC computes outer products, and outer products are pairwise multiplications, the metric only considers second order correlations. Thus, the stimuli that are used must have at most second order correlations. Theoretical analysis has further shown that STC analysis imposes stricter stimulus conditions than the STA. While the STA required that stimuli be described by second order statistics, the STC further requires that the stimuli be Gaussian

(Paninski, 2003). Deviations from these requirements will lead to biased, or incorrect, filter estimates (Sharpee et al., 2004). This problem is significant for natural sounds.

In the auditory system, the STC approach was first used by Lewis and colleagues (Yamada and Lewis, 1999; Lewis et al., 2002a, b). They presented a particularly elegant and clear description of the analysis in (Lewis et al., 2002b). They presented Gaussian white noise while recording from frog auditory nerves that had high characteristic frequencies. They then estimated the STA and the STC filters. The recovered STA did not have significant features, since the high CF neurons could not phase-lock to the white noise waveform. However, the STC analysis did reveal multiple linear filters that described the frequency tuning and spectral sidebands of the associated neurons.

In summary, the STA recovers a single filter. For STRFs that are best described by multiple linear filters, the STC approach can be beneficially applied. Once the additional filters are obtained, the nonlinearities associated with each filter may be recovered from the data if there are only two filters. If there are more than two, then the data requirements will usually be too great, and multidimensional nonlinearities usually cannot be estimated (Fitzgerald et al., 2011). To alleviate this issue, a parametric form for the nonlinearities has been proposed, though it is unclear if this form is appropriate for auditory neurons. The nonlinearities are modeled as a ratio of Gaussian distributions. In the visual system, this parametric model was found to be appropriate for retinal ganglion cells, but not for visual cortical cells (Pillow and Simoncelli, 2006).

Therefore, while STC can recover multiple filters, it also has multiple weaknesses. First, it can only be used with Gaussian stimuli. STC analysis can be modified to apply to non-Gaussian stimuli, though in this extension the stimuli must still be characterized by their mean and variance (Samengo and Gollisch, 2012). When non-Gaussian stimuli with higher than second-order correlations are used, the results may be difficult to interpret, since the approach cannot take into account higher order stimulus correlations. Second, the joint nonlinearity for more than two linear filters cannot usually be empirically estimated, and thus a parametric form for the nonlinearities must be assumed.

The next approach that we discuss, Maximally Informative Dimensions, can be used with a wide range of stimulus ensembles, and can be used to recover multiple filters.

C. Maximally Informative Dimensions (MID)

A very powerful technique for estimating STRFs is the method of Maximally Informative Dimensions (MID; Figure 2). This method can be used with a wide range of broad-band stimulus statistics, since the procedure corrects for all stimulus correlations. It is able to bypass the stimulus requirements of the STA and STC procedure since it uses a different evaluation metric.

STA finds the filter that represents deviations from the mean background stimulus, and STC finds filters that represent changes in the variance of the spike triggered stimulus ensemble. The MID approach supersedes these by finding the filter that maximizes the information between the stimulus and the response. Information operates on the entire stimulus distribution, and thus can take into account all stimulus correlations. The information provided by any filter, v, is estimated as:

$$I(v) = \int dx P_v(x \mid spike) \log_2 \left[\frac{P_v(x \mid spike)}{P_v(x)} \right]$$

In the MID approach, the stimulus space is searched for the filter v that maximizes the information (Figure 2). The filter that maximizes the information is the first maximally informative dimension (MID1).

The nonlinearity is found at the same time as the filter. This can be seen by considering the form of the nonlinearity:

$$P_v(spike \mid x) = P_v(spike) \frac{P_v(x \mid spike)}{P_v(x)}$$

Therefore, up to the scaling constant $P_v(spike)$, the nonlinearity is equivalent to the argument of the logarithm term within the information equation. Hence, when MID1 is estimated, so is the corresponding nonlinearity.

The MID approach has multiple strengths: it can be used with many stimulus ensembles – natural or otherwise; it can be straightforwardly extended to find a second (or more) MIDs that act in parallel to the first filter and further maximize the information; and it simultaneously finds the filters and the associated nonlinearities.

The main weakness of the MID approach is the amount of data that is required. Since the information is calculated using an experimental histogram approach, only a limited number of filters may be estimated (Fitzgerald et al., 2011). In practice, usually two, and at most three, filters are obtainable for cortical neurons. A second possible concern is that the MID search procedure may converge to a local maximum. In practice, however, this problem can be circumvented by using an adequate search algorithm, such as simulated annealing (Sharpee et al., 2004). Model simulations showed that when simulated annealing was combined with random starting guesses, the search procedure converged to the correct filter estimate (Sharpee et al., 2011b). Further evidence for the robustness of the MID approach is that when simulated annealing was compared to another powerful search algorithm, random-restart hill climbing, both converged to the same filter estimate (Andrew Saxe, personal communication).

Therefore, if the STRF can be approximated as a single linear filter, the STA approach is adequate. Alternatively, if one seeks the main stimulus feature that contributes to neuronal stimulus selectivity, the STA will recover that feature if appropriate stimuli are used. When multiple filters are required, STC or MID analyses may be applied. STC analysis can be used with Gaussian stimuli to estimate multiple filters, though the complete multi-dimensional nonlinearity may not be empirically obtained if there are more than two filters. MID analysis can be used with all stimuli, though it usually can recover only two filters and their joint nonlinearity.

Classification Schemes

The different analytical approaches can be classified according to the needs of the user and the details of the approach.

Stimulus Metric

One common theme in STRF estimation is the metric that is used. In the STA approach, an implicit comparison is made between the mean of the distribution of the stimuli that elicited spike (the spike-triggered stimulus ensemble), and the distribution mean of stimuli that did not elicit a spike (the complete stimulus ensemble). If there is no difference between the two distributions, then the STA will be uninformative. When the spike-triggered stimulus ensemble differs from the complete stimulus ensemble, then the STA will describe the average stimulus that excited the neuron to fire.

For the STC approach, the metric is the change in the variance of the spike-triggered and non-spike-triggered stimulus ensembles. If the stimulus induces a change in the variance of the spike-triggered stimulus ensemble, then the STC approach will recover the linear filters that cause the change. In the MID approach, the metric is information. Here, information is calculated as a ratio between the distribution of stimuli that lead to a spike compared to the distribution of all presented stimuli. If the two distributions are similar, then knowing if a spike occurred does not provide information, and significant filters cannot be recovered. If the two distributions diverge, then the information is non-zero, and MIDs may be recovered.

Model Dimensionality

Another theme is the number of dimensions in the model. The number of dimensions is the number of linear filters that comprise the STRF. This is also the number of stimulus features that influence the neuron's spiking output. The STA approach is limited to recover one stimulus dimension. The STC and MID approaches are capable of recovering multiple stimulus dimensions. Directly related to the dimensionality of the model is the ability of the model to recover the nonlinearities. When the filters and nonlinearities are recovered, the LN model is completed. For the STA, as noted earlier, the nonlinearity is easily obtained. For the STC and MID, since no assumptions are made about the nonlinearities, only two nonlinearities may be obtained. This is because the data requirements are generally too large to estimate non-parametric nonlinearities (Rust et al., 2005; Fitzgerald et al., 2011).

III. Stimuli

Auditory stimuli may vary along multiple parameter axes. Among these parameters are carrier structure, envelope structure, temporal modulation frequency, and spectral modulation frequency. For spike-triggered analyses, stimuli need to be designed to probe regions of stimulus space that efficiently affect the responses of a neuron (otherwise, the required sampling and data collection duration become unrealistic). If a stimulus does not adequately probe portions of the stimulus space to which a neuron is tuned, then the resulting STRF estimate may only approximate the true STRF.

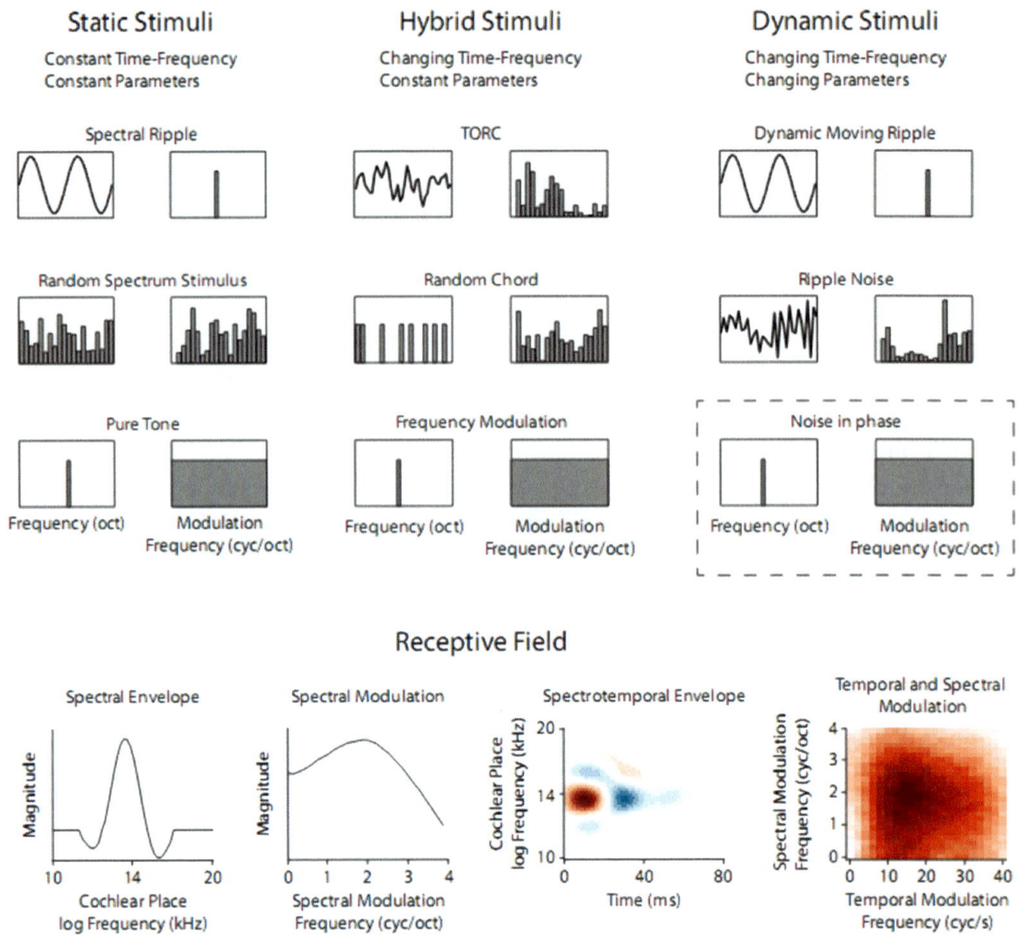

Figure 3. Classification of stimuli. Top: Stimuli can be broadly categorized as Static, Hybrid, and Dynamic. Static Stimuli have a frequency representation which does not change with time. Hybrid stimuli have a frequency representation that changes with time, though the stimulus parameters are constant. Dynamic stimuli have parameters and time-frequency representations that change with time. Hybrid and Dynamic stimuli are appropriate for spike-triggered analysis. Ripple noise is created by adding multiple dynamic moving ripples, each in random spectrotemporal phase. "Noise in phase" is a pathological stimulus that is created by adding dynamic moving ripples that have the same spectrotemporal phase. Bottom: Receptive fields can also be categorized along multiple axes. The spectral envelope describes the frequency tuning of a neuron. Spectral modulation describes the sensitivity of a neuron to changes along the frequency axis. The spectrotemporal envelope of the stimulus can be used to construct an estimate of the STRF. The temporal and spectral modulation frequency preferences of the neuron can be assessed by calculating the modulations within the STRF.

Stimuli may also fall along a continuum from static to dynamic. Static stimuli are those whose parameters do not vary with time. This class of stimuli includes spectral ripples, random spectrum stimuli, and pure tones (Figure 3, first column). Hybrid stimuli have constant parameters and changing time-frequency elements. This class of stimuli includes temporally orthogonal ripple combinations (TORCs), dynamic random chords, and frequency modulated sweeps (Figure 3, second column). Last, dynamic stimuli have both changing parameters and changing time-frequency content. Included in this class of stimuli are dynamic moving ripples (DMRs) and ripple noise (RN) (Figure 3, third column). RN is composed of multiple DMRs that are added together in random spectrotemporal phase. "Noise in phase" stimuli are created by adding together multiple DMRs, each with the same phase. The resulting stimulus is broad-band and has a temporally specific and focused envelope structure (Figure 3, third column, last row). Since this stimulus has limited frequency bandwidth, it is not suitable for spike-triggered analyses.

In the following, we consider stimuli that have the complexity that is necessary for spike-triggered analyses, and that can be used to compute the components of the STRF. Each of the stimuli has been used in STRF analysis, and each has strengths and drawbacks. At present, for a given auditory station, a prototypical stimulus has not been agreed upon by researchers, and therefore each station must be considered individually.

White Noise

Description

White noise is theoretically the ideal stimulus for spike-triggered analyses. It is temporally uncorrelated, its frequency spectrum covers all frequencies with relatively equal energy, and it is capable of eliciting nonlinear interactions. Since the noise is uncorrelated, receptive field estimates are not biased. Ideal white noise cannot be achieved, however, since this would require infinite bandwidth. For experimental and analytical approaches, the bandwidth of white noise can be made to cover the bandwidth of the neuron, which is the fundamental requirement for STRF analyses.

Strength

White noise is the most theoretically unbiased stimulus. It covers the system bandwidth of the neuron, and it is rich in frequency content since it has energy at all frequencies. White noise will have an approximately flat spectrum for long duration samples. A further strength of white noise is that it assumes nothing about the system under study.

Drawback

Though time-domain white noise is theoretically ideal, it has not been used in central auditory system STRF analyses since it suffers from multiple practical deficiencies. First, most central auditory system neurons do not respond well to ongoing, continuous white noise, although many neurons may respond to brief pulses of white noise. Since white noise has energy at all frequencies, it will have significant signal energy in a neuron's inhibitory receptive field subfields. This will cause the neuron to reduce, or eliminate, its spiking response. Additionally, neurons with even moderately high characteristic frequencies cannot phase-lock to the fine structure of the stimulus. Thus, inordinately long samples of white noise must be presented to capture enough spikes to estimate the STRF. In practice, this has made white noise unsuitable for experimental conditions. Therefore, though white noise is theoretically ideal, it is not a fruitful stimulus for central auditory system STRF analyses.

Dynamic Random Chords (DRC)

Description

Dynamic Random Chord (DRC) stimuli are in the family of pure tone stimulation (Figure 4). Single pure tones are used to estimate frequency response areas (FRAs). Single tones of different frequencies and intensities are presented sequentially and positively or negatively modulate the spontaneously occurring activity of a neuron. Low spontaneous activity in many central auditory neurons makes it difficult to probe how stimulation in STRF subfields affects the neuron's response. Two-tone stimuli are those where two pure tones are simultaneously presented, which allows the inhibitory sideband structure of the neuron to be mapped. The FRA and two-tone stimuli can be extended to create a stimulus that has multiple, simultaneously present tones, where the tones are presented at random, interleaved times. This more complex tone stimulus is called a Dynamic Random Chord.

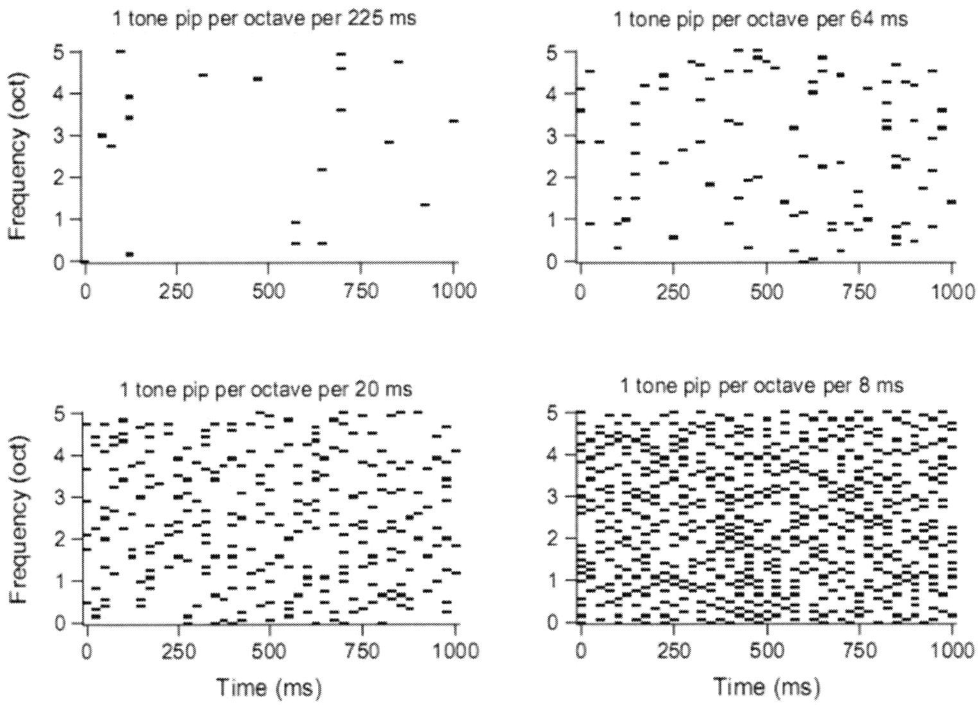

Figure 4. Dynamic Random Chord (DRC) stimuli. DRCs may have different densities. The least dense DRC stimuli are similar to those that are used to estimate frequency response areas. The densest DRCs approach white noise.

The Dynamic Random Chord is controlled by multiple parameters: the overall frequency bandwidth of the set of tones, the logarithmic or linear spacing of the tones, the number of tones along the frequency axis (spectral density), the tone duration, and the nature of the onsets and offsets of each tone. The bandwidth should be set to encompass the bandwidth of the neuron. The frequency spacing is normally logarithmic, which allows equal energy per octave. The temporal resolution of the STRF is determined by the tone duration and the interleaving of the tones (temporal density). Last, the smooth onset and offset of each tone helps to reduce the spectral splatter that would result if the tone was abruptly turned on or off.

Strength

DRCs have been used in multiple studies to uncover spectrotemporal processing. They satisfy many of the requirements of spike-triggered analyses, since they cover the frequency bandwidth of the neuron. The density of the random tones can also be controlled in a random or pseudorandom manner. For the random presentation, the presentation rate of each tone follows a Poisson process. For the pseudorandom sequence, an m-sequence can be used to determine the presentation schedule (Kvale and Schreiner, 1997). Both presentation schemes allow the second order statistics to be explicitly described, and in most cases the stimuli can be designed so that the frequency channels are uncorrelated, which is ideal for spike-triggered analyses.

Drawback

Despite the numerous strengths of DCRs, there are numerous experimenter-dependent choices which need to be made for a given neuron. Also, many of these parameter choices are not independent. For example: choosing the tone duration implicitly determines the density of the stimulus, as does the number of frequency channels.

DRC stimuli have some drawbacks that must be considered. First, the density of the stimulus must be chosen appropriately to provide an adequate sampling of the spectral and temporal STRF dimensions. The density is the number tone pips per octave per ms. Blake and Merzenich (2002) used densities of one tone pip per octave every 720, 225, 64, 20, or 8 ms, while Eggermont and colleagues used densities of one tone pip per octave every 5000, 250, and 24 ms (Valentine and Eggermont, 2004; Norena et al., 2008). Since the density determines how the STRF subfields will be probed, this is a relevant issue and inappropriate parameters can lead to inadequate STRF estimates.

Second, the chosen density is of further significance since it controls the responsiveness of the neuron. As the density increases, the stimulus effectively becomes white noise, which may strongly depress the activity of neurons (Blake and Merzenich, 2002), since slower envelope modulations will be absent. While the tone presentation rate is a proxy for these modulations, it is not an ideal substitute.

Third, the receptive field temporal resolution is determined by the tone duration. Since auditory neurons respond strongly to the onset of a sound, and since the tone duration in DRCs is usually fairly short (e.g., 25 ms), this limits the temporal resolution of the STRF (~ 20 Hz). For neurons that can follow higher modulation rates, this upper limit may not be sufficient. The tone duration can be decreased, but this may have the effect of introducing spectral leakage into adjacent frequency bands, and thus introducing correlations in the stimulus.

Finally, the dynamic random chord contains little structure that is related to the characteristics of natural sounds. No smooth spectrotemporal envelope modulations are present to drive auditory neurons effectively. Thus, though the DRC may cover the bandwidth of the neuron, it may still be inefficient in probing auditory function.

Moving Ripples (MR)

Description

Moving ripple (MR) stimuli are frequently used in STRF analysis (Klein et al., 2000; Depireux et al., 2001; Elhilali et al., 2004; Andoni et al., 2007; Versnel et al., 2009). They are composed of multiple sinusoidal carriers, each of which has random phase. This gives the underlying carrier structure a noise-like quality.

The novel aspect of moving ripples is that the spectrotemporal envelope is characterized by three parameters which do not vary with time. The first, modulation depth, determines the peak-to-trough value in the signal. The other two, temporal and spectral modulation frequency, are also constant. Temporal and spectral modulations are fundamental features of natural sounds. Varying the modulation parameters allows the stimulus to sequentially cover a neuron's modulation preferences.

The spectrotemporal envelope of a moving ripple stimulus is described by a sinusoidal equation (Depireux et al., 2001). For a specific frequency, the envelope is described using:

$$S(t,x) = L\left[1 + \Delta A \sin(2\pi wt + 2\pi\Omega x + \Phi)\right]$$

Here x is the frequency in octaves, and is defined as $x = \log_2(f / f_0)$, where f is the frequency and is the lowest frequency in the stimulus. ω (cyc/s) and Ω (cyc/octave) represent the temporal and spectral modulation parameters. ω is the temporal modulation frequency, and describes how the spectrotemporal envelope varies along the temporal axis. ω can be positive or negative, and its greatest value is determined by the temporal modulation preferences for the system under study (e.g., for anesthetized preparations, in cat midbrain the maximum is usually set to 500 cyc/s, while in cat auditory cortex it is 40 cyc/s). Ω , the spectral modulation frequency, describes the variation of the spectrotemporal envelope along the frequency axis. Φ is a random phase for the envelope, ΔA scales the sinusoidal amplitude, and L determines the depth of the modulation. This equation is similar in form to that used in studies of sinusoidal amplitude modulation, with the only difference being that here the amplitude modulation varies with frequency. Moving ripple stimuli may contain upward or downward frequency modulation (see Figure 5). The upward frequency modulation occurs when ω is negative and downward frequency sweeps occur for positive ω. These characteristics of moving ripple stimuli follow straightforwardly from the mathematical definition. Moving ripple stimuli can also be created so that the envelope amplitude varies on a logarithmic scale. In this case, the stimulus takes the form:

$$A(t,x) = \frac{M}{20}\sin(2\pi wt + 2\pi\Omega x + \Phi) - \frac{M}{20}$$

$$S(t,x) = 10^{A(t,x)}$$

where M represents the modulation depth in dB. The logarithmic amplitude scale has been shown to be more effective than the linear scale for driving midbrain auditory neurons (Escabí and Schreiner, 2002; Escabí et al., 2003).

When the two scales were compared in the midbrain, the logarithmic scale was shown to increase the information carrying capacity of neurons by approximately 50%. This coincides with the amplitude distribution of natural sounds, which also follow a logarithmic distribution.

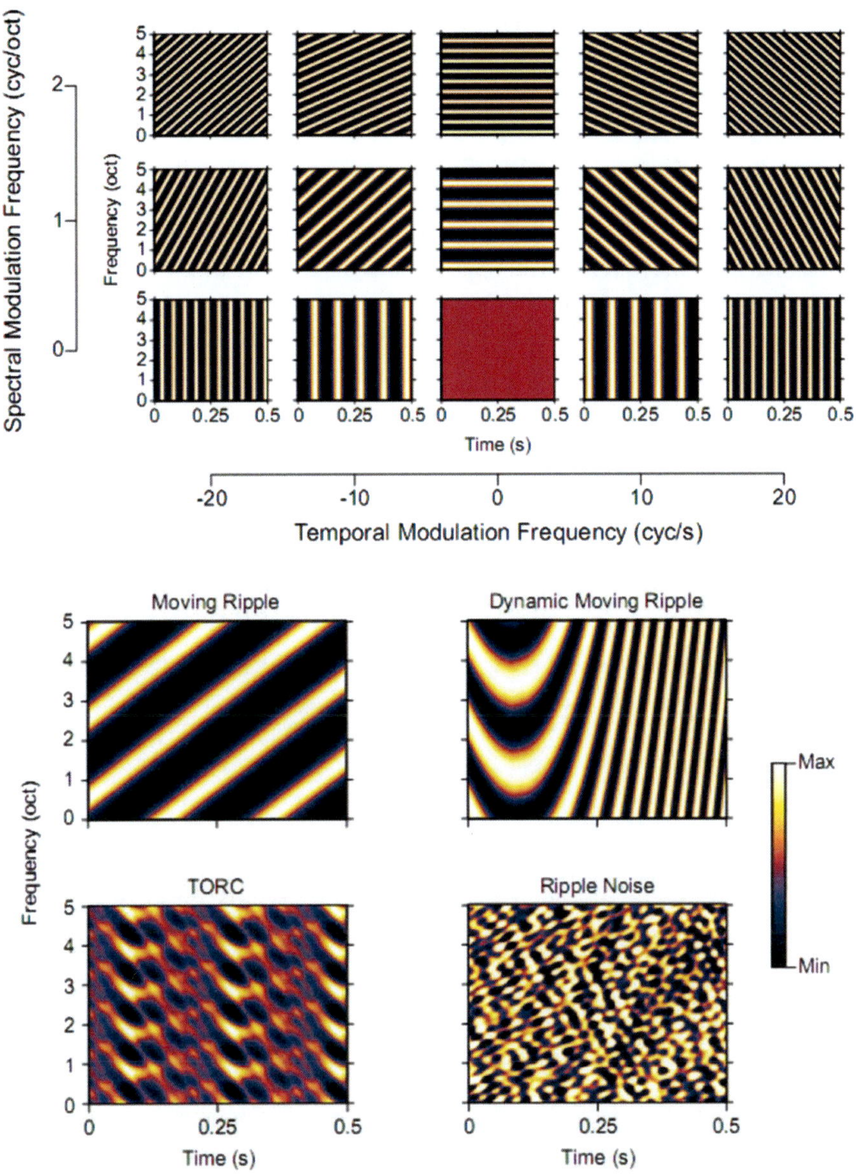

Figure 5. Spectrotemporal representations of ripple stimuli. Top: Moving ripples (MRs) at various temporal and spectral modulation frequencies. The modulation frequencies determine the presence, and orientation, of the frequency modulation in each MR. Bottom: example of a moving ripple (MR), a temporally orthogonal ripple combination (TORC), a dynamic moving ripple (DMR), and a ripple noise (RN) stimulus. TORCs are a sum of MRs, with each constituent MR having a different temporal modulation frequency. DMRs are characterized by temporal and spectral modulation frequencies that change with time. RN is the sum of multiple DMRs.

Strength

Moving ripples have been used extensively in STRF analyses because they have many desirable properties. MRs contain temporal and spectral modulations, which are present in natural sounds. This makes MRs an intermediate stimulus between noise and natural sounds. Moving ripple stimuli also have strong amplitude modulation characteristics, which are sufficient to drive most central auditory system neurons. Finally, since moving ripple stimuli cover the carrier and modulation frequency preferences of auditory neurons, they are suitable for spike-triggered analyses.

Drawback

A main drawback of moving ripple stimuli is that the modulation parameters do not vary across time. Natural sounds, on the other hand, have varying spectrotemporal envelope features. Also, it may be time consuming to present moving ripple stimuli that cover the desired temporal and spectral modulation frequency space. Each moving ripple stimulus usually lasts for approximately 1 second. However, only the steady state response of the neuron can be used to estimate the STRF. Therefore, the response of the neuron to the beginning of each moving ripple stimulus is discarded since it is dominated by adaptation to the onset statistics of the stimulus. This drawback can be mitigated by extending the duration of the MR, though this comes with the tradeoff that fewer stimulus presentations may be available.

Temporally Orthogonal Ripple Combinations (TORCs)

Description

To overcome the sampling issues of moving ripples, a second related stimulus was developed: temporal orthogonal ripple combinations (TORCs; Figure 5). TORCs have been employed in many successful studies by Shamma and colleagues (Fritz et al., 2003; Fritz et al., 2005; Klein et al., 2006; Fritz et al., 2007; David et al., 2012).

TORCs are a sum of multiple (~6) MR stimuli. The spectral modulation frequency values may be chosen by the user. However, none of the MRs have the same temporal modulation frequency. Since the temporal modulation values are different, each component moving ripple stimulus is temporally orthogonal to the others.

Strength

TORCs allow for an efficient probing of modulation space, since multiple static ripples are used to simultaneously sample multiple regions of modulation space. Due to the efficiency of TORC stimulation, they are particularly suited for estimating STRFs in the awake behaving animal, where shorter recording times are common.

Drawback

TORCs still include onsets and offsets, which require that the responses to these stimulus segments be removed. Also, due to these transients, the STRF that is calculated is from a quasi-adapted state; though it is likely that the neuron adapts after a few hundred milliseconds, this is not guaranteed. This downside, however, can be avoided, since TORCs can always be made to have longer durations. Finally, though TORCs do sample the spectrotemporal modulation space in multiple places, their spectrotemporal correlations are reduced, and thus the preferred stimulus correlations of central auditory system neurons may not be present in TORC stimuli.

Natural Sound Temporal Envelope (NSTE)

Description

Natural sounds typically contain envelope modulation frequencies in restricted regions of the temporal and spectral modulation space. The temporal modulation frequency statistics have been shown to have a non-uniform distribution, with a strong bias towards low temporal modulation frequencies. The distribution of temporal modulation frequencies may be approximated by a decaying exponential with a time constant of 20 Hz (Figure 6) (Singh and Theunissen, 2003). Therefore, these characteristics of natural sounds can be mimicked if the temporal modulation frequency statistics of the stimulus follow this distribution.

Stimuli with the temporal envelope distribution of natural sounds (NSTE) are constructed by first filtering white noise using a Gaussian filter bank, which creates a noise carrier. The spacing between the center frequencies of the filters sets the spectral modulation frequency parameter. To obtain the temporal amplitude modulation envelope, white noise is processed through an exponential filter, which produces an envelope that has the temporal modulation frequency distribution of natural sounds. Next, the noise carrier is modulated by the envelope, creating an amplitude modulated signal for that specific frequency band. To obtain the complete stimulus, the amplitude modulated signals in each frequency band are summed together.

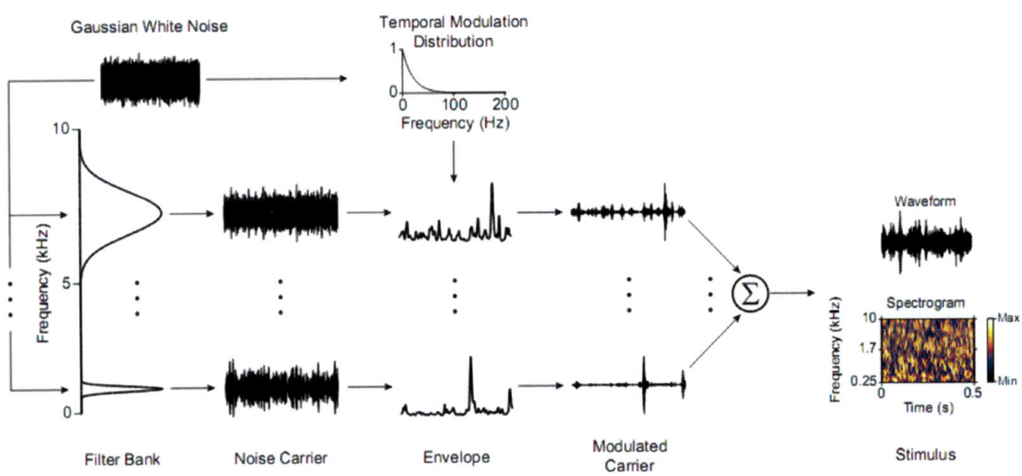

Figure 6. Natural Sound Temporal Envelope (NTSE) stimuli. NTSEs are created by sending Gaussian white noise through a filter bank, which creates the noise carrier for each frequency channel of the stimulus. Gaussian noise is also filtered using an exponential shaped filter to create a temporal modulation envelope for each frequency channel. The exponential shape is meant to approximate the temporal modulation frequency distribution of natural sounds. The carriers and envelopes are multiplied, and then summed, to create the stimulus. Adapted from (Kim and Doupe, 2011).

Strength

NSTE stands at an intermediate point between white noise and natural sounds. The carrier structure of NSTE is noise, but the temporal envelope statistics are chosen from those of the natural sound distribution in the biotope of the organism under study. Further, the filter that produces the temporal modulation envelope can be adjusted for each station, giving this stimulus added utility. Also, since each frequency channel is modulated independently, there are minimal across frequency correlations. The noise-like characteristics make NSTE stimuli appropriate for spike-triggered analyses.

Drawback

Since the carrier structure is determined from bandpass filtering noise, the frequency resolution of the signal is limited by the bandwidth of the filters in the filter bank. One important aspect that is not controlled by NSTE is spectral modulation. Communication sounds have spectral modulations that vary with time, though NSTE stimuli rely on energy fluctuations within each frequency channel to probe the spectral modulation preferences of the neuron. Additionally, the temporal modulation statistics of NSTE are not white. They are biased towards low modulation values. Thus, though NSTE is ethologically motivated, it may not include the moderate to high temporal modulation frequencies that brainstem, midbrain, and thalamic neurons can respond to. The range of temporal modulation frequencies can be adjusted, though a bias toward low temporal modulation frequencies will persist. This bias may have detrimental effects on spike-triggered analyses. Because of the non-white nature of the spectrum, the autocorrelation matrix of the stimuli will be undersampled. In turn, this means that inverting the autocorrelation matrix will result in the amplification of noise. This effect may be corrected by estimating the pseudoinverse, and removing components of the pseudoinverse that do not contribute significantly to the numerical solution. However, choosing the particular cutoff value for the inversion is not a defined solution and thus will be left to the experience and taste of the experimenter (Theunissen et al., 2000; Machens et al., 2004; Lesica and Grothe, 2008; Kim and Doupe, 2011). Many of these problems may be circumvented if the bandwidth of the temporal modulation frequencies is large enough to cover the stimulus preferences of any encountered neuron. This will grant greater stability for STRF estimation, since the larger bandwidth will ensure that the stimulus preferences of each encountered neuron are covered.

Dynamic Moving Ripple (DMR)

Description

Dynamic moving ripple stimuli have been used extensively for STRF analyses (Miller and Schreiner, 2000; Miller et al., 2001b; Miller et al., 2001a; Escabí and Schreiner, 2002; Miller et al., 2002; Escabí et al., 2005; Atencio and Schreiner, 2008; Atencio et al., 2008, 2009; Atencio and Schreiner, 2010a, b, 2012). They are controlled by the same parameters as MR stimuli. However, the difference between the DMR and the MR is that in the DMR the temporal and spectral modulation frequency parameters are allowed to randomly vary. Thus, the stimulus is continuous, which allows for dynamic changes in the spectrotemporal domain. The carrier structure of the DMR can be linear, though in most applications the spacing is logarithmic, which allows for an equal amount of energy per octave. The carriers are given random phase, which gives the DMR a noise-like quality. Also, while there are short-term local correlations in the DMR, the long term auto-correlation of the stimulus is a delta function, indicating that the DMR is globally uncorrelated (Escabí and Schreiner, 2002; Sharpee et al., 2011a). This makes the DMR an excellent choice for spike-triggered analyses.

Strength

The DMR is a parametric stimulus, and thus the characteristics of the DMR can be set by the experimenter. This implies that while the DMR has characteristics of natural sounds, the composition and correlations in the stimulus can be controlled. Additionally, the DMR is a continuous stimulus, and thus it does not contain the onsets and offsets that may cause short time adaptation effects in auditory neurons. Since the stimulus is continuous, and in most applications lasts over 5 minutes, the neuron is in a fairly constant adapted state. This in turn helps to reduce the oscillatory effects that may be present with shorter-lasting stimuli, and keeps the network in a dynamic state resembling that observed in alert animals (Miller and Schreiner, 2000). Also, the randomly varying temporal and spectral modulation frequency parameters are two of the main components of natural sounds. By allowing these parameters to randomly vary, the dynamic changes that are present in natural sounds can be modeled effectively.

Drawback

Since the parameter space is continuously explored, care must be taken to create DMRs that last long enough to cover the stimulus preferences of the neural system under study. Unlike the MR, where multiple stimuli may be chosen to cover the temporal and spectral modulation space, the DMR achieves this covering through a random walk through the temporal and spectral modulation parameters. Hence, the duration of the DMR must be long enough to ensure sufficient coverage of the necessary parameter space. In practice, DMRs on the order of a few minutes or more will satisfy this requirement. As a parametric sound, the DMR lacks some of the characteristics of natural sounds: it has neither onsets/offsets nor significant higher-order correlations (Voss and Clarke, 1975, 1978; Garcia-Lazaro et al., 2006, 2011). Thus, the DMR does not contain transient temporal dynamics, which are characteristic of natural sounds.

Spectrotemporal White Noise (STWN)/Ripple Noise (RN)

Description

Spectrotemporal white noise (STWN) and Ripple Noise (RN) are the most complex of the stimuli that are based on temporal and spectral modulation parameters (Escabí and Schreiner, 2002; Klein et al., 2006; Atencio et al., 2008). In addition to being the most complex, they are also the most unbiased. STWN and RN are created to contain the temporal and spectral modulation frequencies under study. STWN flow from the moving ripple/TORC framework: they are made by adding moving ripple stimuli that cover a large range of modulation frequencies. RN comes from the DMR framework: it is created by adding many (~15) DMRs together so that the modulation space is adequately covered in any time window.

Viewed in the spectrotemporal plane, the stimuli have no short-term or long-term correlations (Figure 5). One difference between STWN and RN stimuli is that STWN will repeat after a sufficient amount of time, since the constituent MRs repeat. RN stimuli, however, do not repeat.

Strength

STWN and RN stimuli are unbiased in their statistics. They cover the bandwidth of the system under study, and they make no assumptions about the modulation preferences of the neuron: they include the range of modulation preferences of the neuron. Additionally, the stimuli are uncorrelated in the spectrotemporal domain, and therefore no corrections are necessary when an STRF component is estimated using STA analysis. Further, their durations can be adjusted to be either short or long, and thus they can be modified to fit the conditions of each experiment.

Drawback

The main downside to these stimuli is that they lack strong correlations, and thus they may not sufficiently drive auditory neurons. Since there is no local correlation structure, any neuron that is tuned to these characteristics, as might be expected for neurons that are tuned to the characteristics of natural stimuli, will not be optimally responsive. However, to date, the STAs derived from these stimuli are in general accord with those derived using alternative stimulation (see below for further discussion) (Escabí and Schreiner, 2002; Klein et al., 2006; Atencio et al., 2008).

In only a few cases in the midbrain have RN stimuli been shown to produce STAs that diverge from those derived from DMR stimuli. Last, since these stimuli are white in the spectrotemporal domain, they are dense, and thus they will simultaneously probe excitatory and inhibitory receptive field subfields. This may cause neurons to reduce their firing since stimulating inhibitory subfields may suppress spiking responses, similar to traditional white noise stimuli.

Natural Sounds (NS)

Description

Natural sounds are signals that are experienced in the habitat of biological organisms. As such, they may be from environmental sources, such as rain or water (Lesica and Grothe, 2008), may originate from communication between non-human subjects (Wang et al., 1995; Woolley et al., 2005), may be used for communication between humans, or they may be products of human culture, such as music and voice.

In these cases, a parametric model is not used to create the sounds. The underlying generating model can be approximated, but the characteristics of the source are not known completely. This makes natural sounds difficult to characterize, since the features that make them biologically important may only be surmised. Thus, one of the larger goals in neuroscience is to characterize natural sounds and to understand their statistical properties.

An alternative approach is to create stimuli with the characteristics of natural sounds. These artificial sounds approximate natural sounds to varying degrees and their "naturalness" can be assessed using psychophysical procedures. It is hoped that if we can parametrically describe these "naturalistic" sounds, then we may gain insight into which features give natural sounds their behavioral salience and perceptual qualities. In auditory neuroscience, this process has been applied to texture sounds with stationary statistics (Lesica and Grothe, 2008; Geffen et al., 2011; McDermott and Simoncelli, 2011).

Strength

The strength of natural sounds as a stimulus rests on the knowledge that these signals are extensively experienced in the lives of organisms. Therefore, it is assumed that the auditory systems of these organisms are especially tuned to process natural sounds. And because of this tuning, these sounds may be especially effective at driving auditory responses. Further, since these sounds contain features that usually are not present in parametric sounds, they may provide better estimates of receptive fields, since they will be able to probe aspects of the neural system that artificial sounds cannot. Thus, without knowing the stimulus selectivity of the system under study, natural sounds may be the most parsimonious choice for stimulation.

Drawback

Though natural sounds appear to be ideal for receptive field analyses, multiple aspects should give researchers pause. First, we currently do not have a complete understanding of the features of natural sounds that neurons are sensitive to. Since models can only approximate natural sounds, we do not have sufficient knowledge of the essential features of these sounds (McDermott and Simoncelli, 2011). Second, and more importantly, natural sounds cannot be used with the majority of spike-triggered analysis techniques. Most techniques can correct for correlations at or below second-order, but any higher order correlations cannot be removed (Paninski, 2003). Thus, the natural-sound based receptive fields for most techniques will be biased estimates, and will not be true estimates of the receptive fields (Sharpee et al., 2004). Third, because natural sounds have characteristic fine structure and envelope features, constructing receptive field estimates based only on the spectrotemporal envelope may be incomplete, since the fine structure is also important (Smith et al., 2002). Signals such as the MR, TORCs, or DMR have a noise carrier, and thus this effect may be reduced. In natural sounds, however, carrier and envelope both carry information. Therefore, though natural sounds appear to be a logical choice for a stimulus, their complexity and the inadequacy of most analytical approaches in correcting for correlations must caution anyone who wishes to employ them (Andoni and Pollak, 2011). Finally, it is difficult to quantify the true biotope of an organism. For the most prevalent experimental subjects, vocalizations can be studied, but these sounds are often simple in structure (e.g., mouse, rat, cat vocalizations). Determining the additional sounds that the organism encounters in its habitat requires an extensive ethological characterization that has seldom been attempted.

Since natural sounds are attractive, and their use may be motivated by theoretical considerations, it is important to note the sets of analysis procedures that may be used. STA and STC analyses are not appropriate, since they cannot correct for the higher-order correlations in most natural sounds, though if the correlations can be determined to be limited to second-order, then these techniques may be used. MID analysis can be used with natural sounds, and at present this analysis represents the most theoretically sound methodology for estimating receptive fields from naturalistic stimulation.

IV. Stimulus Representations

Implicit to any spike-triggered analysis is how the stimulus is represented. Though this issue is important, it is rarely considered. Therefore, the two main topics that are considered in experiments are usually the analysis technique and the stimulus. However, the representation of the stimulus that is used may significantly determine the validity and interpretation of the results.

Two commonly used spectrotemporal representations are the Wigner distribution and the spectrogram. They provide time-frequency representations in conceptually different ways. For the Wigner distribution, the signal is correlated with a time reversed version of itself. The frequency distribution of this correlated signal is then used to give the time-frequency representation. For the spectrogram, the signal is multiplied by a window, and then the frequency content is obtained. Then the magnitude of the result is squared and displayed. Thus, for these distributions, the order of the operations is fundamentally different: for the Wigner distribution, the signal is correlated with itself, and then the frequency representation is obtained, while for the spectrogram the frequency content is obtained and then squared. The difference in the order of these operations has fundamental implications for time-frequency analysis. (Note: The Time-Frequency Toolbox, by F. Auger, P. Flandrin, P. Gonçalvès, and O. Lemoine, located at http://tftb.nongnu.org/, is a very helpful Matlab suite for experimenting with time-frequency analyses).

The Wigner distribution has many positive qualities, though one negative quality has limited its utility (Eggermont and Smith, 1990; Kim and Young, 1994). The time-frequency transform produces artifacts in the resulting time-frequency plot. These artifacts are not related to the signal, but result from the signal multiplication that takes place when the transform is calculated. For the Wigner distribution, the artifacts result from nonlinear interactions between different frequency components. The artifacts are unavoidable, since they are implicit in the definition of the Wigner distribution. Thus, they are inherent to the distribution. If the STRF is calculated using the Wigner distribution, it will include these artifacts. Because of this, the results will often be difficult or even impossible to interpret, since trying to smooth out or remove the artifacts requires a priori experimenter assumptions regarding the structure of the time-frequency representation of the stimulus or the STRF. This is an unappealing procedure upon which to base receptive field analysis. Therefore, the Wigner distribution has been seldom used in the STRF literature.

The spectrogram is based on the short-time Fourier transform (STFT), and can be viewed in two equivalent ways. In the first, a sliding window moves over a time-domain signal, and the Fourier transform of each segment is computed. Each transform represents the frequency distribution at the time of the center of the window. Each segment is appended to another in the form of a matrix, with each column representing a time point and the rows representing the frequency distribution. Once the process is completed, the squared magnitude of the transform is taken, giving the spectrogram. The spectrogram is subject to time-frequency tradeoffs: as the temporal resolution becomes greater, the frequency resolution decreases, and vice-versa. Since the frequency resolution of the spectrogram depends on the window, different windows may be chosen to limit smearing of the signal in the time-frequency plane.

The second way to view the spectrogram is as a filter bank (Allen and Rabiner, 1977). The frequency resolution of the spectrogram is provided by a bank of filters, each of which filters the time domain signal. The outputs of the filters across time show the frequency content of the signal; since the outputs vary with time, the temporal dimension is implicit in this interpretation.

Because of the straightforward nature of the spectrogram, the spectrogram remains one of the most utilized time-frequency distributions in STRF analysis. One drawback of the spectrogram is that in applications the magnitude of the envelope is used to obtain the STRF. Because of this, the phase information in the signal is lost, and therefore the stimulus fine structure is not retained. This implies that the spectrotemporal envelope that is obtained from the spectrogram, and that is used in STRF construction, contains less information than the original signal.

Related to the spectrogram is the cochlear filter bank representation (de Boer, 1975; de Boer and de Jongh, 1978; Patterson et al., 1992; Slaney, 1993). (The Auditory Toolbox by Malcolm Slaney is a Matlab suite that implements cochlear filter banks and may be found at https://engineering.purdue.edu/~malcolm/interval/1998-010/). The cochlear filter bank representation has been used in multiple auditory cortical studies (Elhilali et al., 2004; Szymanski et al., 2011).

Here the experimenter seeks a time-frequency representation that resembles the time-frequency processing in the cochlea. Much recent work has uncovered the characteristics of cochlear filtering, and these filter bank models have been used extensively in auditory scene analysis. In these approaches a cochlear filter bank model processes the signal, and the output of the filter bank is then used as the input to spike-triggered analyses.

To avoid the time-frequency resolution tradeoffs that are inherent in the spectrogram, the experimenter may parametrically create the signal. Because the envelope is under experimental control it avoids time-frequency tradeoffs. This is ideal, since the spectral and temporal axes can be specified to arbitrary precision. Approaches that use parametric sounds, which create a spectrotemporal envelope, include all ripple stimuli. Thus, these representations are free of distribution artifacts and time-frequency tradeoffs.

V. Survey

The literature is replete with studies that used diverse stimuli and analytical approaches. In these studies, the approaches, the results, and the interpretations need to be viewed within a coherent framework if the findings are to inform across specialized research platforms. As mentioned above, this framework requires understanding the stimulation requirements for Volterra systems: covering the bandwidth/stimulus preferences of the neurons and having the ability to correct for correlations in the stimulus ensemble.

Deviations from these requirements necessarily mean that the results of the study become difficult to interpret and generalize. This ensues because of the many ways in which neural processing can vary for nonlinear neural systems. Choosing different stimulus parameters and characteristics can fundamentally change the estimated STRF, and therefore confound any conclusions that are drawn if the conceptual framework is not valid.

When the correct approach is applied with appropriate stimuli, then the signal processing of the neuron can be effectively assessed. From these well-planned experiments, general theories of neural coding and information processing can be developed, helping to give insight into the function of various aspects and elements of auditory processing. When the core requirements are not met, the impact of such studies is greatly diminished and other insights must be salvaged.

We note that the estimated STRFs may vary when stimulus bandwidth, stimulus type, stimulus density, and animal behavioral state are varied. However, these effects on STRFs may be reasonably predictable if we understand the stimulation and analysis requirements of neural systems in their various states. In the following, we examine multiple studies, and discuss how they fit into the STRF modeling framework. We point out the places where a study met the requirements of systems analysis, and where it may have fallen short. We then describe the utility of the results for each approach.

STRF Dependence on Stimulus Bandwidth

Eggermont and colleagues have studied how changing the stimulus bandwidth affects cortical STRFs (Gourevitch et al., 2009; Eggermont, 2011). To estimate STRFs, they presented random, dynamic chord stimuli. These broadband stimuli covered seven octaves, with 16 frequencies per octave. The random chord stimuli were then divided into two sections, each having a 2 octave bandwidth that overlapped by 1 octave. The main findings were that spurious peaks were found in the STRFs that were derived for the stimuli with limited bandwidths. The conclusion of the study was that the STRF differences were the result of a release from inhibition under narrowband stimulation conditions.

Within the Volterra systems framework, the band-limited stimuli did not cover the bandwidth of the neuron and, consequently, the true system function could not be recovered. The results will likely reflect nonlinear processing that has only been partially captured by the analysis procedure. Thus, within this framework, deviations between full-bandwidth and limited-bandwidth results are expected, since using narrow-band stimuli violates an important principle of neural system modeling. However, the nature of the deviations are difficult to interpret, since the different STRFs could reflect any type of nonlinear processing which cortical neurons perform.

STRF Dependence on Stimulus Type

Given our reasoning regarding analytical procedures and stimulus types, STRFs will be expected to vary when the conditions for analysis are violated by inappropriate stimulus choices. Earlier work was perhaps not as clear on the necessity of maintaining these principles, and thus many of those studies combined linear receptive field construction with stimuli that were fraught with higher ordered correlations.

Initially, Aertsen and colleagues showed that the STRF was dependent on the stimulus ensemble (Aertsen et al., 1981). They used natural and tonal stimuli, two entirely different sets of stimuli, and which require very different analysis techniques. In this case even making the bandwidth of the natural sound as broad as possible did not alleviate the STRF differences. This is expected since an unbiased STRF cannot be recovered from natural sounds when simple reverse correlation is used.

The differences that Aertsen et al. uncovered when applying the two types of stimuli were numerous. STRFs could have spectrally well-defined regions with short latencies, or the STRFs could have less well defined spectral region with longer latencies. The duration of the regions could also vary considerably. For some neurons, the natural stimulus ensemble led to an STRF that was similar to the STRF from tonal stimuli. In other cases, however, the STRFs were markedly different.

The results point to the fact that using stimuli with an inappropriate analytical procedure may not provide interpretable results. Since natural stimuli were used, and no procedure was applied to correct for the stimulus correlations, the STRFs were likely biased. Also, despite the attempt to include a realistic biotope of sounds, it is unlikely that the system bandwidth of the neuron was covered. Therefore, it is probable that the neurons were not properly stimulated, which makes it challenging to recover the STRF.

STRFs have been extensively used in work with zebra finches. Work by Theunissen and colleagues has been at the forefront of this field (Theunissen et al., 2000). They found in earlier studies that the STRFs of field L neurons in zebra finches were different when natural sounds and random tone pips were used. The STRFs from natural sounds were better at predicting the response to novel sounds. This result is not unexpected, since it allows multiple interpretations. First, the procedure used to derive STRFs relies on correcting for stimulus autocorrelations, which are only second order corrections. Thus, the STRF may still be biased. Second, the two types of stimuli are different: natural sounds have strong correlations, while randomly presented tone pips do not. Third, the nature of the sounds themselves are divergent. Natural sounds have continuous portions, and contain strong temporal and spectral modulations. Tone pips, on the other hand, are largely discontinuous, and are characterized by strong onsets and offsets, which can produce markedly strong effects in auditory neurons. Thus, the analysis technique and the nature of the sounds were different and necessarily led to conflicting results.

Further work by (Woolley et al., 2006) showed differences between stimulation types for STRFs in the bird auditory midbrain. They used STRFs to measure modulation processing. The stimuli that were used were natural sounds and modulation limited noise that matched the spectrotemporal modulation and power characteristics of natural birdsong. They found that 91% of midbrain neurons displayed differences in spectrotemporal tuning for these two types of stimuli.

This result can also be viewed within the framework that we presented. If the modulation matched noise contained no higher than second order correlations, then the STRF that was estimated would be expected to be a reasonable approximation to the STRF. In this case, the correlations in the stimulus could be corrected for. For natural sounds, the STRF remains biased since the correlations in the stimulus cannot be removed using the STA procedure.

This study may also point to the importance of stimulus representations as we discussed in Section IV. Since the spectrotemporal envelopes of both stimuli were similar, and their bandwidths were similar, the underlying carrier structure may have been important in evoking neural responses. However, the spectrogram representation cannot reveal these differences, since it represents the spectrotemporal envelope, and not the fine structure. Thus, while the STRF is estimated from the spectrogram representation, the neural response comes from the total time domain signal, of which the spectrogram is an incomplete representation. Therefore, it may be that the auditory midbrain is capable of responding to the fine structure, which cannot be accounted for by the analysis approach that was used.

Natural sounds have also been used in rat auditory cortex. Machens and colleagues combined in vivo whole-cell recordings in the rat with natural sound stimulation (Machens et al., 2004). The complex sounds that were used included samples from various animals, the tropical rain forest, recordings from the great smoky mountains, spectacular artificial sound effects, and some samples from Jimi Hendrix's "purple rain". Multiple analytical controls were applied, though the analysis procedure is not guaranteed to succeed due to the non-Gaussian nature of the stimuli that were used. The study is strong, however, in providing a rigorous application of Ridge Regression. The analysis elucidated the tradeoffs that must be made when this technique is used with stimuli that have higher than second order correlations. Different performance levels were achieved based on different, user-supplied parameter values in the regression analysis. Additionally, the sound representation that was used may have led to the poor predictions.

In another approach, David and colleagues estimated STRFs using three types of sounds (David et al., 2009). They used TORCs, speech, and TORCs that were multiplied by the envelopes of speech sounds (SPORCs). Thus, SPORCs are similar to natural sound temporal envelope (NSTE) stimuli, though the envelopes may not be Gaussian distributed. A machine learning procedure, Boosting, was used to estimate the STRFs for the three types of stimuli (David et al., 2007). When boosting was compared to the STA, it was found to produce STRFs with smaller subfields than the STA. Though the accuracy of boosting has not been tested on a model cell, it does result in greater predictive power compared to the STA for natural stimuli. This is expected, since the STA is strongly biased for natural sounds. When boosting was used for the three stimuli, two-thirds of the neurons had similar STRFs. For the remaining neurons, differences were found for inhibitory subfield structure and gain in the STRF. Since the different stimuli revealed STRF differences, the stimuli revealed nonlinear processing. Further, since the STRFs were different, this indicates two possibilities. First, the different stimuli may have probed different areas of the stimulus parameter space, and thus produced nonlinear interactions. Second, the STRF estimation technique may not have been able to produce sufficiently accurate receptive fields, and thus may have been influenced by the different correlation structures in the stimuli.

Andoni and Pollak studied bat midbrain neurons using MR and natural sound stimulation (Andoni et al., 2007; Andoni and Pollak, 2011). First, they focused on MRs, from which they estimated STAs and were able to predict the responses to a small set of natural calls. The nonlinearity that was employed was a simple rectification, and thus the predictions are likely to be a lower bound since a data derived nonlinearity would increase the predictive power (Sharpee et al., 2008).

In the second study, they presented bat social communication calls, and then constructed STRF components using STA and STC analysis. They found multiple components for bat midbrain neurons (Andoni and Pollak, 2011). By applying information analysis, they were able to order the STRF components according to the amount of information that each component conveyed (Pillow and Simoncelli, 2006). Of note is that when multiple features were found, the STA was not the most informative dimension. Though an STA was present, the features from the STC analysis bore more information. In many cases two STC components were found, indicating that neurons could respond to stimulus features in a phase invariant manner.

It is unknown whether the features from the combined STA/STC analysis were able to produce unbiased estimates, since natural sounds have inherent higher-order correlations. A whitening process was used to remove second order envelope correlations, and a check using the spectrogram was provided, though these can only assess envelope processing, and they neither relate to the presence of higher-order correlations nor to the signal that the neuron encounters, which is the complete time domain waveform. Also, in the first study, when an STA could be obtained, it could be used to predict the responses for 73% of the neurons, implying that the STA accounted for a large proportion of the information processing (Andoni et al., 2007). Alternatively, in the second study the STA was the most informative stimulus feature for only 13% of the neurons (Andoni and Pollak, 2011). This may imply that using natural sounds changed the dominant processing mode: for MR stimuli it was the STA, while for natural sounds it was the STC derived filters. Additionally, using natural sounds may have resulted in biased STA and STC filters, which resulted in incorrect information estimates. Since different populations of neurons were sampled in the two studies, a direct comparison is difficult. A fruitful approach would be to present both MR stimuli and natural sounds, and then estimate filters, so that the effects of stimulus type can be better assessed.

The two most significant studies of STRF dependence on stimulus identity were performed by Escabí and colleagues and by Klein and colleagues (Escabí and Schreiner, 2002; Klein et al., 2006). Each study used the STA to estimate the STRF. The study by Escabí and colleagues was performed in the auditory midbrain. The key to their approach was contrasting dynamic moving ripple stimuli and ripple noise stimuli. These continuous stimuli were presented for approximately 15 minutes, allowing the system to settle into steady state, and thus limiting the effects of strong adaptation on STRF structure. The stimuli are also similar in their carrier structure, with each stimulus composed of the same number of tonal carriers, and with the carriers each spaced on a logarithmic axis. The only difference between the stimuli was the spectrotemporal envelope: for the dynamic moving ripple, the envelope contained local correlations, while the ripple noise contained no correlations. STRFs for both types of stimuli were highly similar: the main STRF subfields were highly correlated. For a small subset of neurons, it appeared that the DMR produced an STRF while the ripple noise did not, though later examination revealed that even in these cases the RN produced an STRF, though the subfields of the STRF were significantly reduced in magnitude. Buttressing this result, in a study of multidimensional STRFs in auditory cortex, Atencio and colleagues found that the STRFs for DMR and RN were well-correlated (Atencio et al., 2008).

The study by Klein was designed to show how changes in the spectrotemporal envelope changed estimated STRFs (Klein et al., 2006). Three different stimuli were used: moving ripples, spectrotemporal white noise, and TORCs. These stimuli shared the same carrier structure and differed only in their spectrotemporal envelope statistics. Though each type of stimulus produced a different number of successful STRFs, for each neuron that produced an STRF to the three stimuli, the STRFs were highly similar. This result is remarkable since these stimuli last only a few seconds, and thus the neurons may not be in steady state. Despite this, the STRFs were in agreement. Further, the envelope characteristics were markedly different, ranging from strong local correlations to no local correlations. Therefore, when stimuli are appropriate for spike-triggered analyses, and though the stimuli have drastically different correlation structures, in both the midbrain and the auditory cortex the STRFs were moderately to highly similar. This highlights the need to carefully design stimuli for experiments, and to match the analysis approach to the stimuli that are employed.

STRF Dependence on Stimulus Density

When dynamic random chord (DRC) stimuli are used, experimenter decisions may influence the results. For each DRC stimulus the experimenter must choose the appropriate density of the pips. Choosing a low density is similar to presenting frequency response area stimuli and may not allow inhibitory sidebands to be explored. Choosing a density that is too high, however, produces unmodulated noise, which drastically reduces the responsiveness of many cortical cells.

Blake and Merzenich (2002) presented dynamic random chord stimuli with different densities to awake owl monkeys (Blake and Merzenich, 2002). The different densities produced different cortical STRFs. STRFs obtained with high density stimuli had subfields that were reduced in strength and had much lower firing rates than those for low-density stimuli.

Similar results were found by Valentine and Eggermont (2004) in the auditory cortex of the cat, where changes in STRF bandwidth and response rate varied with the density of the random chords (Valentine and Eggermont, 2004). Consistent with the Blake and Merzenich study, increasing tone pip density reduced the STRF strength. Thus, for dynamic random chords, care must be taken in choosing appropriate stimulus parameters so that comparisons may be made to results obtained with other stimulus paradigms.

STRF Dependence on Behavior

One further aspect that needs to be addressed is the behavioral context in which STRFs are computed. Anesthetized studies have the strength that the behavioral condition is fairly stable and uniform, allowing for adequate data sampling.

However, awake, and behaving, conditions are more realistic for real-world listening situations. Shamma and his group have pioneered the combined use of behavioral performance and STA/STRF estimation. They have shown that rapid task-related STRF changes occur in AI of the behaving ferret (Fritz et al., 2003). In tone detection and two-tone discrimination tasks, the STRF shape changed in comparison to passive listening conditions (Fritz et al., 2005).

Since the STRF changes occur at the network and single-unit level, it is important to determine the time constant of the changes. The duration of the changes needs to be assessed since this will place a bound on the time over which the neural system is non-stationary. David and colleagues accomplished such an evaluation (David et al., 2012). They first showed that positive or negative reinforcement paradigms led to differential STA/STRF changes.

Thus, the behavioral task influenced the changes in the STRF. They then found that after behavior ceased, the STRF returned to baseline levels. This implies that the return to baseline in the STRF occurred just as quickly after behavior ended as it did when behavior ensued. This has important implications: even though appropriately estimated STRFs may change during behavior, they are relatively stable entities and thus are adequate and reliable measures of system function (Elhilali et al., 2007).

Conclusion

The stimulus choices for spike-triggered analyses are dictated by two main principles. First, the stimuli must cover the bandwidth of the neuron and they should contain the spectrotemporal features to which the neuron is tuned. Second, the stimulus must be appropriate for the analysis technique that is applied. If either of these principles is violated, then the receptive field estimates will be difficult to interpret and will be challenging to compare with other studies. Much time and effort has been expended in the past on approaches that have violated some of these considerations, and thus the usefulness of the results has been diminished.

Many spike-triggered analytical approaches have been applied to auditory data. The most prevalent is the spike-triggered average approach. For most neurons, the STA represents the main response mode, or stimulus feature, to which a neuron is tuned. Thus, it is the linear filter that captures the most information between the stimulus and the response. A limitation of STA analysis is that it can only be used when stimuli have at most second-order correlations. Higher-order stimulus correlations will result in biased STA estimates. A second approach, STC analysis, is sensitive to pairwise multiplicative interactions in the stimulus ensemble, and it can be used to obtain multiple spectrotemporal features. STC is computationally simple, and produces a set of orthogonal filters. STC analysis also suffers from the same stimulus limitations as STA: it cannot be used with stimuli that have higher than second-order correlations. If it is applied with such stimuli, the results may be biased. Finally, we outlined MID analysis, which can be used with any stimulus type. It is the most general of the analytical approaches, and it can recover two filters. MID analysis is limited, however, to recovering two filters, and not more, due to data requirements.

Different classes of stimuli may be used with each analytical technique. For STA analysis, the family of ripple stimuli – MR, TORC, DMR, and RN – may be applied. NSTE stimuli may also be used, and they are attractive because these stimuli have the temporal modulation envelope statistics of natural sounds. For STC, these stimuli may also be applied, as long as the particular instantiation of each stimulus is Gaussian. For non-Gaussian stimuli that are characterized by no more than second-order correlations, modifications to the STC analysis can be made (Samengo and Gollisch, 2012). For MID analysis, any of the stimuli that we described may be used.

Caution is advised when stimuli are used with analytical procedures that cannot support them. Recent work has shown that nonlinear processing may result in STAs that contain artifacts due to the processing of the stimulus by a neural system (Ahrens et al., 2008). The artifacts result from multiplicative interactions between components in the stimulus, similar to the way in which two-tone stimulation can elucidate nonlinear frequency interactions. In practice, when the STA and the MID technique were applied, the resulting filters were in concord, indicating that for auditory midbrain and cortical neurons the effects of these artifacts may be minimized for DMR stimulation (Atencio et al., 2008, 2009, 2012). For other samples of neurons, however, this concern must always be kept in mind.

Therefore, every stimulus choice involves tradeoffs. First, since recording times are limited, we cannot present every parameter of interest. Stimulus parameter regimes must be chosen carefully for each auditory station. Second, we must correctly choose the appropriate frequency extent, dynamic range, and statistical distribution of each stimulus. And third, we must consider the data-record that is required to make the STRF estimate. This implies that we must estimate the number of spikes that are needed to approximate the receptive field.

For each analytical approach that is chosen, we advocate the following sequence once the appropriate stimulus is identified. The first step is to set the stimulus bandwidth so that it encompasses the bandwidth of the neuron. The second step involves parameters that are particular to each type of stimulus. These parameter choices must be held in tension and adjusted inter-dependently. First, with the bandwidth chosen, additional statistics may be chosen that are based on the analysis approach that will be used. These include the temporal and spectral modulation frequency content, stimulus density, and the correlation structure of the stimulus. For each of these parameters, the range of the parameters must be chosen to cover the neural system's bandwidth for that particular parameter. Second, the stimulus duration must be chosen to ensure an adequate sampling of responses. This applies first to the overall stimulus duration, and second to the types of responses that are desired. For example, if TORC stimuli are used and steady-state responses are desired, then the stimuli must be made long enough so that the effects of onset/offset adaption are minimized.

The representation of the signal is usually not considered. However, it is implicit to each approach. The spectrogram needs care, since it is a nonlinear (squaring) transformation of the input signal. It is also not a complete representation of the input signal. Information is lost since the spectrogram does not include signal phase. For parametric signals, where the envelope is specified by the user, the spectrotemporal envelope may avoid the nonlinear transformation that is inherent to the spectrogram. However, even in this case, information is lost, since the spectrotemporal envelope does not contain information about the temporal fine structure of the signal.

Since it is challenging to discern the stimulus features to which neurons are tuned, some approaches have transformed the input signal to determine the parameter regimes to which neurons are sensitive. One approach estimated the nature of transients in the spectrotemporal representation, and this new representation was termed "surprise". STAs for bird neurons were constructed, showing that the bird auditory system may be sensitive to surprising features in the auditory signal (Gill et al., 2008). Also, methods that consider the contrast of the auditory signal may be used (Shechter and Depireux, 2012). For contrast analysis, a filter is estimated from the original spectrogram, and a second filter is estimated using a transformed version of the spectrogram that represents spectrotemporal contrast.

These input transform methods represent challenges and provide important insights into auditory stations. On one hand, these methods may result in interpretational difficulties, since they imply an additional nonlinear transformation of the input signal, beyond that provided by the spectrogram. This may be pertinent since performing a nonlinear transformation before the dynamics of a system, which in this case is the transformation of the signal before the system is estimated, may result in modeling difficulties (Marmarelis, 1997). On the other hand, these approaches may bring to light aspects of the signal that are pertinent for each station, and would otherwise be unknown. Once these information bearing aspects of the signal are understood, further stimulus classes may be designed that incorporate these features, which will allow more efficient probing of the auditory station and better receptive field estimation.

The discussion in the previous sections indicates that the use of spike-triggered receptive field analyses is rigorous and theoretically sound. Therefore it is feasible and useful to compare studies that applied different analysis methods and stimulus configurations.

However, the discussion also illustrated that great care must be taken to stay within the boundaries of each methodology, and to select appropriate stimulus conditions, so that experimental findings, interpretations, and conclusions may be generalized and compared across approaches.

References

Aertsen AM, Olders JH, Johannesma PI (1981) Spectro-temporal receptive fields of auditory neurons in the grassfrog. III. Analysis of the stimulus-event relation for natural stimuli. *Biol. Cybern* 39:195-209.

Ahrens MB, Linden JF, Sahani M (2008) Nonlinearities and contextual influences in auditory cortical responses modeled with multilinear spectrotemporal methods. *J. Neurosci.* 28:1929-1942.

Allen JB, Rabiner LR (1977) A Unified Approach to Short-Time Fourier Analysis and Synthesis. *P Ieee* 65:1558-1564.

Andoni S, Pollak GD (2011) Selectivity for spectral motion as a neural computation for encoding natural communication signals in bat inferior colliculus. *J. Neurosci.* 31:16529-16540.

Andoni S, Li N, Pollak GD (2007) Spectrotemporal receptive fields in the inferior colliculus revealing selectivity for spectral motion in conspecific vocalizations. *J. Neurosci.* 27:4882-4893.

Atencio CA, Schreiner CE (2008) Spectrotemporal processing differences between auditory cortical fast-spiking and regular-spiking neurons. *J. Neurosci.* 28:3897-3910.

Atencio CA, Schreiner CE (2010a) Columnar connectivity and laminar processing in cat primary auditory cortex. *PLoS One* 5:e9521.

Atencio CA, Schreiner CE (2010b) Laminar diversity of dynamic sound processing in cat primary auditory cortex. *J. Neurophysiol.* 103:192-205.

Atencio CA, Schreiner CE (2012) Spectrotemporal processing in spectral tuning modules of cat primary auditory cortex. *PLoS One* 7:e31537.

Atencio CA, Sharpee TO, Schreiner CE (2008) Cooperative nonlinearities in auditory cortical neurons. *Neuron* 58:956-966.

Atencio CA, Sharpee TO, Schreiner CE (2009) Hierarchical computation in the canonical auditory cortical circuit. *Proc. Natl. Acad. Sci. USA* 106:21894-21899.

Atencio CA, Sharpee TO, Schreiner CE (2012) Receptive field dimensionality increases from the auditory midbrain to cortex. *J. Neurophysiol.* 107:2594-2603.

Bialek W, de Ruyter van Steveninck R (2005) Features and dimensions: Motion estimation in fly vision. http://arxiv.org/abs/q-bio/0505003.

Blake DT, Merzenich MM (2002) Changes of AI receptive fields with sound density. *J. Neurophysiol.* 88:3409-3420.

Boyd S, Chua LO (1985) Fading memory and the problem of approximating nonlinear operators with Volterra series. *IEEE Trans Circ. Syst.* CAS-32:1150-1161.

Chichilnisky EJ (2001) A simple white noise analysis of neuronal light responses. *Network* 12:199-213.

David SV, Mesgarani N, Shamma SA (2007) Estimating sparse spectro-temporal receptive fields with natural stimuli. *Network* 18:191-212.

David SV, Fritz JB, Shamma SA (2012) Task reward structure shapes rapid receptive field plasticity in auditory cortex. *Proc. Natl. Acad. Sci. USA* 109:2144-2149.

David SV, Mesgarani N, Fritz JB, Shamma SA (2009) Rapid synaptic depression explains nonlinear modulation of spectro-temporal tuning in primary auditory cortex by natural stimuli. *J. Neurosci.* 29:3374-3386.

de Boer E (1975) Synthetic whole-nerve action potentials for the cat. *J. Acoust Soc. Am.* 58:1030-1045.

de Boer E, Kuyper P (1968) Triggered correlation. *IEEE Trans Biomed Eng* 15:169-179.

de Boer E, de Jongh HR (1978) On cochlear encoding: potentialities and limitations of the reverse-correlation technique. *J. Acoust Soc. Am.* 63:115-135.

deCharms RC, Blake DT, Merzenich MM (1998) Optimizing sound features for cortical neurons. *Science* 280:1439-1443.

Depireux DA, Simon JZ, Klein DJ, Shamma SA (2001) Spectro-temporal response field characterization with dynamic ripples in ferret primary auditory cortex. *J. Neurophysiol.* 85:1220-1234.

DiCarlo JJ, Johnson KO, Hsiao SS (1998) Structure of receptive fields in area 3b of primary somatosensory cortex in the alert monkey. *J. Neurosci.* 18:2626-2645.

Draper NR, Smith H (1981) Applied Regression Analysis, Second Edition. New York: John Wiley & Songs.

Eggermont JJ (2011) Context dependence of spectro-temporal receptive fields with implications for neural coding. *Hear Res.* 271:123-132.

Eggermont JJ, Smith GM (1990) Characterizing auditory neurons using the Wigner and Rihacek distributions: a comparison. *J. Acoust Soc. Am.* 87:246-259.

Elhilali M, Fritz JB, Chi TS, Shamma SA (2007) Auditory cortical receptive fields: stable entities with plastic abilities. *J. Neurosci.* 27:10372-10382.

Elhilali M, Fritz JB, Klein DJ, Simon JZ, Shamma SA (2004) Dynamics of precise spike timing in primary auditory cortex. *J. Neurosci.* 24:1159-1172.

Escabí MA, Schreiner CE (2002) Nonlinear spectrotemporal sound analysis by neurons in the auditory midbrain. *J. Neurosci.* 22:4114-4131.

Escabí MA, Miller LM, Read HL, Schreiner CE (2003) Naturalistic auditory contrast improves spectrotemporal coding in the cat inferior colliculus. *J. Neurosci.* 23:11489-11504.

Escabí MA, Nassiri R, Miller LM, Schreiner CE, Read HL (2005) The contribution of spike threshold to acoustic feature selectivity, spike information content, and information throughput. *J. Neurosci.* 25:9524-9534.

Fitzgerald JD, Rowekamp RJ, Sincich LC, Sharpee TO (2011) Second order dimensionality reduction using minimum and maximum mutual information models. *PLoS Comput Biol.* 7:e1002249.

Fritz J, Shamma S, Elhilali M, Klein D (2003) Rapid task-related plasticity of spectrotemporal receptive fields in primary auditory cortex. *Nat Neurosci* 6:1216-1223.

Fritz JB, Elhilali M, Shamma SA (2005) Differential dynamic plasticity of A1 receptive fields during multiple spectral tasks. *J. Neurosci.* 25:7623-7635.

Fritz JB, Elhilali M, Shamma SA (2007) Adaptive changes in cortical receptive fields induced by attention to complex sounds. *J. Neurophysiol.* 98:2337-2346.

Garcia-Lazaro JA, Ahmed B, Schnupp JW (2006) Tuning to natural stimulus dynamics in primary auditory cortex. *Curr. Biol.* 16:264-271.

Garcia-Lazaro JA, Ahmed B, Schnupp JW (2011) Emergence of tuning to natural stimulus statistics along the central auditory pathway. *PLoS One* 6:e22584.

Geffen MN, Gervain J, Werker JF, Magnasco MO (2011) Auditory perception of self-similarity in water sounds. *Frontiers in integrative neuroscience* 5:15.

Gill P, Woolley SM, Fremouw T, Theunissen FE (2008) What's that sound? Auditory area CLM encodes stimulus surprise, not intensity or intensity changes. *J. Neurophysiol.* 99:2809-2820.

Gourevitch B, Norena A, Shaw G, Eggermont JJ (2009) Spectrotemporal receptive fields in anesthetized cat primary auditory cortex are context dependent. *Cereb. Cortex* 19:1448-1461.

Joris PX, Schreiner CE, Rees A (2004) Neural processing of amplitude-modulated sounds. *Physiol Rev* 84:541-577.

Kim G, Doupe A (2011) Organized representation of spectrotemporal features in songbird auditory forebrain. *J. Neurosci.* 31:16977-16990.

Kim PJ, Young ED (1994) Comparative analysis of spectro-temporal receptive fields, reverse correlation functions, and frequency tuning curves of auditory-nerve fibers. *J. Acoust Soc. Am.* 95:410-422.

Klein DJ, Depireux DA, Simon JZ, Shamma SA (2000) Robust spectrotemporal reverse correlation for the auditory system: optimizing stimulus design. *J. Comput. Neurosci.* 9:85-111.

Klein DJ, Simon JZ, Depireux DA, Shamma SA (2006) Stimulus-invariant processing and spectrotemporal reverse correlation in primary auditory cortex. *J. Comput. Neurosci.* 20:111-136.

Kvale M, Schreiner CE (1997) Perturbative m-sequences for auditory systems identification. *Acustica* 83:653-658.

Lesica NA, Grothe B (2008) Dynamic spectrotemporal feature selectivity in the auditory midbrain. *J. Neurosci.* 28:5412-5421.

Lewis ER, Henry KR, Yamada WM (2002a) Tuning and timing in the gerbil ear: Wiener-kernel analysis. *Hear Res.* 174:206-221.

Lewis ER, Henry KR, Yamada WM (2002b) Tuning and timing of excitation and inhibition in primary auditory nerve fibers. *Hear Res* 171:13-31.

Machens CK, Wehr MS, Zador AM (2004) Linearity of cortical receptive fields measured with natural sounds. *J. Neurosci.* 24:1089-1100.

Marmarelis VZ (1989) Signal transformation and coding in neural systems. *IEEE Trans. Biomed. Eng.* 36:15-24.

Marmarelis VZ (1997) Modeling methodology for nonlinear physiological systems. *Ann. Biomed. Eng.* 25:239-251.

Marmarelis VZ (2004) Nonlinear dynamic modeling of physiological systems. New York: Plenum Publishers.

Marmarelis VZ, Juusola M, French AS (1999) Principal dynamic mode analysis of nonlinear transduction in a spider mechanoreceptor. *Ann. Biomed. Eng.* 27:391-402.

McDermott JH, Simoncelli EP (2011) Sound texture perception via statistics of the auditory periphery: evidence from sound synthesis. *Neuron* 71:926-940.

Miller LM, Schreiner CE (2000) Stimulus-based state control in the thalamocortical system. *J. Neurosci.* 20:7011-7016.

Miller LM, Escabí MA, Schreiner CE (2001a) Feature selectivity and interneuronal cooperation in the thalamocortical system. *J. Neurosci.* 21:8136-8144.

Miller LM, Escabí MA, Read HL, Schreiner CE (2001b) Functional convergence of response properties in the auditory thalamocortical system. *Neuron* 32:151-160.

Miller LM, Escabí MA, Read HL, Schreiner CE (2002) Spectrotemporal receptive fields in the lemniscal auditory thalamus and cortex. *J. Neurophysiol.* 87:516-527.

Norena AJ, Gourevitch B, Pienkowski M, Shaw G, Eggermont JJ (2008) Increasing spectrotemporal sound density reveals an octave-based organization in cat primary auditory cortex. *J. Neurosci.* 28:8885-8896.

Palm G (1979) Representation and Approximation of Non-Linear Systems. 2. Discrete-Time. *Biological Cybernetics* 34:49-52.

Paninski L (2003) Convergence properties of three spike-triggered analysis techniques. *Network* 14:437-464.

Patterson RD, Robinson K, Holdsworth JW, McKeown D, Zhang C, Allerhand M (1992) Complex sounds and auditory images. In: Auditory Physiology and Perception (Cazals Y, Demany L, Horner K, eds), pp 429-446. Oxford: Pergamon.

Pienkowski M, Shaw G, Eggermont JJ (2009) Wiener-Volterra characterization of neurons in primary auditory cortex using poisson-distributed impulse train inputs. *J. Neurophysiol.* 101:3031-3041.

Pillow JW, Simoncelli EP (2006) Dimensionality reduction in neural models: an information-theoretic generalization of spike-triggered average and covariance analysis. *J. Vis.* 6:414-428.

Rust NC, Schwartz O, Movshon JA, Simoncelli EP (2005) Spatiotemporal elements of macaque v1 receptive fields. *Neuron* 46:945-956.

Samengo I, Gollisch T (2013) Spike-triggered covariance: geometric proof, symmetry properties, and extension beyond Gaussian stimuli. *J. Comput. Neurosci.* 34(1):137-161.

Schwartz O, Pillow JW, Rust NC, Simoncelli EP (2006) Spike-triggered neural characterization. *J. Vis.* 6:484-507.

Sharpee T, Rust NC, Bialek W (2004) Analyzing neural responses to natural signals: maximally informative dimensions. *Neural Comput* 16:223-250.

Sharpee TO, Miller KD, Stryker MP (2008) On the importance of static nonlinearity in estimating spatiotemporal neural filters with natural stimuli. *J. Neurophysiol.* 99:2496-2509.

Sharpee TO, Atencio CA, Schreiner CE (2011a) Hierarchical representations in the auditory cortex. *Curr. Opin. Neurobiol* 21:761-767.

Sharpee TO, Nagel KI, Doupe AJ (2011b) Two-dimensional adaptation in the auditory forebrain. *J. Neurophysiol.* 106:1841-1861.

Shechter B, Depireux DA (2012) Contrast tuned responses in primary auditory cortex of the awake ferret. *Eur. J. Neurosci.* 35:550-561.

Singh NC, Theunissen FE (2003) Modulation spectra of natural sounds and ethological theories of auditory processing. *J. Acoust Soc. Am.* 114:3394-3411.

Slaney M (1993) An efficient implementation of the Patterson-Holdsworth auditory filterbank. *Apple Computer Technical Report* #35.

Smith ZM, Delgutte B, Oxenham AJ (2002) Chimaeric sounds reveal dichotomies in auditory perception. *Nature* 416:87-90.

Szymanski FD, Rabinowitz NC, Magri C, Panzeri S, Schnupp JW (2011) The laminar and temporal structure of stimulus information in the phase of field potentials of auditory cortex. *J. Neurosci.* 31:15787-15801.

Theunissen FE, Sen K, Doupe AJ (2000) Spectral-temporal receptive fields of nonlinear auditory neurons obtained using natural sounds. *J. Neurosci.* 20:2315-2331.

Touryan J, Lau B, Dan Y (2002) Isolation of relevant visual features from random stimuli for cortical complex cells. *J. Neurosci.* 22:10811-10818.

Valentine PA, Eggermont JJ (2004) Stimulus dependence of spectro-temporal receptive fields in cat primary auditory cortex. *Hear Res.* 196:119-133.

Versnel H, Zwiers MP, van Opstal AJ (2009) Spectrotemporal response properties of inferior colliculus neurons in alert monkey. In: *J. Neurosci.*, pp 9725-9739. United States.

Voss RF, Clarke J (1975) 1-F-Noise in Music and Speech. Nature 258:317-318.

Voss RF, Clarke J (1978) "1/f Noise in Music": Music from 1/f Noise. *Journal of the Acoustical Society of America* 63:258-263.

Wang X, Merzenich MM, Beitel R, Schreiner CE (1995) Representation of a species-specific vocalization in the primary auditory cortex of the common marmoset: temporal and spectral characteristics. *J. Neurophysiol.* 74:2685-2706.

Westwick DT, Kearney RE (1998) Nonparametric identification of nonlinear biomedical systems, part 1: theory. *Critical reviews in biomedical engineering* 26:153-226.

Woolley SM, Gill PR, Theunissen FE (2006) Stimulus-dependent auditory tuning results in synchronous population coding of vocalizations in the songbird midbrain. *J. Neurosci.* 26:2499-2512.

Woolley SM, Fremouw TE, Hsu A, Theunissen FE (2005) Tuning for spectro-temporal modulations as a mechanism for auditory discrimination of natural sounds. *Nat. Neurosci.* 8:1371-1379.

Yamada WM, Lewis ER (1999) Predicting the temporal responses of non-phase-locking bullfrog auditory units to complex acoustic waveforms. *Hear Res.* 130:155-170.

In: Handbook of Modern Techniques in Auditory Cortex
Editors: Didier A. Depireux and Mounya Elhilali
ISBN: 978-1-62808-894-6

Chapter 4

Uncovering Non-Linear Coding in the Primary Auditory Cortex

Didier A. Depireux and Barak Shechter
Institute for Systems Research, University of Maryland,
College Park, Maryland, US

Abbreviations

AI – primary auditory cortex
MTF – modulation transfer function
RMS – root-mean-square
SNR – signal-to-noise
STRF – spectro-temporal receptive field
TORC – temporally orthogonal ripple combination

Introduction

Neural coding of natural stimuli in sensory systems is often modeled by a linear system. This is natural first step, since it is the simplest approach and the mathematics involved are well-established. This first order approximation is computed by reverse correlating a certain aspect of the stimulus with the neural spike train it evokes. It was used by de Boer et al (de Boer 1967; de Boer and De Jongh 1975; Moller 1983) to study the "impulse response function" of structures in the early auditory pathway, by computing a reverse correlation between the stimulus (i.e., the waveform) and the spike trains the stimulus elicits. This method is particularly effective at the level of the auditory nerve, where responses are robust and reliable, and can follow temporal features of the stimulus with great precision. This is in stark contrast to the activity observed in auditory cortex, in which at best the neural firing can be seen to phase-lock to amplitude modulations rather than to the physical waveform itself. While at some level, the underlying theoretical model is the same, the practical or phenomenological study of nonlinearities at the level of the auditory nerve leads to a very different set of methods than those presented in this chapter. See for instance (Zhang, Heinz et al. 2001; Tan and Carney 2003) among many others.

The spectro-temporal receptive field (STRF) is a generalization of this procedure which characterizes processing in the auditory pathway in both frequency and time. In this aspect of containing two dimensions of space and time, it is not the typical concept of linear system found in most mathematical treatises about linear systems. In auditory cortex, it is calculated as the average spectro-temporal envelope before a spike. Because the stimulus has dimensions of spectrum and time, but the neural response has a dimension of time only (the timing of the spikes), the STRF really is a collection of parallel linear systems, one for each frequency band. Used as a predictive tool, the outputs of each linear system, corresponding to each frequency band, are linearly added together to result in a probability density of neural firing.

The STRF performs surprisingly well in predicting the overall course of the response to novel broadband stimuli, considering there is no real *a priori* reason to believe it would. By construction, it is unable to account for aspects of neural activity which are inherently nonlinear. Some of these nonlinearities are obvious: spikes are events which are discrete, and spike rates cannot be negative. Other nonlinearities are less obvious, but more interesting and relevant to understanding neural processing in auditory cortex: for instance, we have found that a (linear) STRF followed by an instantaneous nonlinearity accounted for much of the variance unexplained by the STRF alone, if the nonlinearity was quadratic (i.e. a second order polynomial). But what sort of computational advantage can be achieved by a static nonlinearity, particularly a quadratic one?

- First, a squared output can encode a phase-specific component of Fourier energy in a local (time and frequency-wise) region of the stimulus. This may be an ideal way of preserving both local amplitude and phase information, as first proposed by Pollen and Ronner (Pollen and Ronner 1982).
- Second, squaring enhances stimulus selectivity: tuning of cells for stimulus parameters becomes narrower, and edges steeper.
- Third, and probably most relevant, the squared outputs of linear filters are the building blocks for an energy model: combining the squared output of cells, all encoding the same region of the tonotopic axis and tuned to the same range of spectral densities and temporal periodicities, results in responses whose characteristics are the auditory equivalent of the complex cell of visual cortex. In the standard model of building a complex V1 cell from simple cells, the squared outputs of linear cells, which respond to subregions of the responsive region of the complex cell, are added together. Since neighboring simple cells in V1 tend to have receptive fields in quadrature, the resulting sum has the characteristics needed to generate the response properties of complex cells (Watson and Ahumada 1985; Ohzawa, DeAngelis et al. 1990; Rust, Schwartz et al. 2005).

These simple arguments show that even a simple instantaneous non-linearity, as detailed in the following, can provide a significant insight into neural processing.

Background

Linear STRF (Brief Recap of Chap. 2)

The natural, real-life auditory environment is complex, multi-source and usually noisy. This impacts normal hearing and the ability to help the hearing-impaired. For instance, speech intelligibility decreases nonlinearly with reductions in signal to noise ratios or modulation depth (Drullman, Festen et al. 1994; Chi, Gao et al. 1999; Deller JR., Hansen et al. 2000). In a noisy environment, a healthy listener can easily attend a specific stream and perceive its content. However, there is a heightened sensitivity to masking following bilateral auditory cortex strokes (Tramo, Bharucha et al. 1990; Tramo, Shah et al. 2002). Patients with damage to AI describe having difficulty extracting low-contrast features. These studies implicate the role of higher stations of the auditory pathway, including AI, in signal detection and enhancement. Thus, the processing that occurs as early as AI likely reflects the nonlinear aspects of competing sound envelopes, maskers and simple envelope contrast. Intelligibility of speech in noise is dependent on contrast between the spectral peaks and the background, and a complex spectral enhancement is key for a sound analysis of the auditory scene.

Few studies have characterized in the awake animal the nonlinear processing components involved in the analysis of competing sound envelopes and the relevant neural circuitries. In both anesthetized and awake animals, phase-locked responses to the sound envelope can deviate from linear predictors; these are considered nonlinearities, and may arise from both trivial and non-trivial sources. Even from purely physical constraints on neurons, we expect nonlinear responses. We define response nonlinearity that arises due to physical properties of neurons to be trivial: there are absolute bounds imposed on the neural response by metabolic processes. The firing rate of a neuron has a maximum possible value, or saturation rate, and inhibition of its firing cannot induce a negative firing rate. While these nonlinearities are trivial or at least expected, they still contribute to the essential processing of the auditory scene. In addition to our expectation of trivial nonlinearities, there is neurophysiological evidence that more complex output processing occurs in cortex beyond that of thresholding and saturation, such as circuit convergence and delay patterns (Schnupp, Mrsic-Flogel et al. 2001; Fishbach, Yeshurun et al. 2003). Such nonlinearities, which arise due to network properties, and not purely physical properties of the neurons, are nontrivial nonlinearities. For instance, the average firing rates in cortex drop in magnitude from earlier stages in the pathway. An input-output nonlinearity at such a stage would enable a nonlinear compression scheme whereby essential information of the auditory scene is preserved—perhaps even enhanced—and features of lesser relevance are degraded or discarded. When trivial nonlinearities are included in models used to predict A1 responses to complex sound, the prediction success can be improved (Shechter and Depireux 2007); however these do not sufficiently describe the output nonlinearity (Machens, Wehr et al. 2004; Young 2008) .

At the level of cortex, processing is believed to be well *approximated* by linear systems, but having a nontrivial nonlinear component to responses (Calhoun and Schreiner 1998; Theunissen, Sen et al. 2000; Schnupp, Mrsic-Flogel et al. 2001; Sen, Theunissen et al. 2001; Sahani and Linden 2002; Machens, Wehr et al. 2004). Neurons in auditory cortex are tuned to extract specific aspects of the spectro-temporal content of sounds. The spectral profile encoded by these neurons is built up from features extracted in subcortical input neurons. The cortical representation of spectro-temporally rich, well parameterized sounds has been the subject of intense research (Schreiner and Calhoun 1994; Versnel, Kowalski et al. 1995; Kowalski, Depireux et al. 1996; Kowalski, Depireux et al. 1996; Depireux, Simon et al. 2001; Linden, Liu et al. 2003). While details vary considerably between methods, auditory cortical processing can be modeled by linear systems which transform an input sound stimulus to a predicted neural response. These linear spectro-temporal receptive fields (STRFs) are useful as a first approximation in that they generally capture the overall trend of the response. However, by definition, they cannot provide a construct to characterize nonlinear processing. A well-established method of obtaining a preliminary characterization of the output nonlinearity is to relate the neural response to its linear receptive field by a static input/output function (Lee and Schetzen 1965; Marmarelis 1993).

In this chapter, we examine and classify the static output nonlinearities observed in cortical responses. Are these nonlinearities trivial in the sense that they are predetermined by physical constraints of the individual neurons? Or do they perform a computation on the input thereby enhancing features important to processing the auditory scene. Is a static output nonlinearity (either trivial or nontrivial) sufficient to account for the complex output processing of neurons in primary auditory cortex? To address these questions, we quantify the degree of linearity of responses in AI. We show that these neurons employ nontrivial nonlinearity in their computations, which reflects the extraction of spectro-temporal contrast.

Possibilities

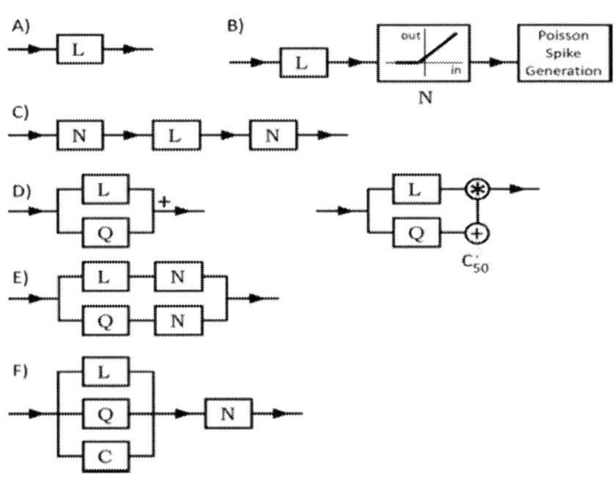

Figure 1. Nonlinear extensions: the STRF, shown as a black box labeled L (for Linear) in A), transforms the acoustic input into a neural output. Implicit in the STRF model is the model shown in B): namely, the STRF is followed by a partial rectification, i.e. the neuron has a spontaneous rate of firing, which can be lowered but cannot be less than zero; the output of this trivial nonlinearity then drives a non-homogeneous Poisson process. C) In further non-linear extensions of the model, more general but still instantaneous non-linearities can be placed on the input to and the output from the STRF. D) The next data-driven extension of the model in C) consists in measuring the coding of "contrast" (Q, for quadratic) by cortical neurons. The left model turns out to be the successful one, though it was initially inspired by the model on the right, used in vision (Bonin and Carandini, nonlinear processing in LGN neurons). E) The most complete model developed in this chapter. F) would be an even more complete model, with a box labeled C for Cubic (third order). We found that the (noisy) nature of our neural data is such that no consistent picture emerges for any coding of the "cube" of the spectro-temporal envelope in auditory cortex.

Experimental Procedures

We measured the response of neurons in the primary auditory cortex (AI) of awake ferrets using spectro-temporally modulated auditory gratings[1], or ripples. The ferrets were surgically implanted with chronic multi-electrode arrays. A detailed description of recording and surgical procedures can be found in (Dobbins, Marvit et al. 2007). All procedures were approved by the U of Md Animal Care and Use Committee and in accord with NIH Guidelines on care and use of lab animals.

STRF Computation

For the rest of this chapter, cells were characterized by measuring their spectro-temporal receptive field. These stimuli, known as auditory gratings or ripples are described in full details in the previous 2 chapters. Each have a spectro-temporal profile modulated sinusoidally in spectrum and in time. The modulation of a grating is characterized in spectrum by its spectral density (cycles/octave), in time by its angular frequency w (Hz), and in amplitude by its excursions away from the mean level of the stimulus (modulation depth ΔA, % of mean). The amplitude $S(x,t)$, corresponding to frequency f, where and the lower edge of the spectrum, is then adjusted at time t as

$$S(x,t) = L[1 + \Delta A \cdot \cos(2\pi(\Omega \cdot x + w \cdot t) + \phi)], \quad (1)$$

for a linear modulation. *S* defines the spectro-temporal envelope of the stimulus. *L* is the average level of the stimulus (measured as the RMS of the stimulus with reference to a 1kHz sine tone) and is the starting phase of the grating. Since the 100 tones per octave that make up a grating are logarithmically spaced, it does not elicit the perception of a pitch.

The spectral and angular densities of the stimulus set ranged from -5 to 5 cyc/oct and from 4 to 48 Hz, respectively. Each stimulus had a duration of 3 seconds and was presented with at least 4 repetitions at 65 dB SPL and at 90% modulation. The derivation of the steady state STRF follows (Klein, Depireux et al. 2000). Briefly, a reverse correlation with the stimulus spectro-temporal envelope is used to obtain the STRF from the spike train elicited by the stimulus.

The responses were binned into time windows as determined by the periodicity of the stimulus set. Bin width was chosen such that the maximal angular frequency was below the Nyquist frequency (from 10-15 msec, depending on *w*). All further spike rates for a particular cell used the same time resolution. In order to allow the response to reach a steady-state, the analysis was started at 250 msec post stimulus onset, thereby removing the effect of level transients present at the onset of the stimulus. We also measured the *evoked spike rate* elicited by the mean level of the stimulus (away from which the spectro-temporal envelope is modulated). The STRF measures the neural response to the stimulus modulations, whereas the evoked spike rate measures the response to the noise carrier, i.e., to a broadband noise of equivalent level as the grating stimulus. These measures are in contrast to the spontaneous

[1] We prefer the term "grating", as it is a better description of the shape of the spectro-temporal envelope, and it makes the connection to the gratings used in vision research clearer. The original term "ripple" is equivalent.

rate of firing, which exists in the absence of any stimulus. This measure of the *evoked spike rate* r_0 will be explored in much greater details later in this chapter.

SNR Computation

To determine the reliability of the STRF measured for the steady state response, we computed a signal-to-noise ratio (SNR) of the corresponding modulation transfer function (MTF, the 2-dimensional Fourier transform of the STRF). The MTF is the dual representation of the STRF, where each point is a complex number which represents the response of the neuron to an auditory grating with spectral density (cycles/octave) and angular frequency (Hz), see Eq.1.

The amplitude of the complex number is the corresponding amplitude of the response and the phase is the corresponding phase lag between stimulus and response. 50 bootstrap estimates were generated for each point of the MTF by choosing with repetition from the entire set of responses obtained. The SNR of each point ($\mathrm{SNR}_{\Omega,w}$) was taken to be the average power divided by the variance of the estimates. The SNR of the STRF was computed as the power-weighted mean of the SNR at each point. is the power of the MTF at the point (Ω, w).

$$\mathrm{SNR}_{\Omega,w} = \frac{\left|\sum_{bootstraps} \psi(\Omega, w)\right|^2}{N_{bootstraps} \cdot \sigma_{\psi}^2} \tag{2}$$

$$\mathrm{SNR} = \frac{\sum_{\Omega,w} P_{\Omega,w} \cdot \mathrm{SNR}_{\Omega,w}}{\sum_{\Omega,w} P_{\Omega,w}} \tag{3}$$

For a cell to be included in the subsequent analyses, we required that its SNR be greater than 1. Computing 50, 75, and 100 bootstrap estimates for a subset of recordings resulted in statistically equivalent SNRs; we therefore chose to compute SNR using 50 bootstrap estimates throughout.

Computation of Static Output Nonlinearities

The STRF can be used to predict responses to novel stimuli with complex spectro-temporal envelopes. This is achieved by convolving in time a spectro-temporal envelope with the STRF, and summing across all frequency bands. A predicted response spike rate to a stimulus with spectro-temporal envelope is therefore computed as

$$r_{lin}(t) = \int \int STRF(x,\tau) \cdot S(x, t-\tau)\, d\tau dx \tag{4}$$

Using the derived receptive fields, we computed the predicted responses to the stimuli used in measurement of the STRF (Figure 2). We characterized the relationship between predicted and actual response by means of a parameterized fit.

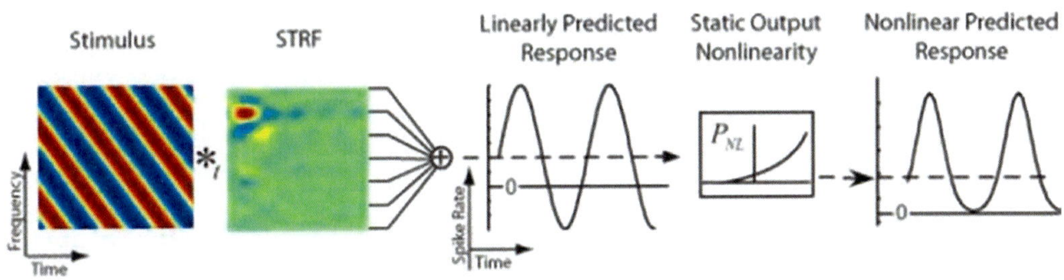

Figure 2. Linear-Nonlinear STRF Model. Using the spectro-temporal receptive field (STRF) derived by reverse correlation, a linear predicted response rate is obtained by convolution of stimulus and STRF in time and summation across frequency. The nonlinear prediction is obtained by applying the polynomial static output nonlinearity function to the linearly predicted response. A squaring output nonlinearity can enhance stimulus selectivity, demonstrated by narrower peaks and steeper edges in the response.

Degree of Linearity

In order to measure the *degree of linearity* in the response, we measured the power of the relationship between predicted response and actual response: $r_{act}(t) \propto r_{lin}(t)^{\alpha}$. The exponent was found by finding the slope of a linear fit *on a logarithmic scale*. Specifically, the evoked spike rate was added to the predicted response; the logarithm of this sum and the logarithm of the actual response were calculated for positive values; and the least squares linear fit was computed between both logarithms. The slope of this fit was α. A value of 1 implies a linear relationship between stimulus and response, whereas values different than 1 implies the existence of higher order processing.

α is the simplest measure that enables us to measure some degree of linearity in auditory responses with a single quantity. Good as a first approximation, it provided a concise descriptor for comparing all recorded cells. After measuring the degree of linearity with α, we can characterize in more detail the functional relationship between the linear prediction and the recorded responses. In our hands, inspection of our entire dataset (as shown in Figures 2,3) showed no rate saturation, as would occur from the neurons reaching a maximal firing rate. Rate saturation would be indicated by a leveling-off of actual response when plotted as a function of the linearly predicted response (similar to a sigmoid function). Given that we did not observe saturation in any of our recordings, (even though it is usually found when measuring rate-level functions in the onset response to different kind of stimuli, such as pure tones (Heil 1997)), and because of the highly general quantitative power offered by polynomial approximations, we then computed the static output nonlinearity as the 3rd order polynomial which minimized the squared error between the predicted response and the actual response (Figure 1). This allowed us to characterize the nonlinearity arbitrarily in terms of a power series, without over-emphasizing lower spike rates.

$$r_{poly}(t) = P_{NL}[r_{lin}(t)]. \tag{5}$$

In order to measure the efficacy of the computed static output nonlinearity, we recorded responses to new test stimuli. These stimuli, called temporally orthogonal ripple combinations (TORCs), had complex spectro-temporal envelopes defined as the sum of multiple auditory gratings (Klein, Depireux et al. 2000). Each of the grating components comprising a TORC had the same spectral density and depth, but differed in angular frequency. Their initial phases were "optimized", in the sense that their values were randomly selected so as to minimize the "peakiness" of the envelope, as measured by the peak to RMS ratio. The STRF was used to compute the linear predicted response r_{lin}, and in conjunction with P_{NL}, also the prediction r_{poly}. We measured the RMS error between predictions and actual responses obtained.

Examples:

We show some example cells (meeting the requirement of $SNR > 1$). Figures 3 & 4 demonstrate cells for which the analyses described above were computed. The STRF of each cell is depicted alongside the relationship observed between the linear predicted responses and the actual responses.

Quantifying the Degree of Linearity

We measured the power (α) of the regression between predicted response and actual response by computing the slope of a linear regression analysis performed on a logarithmic scale. This value characterizes the degree of linearity these neurons showed in their responses. The data shown in Figure 3 are from neurons which responded linearly, except for a trivial rectifying nonlinearity ($\alpha \approx 1$). Those in Figure 4 responded with nontrivial output nonlinearities ($\alpha > 1$).

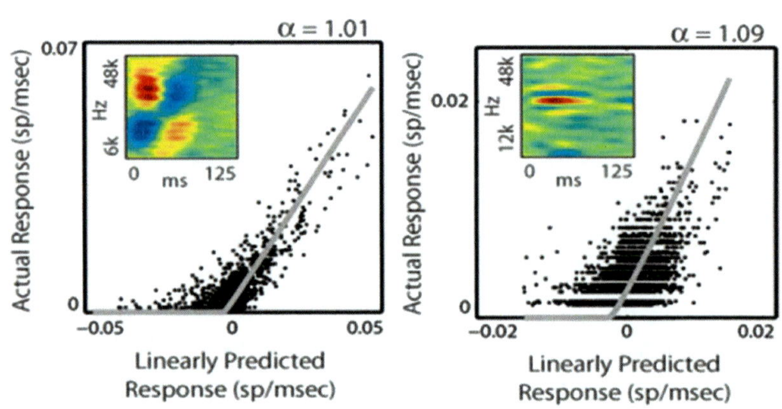

Figure 3. Example Linear Responses of neurons whose outputs were linear with respect to modulations in the stimulus spectro-temporal envelopes. Each point represents a point in time at which the actual response rate was sampled and a predicted response rate was computed. Values of which were near 1 signified linearity. The STRF of each neuron is inset.

Across all cells we recorded in AI, the mean of all measured α's was 1.92 ± 0.76. Thus, the relationship between predicted linear response and actual response was nontrivial for most cells, with a power close to 2 (squaring).

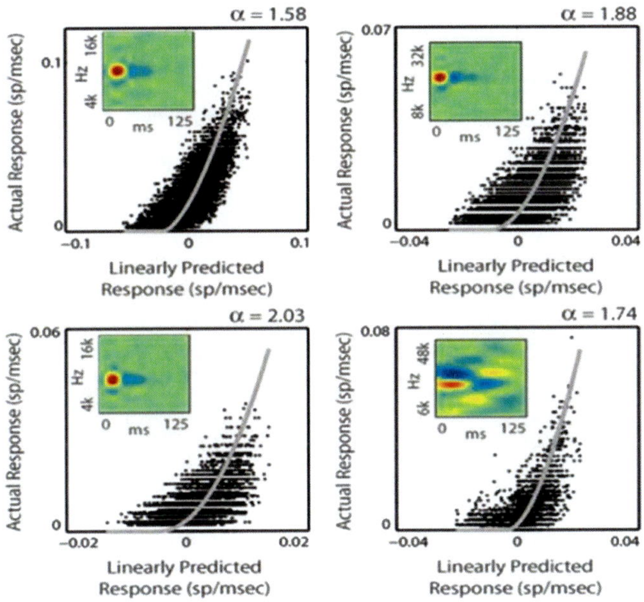

Figure 4. Nonlinear Responses. The responses of four neurons whose outputs were nonlinear with respect to modulations in spectro-temporal envelopes. Each point represents a point in time at which the actual response rate was sampled and a predicted response rate was computed. Values of which were different than 1 signified nonlinearity. The STRF of each neuron is inset.

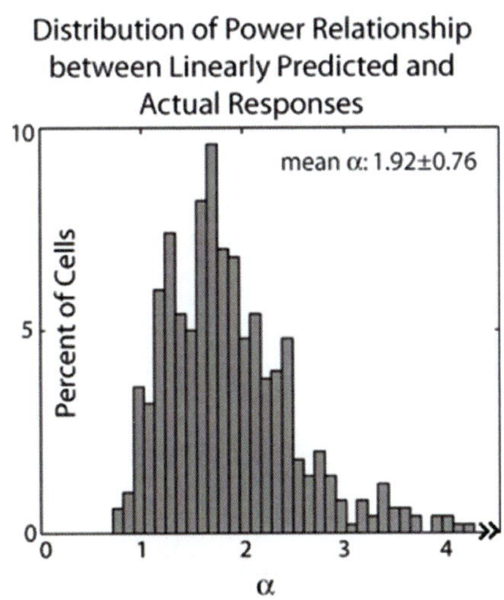

Figure 5. Distribution of α. The degree of linearity was measured by computing the slope of a linear fit between linearly predicted response and actual response on a logarithmic scale. The mean value of was 1.92 ± 0.76, implying the existence of a squaring output nonlinearity for most cells in AI.

Characterization of the Nonlinearity

Using the instantaneous nonlinearity just described, we can quantify the relation between predicted output from the STRF and the actual responses recorded for each neuron. We found it most practical to use a 3rd order polynomial fit to minimize the squared error between predicted and actual responses, using a goodness-of-fit test. To obtain a *predicted* response, we evaluate the polynomial on the output of the STRF (Eqs. 4,5). In order to determine the utility of P_{NL}, we quantified the error when used to predict responses to *new sounds* (i.e., not those used to construct the STRF and P_{NL}). With respect to the TORC stimuli described in chapter 2, we measure RMS error between both linear and nonlinear predictions and the actual responses obtained during the recording session. In (Shechter and Depireux 2010), we show for individual cells that using the non-linearity improves the prediction of response to new sounds, as well as reduce the variability of the predicted values. In Figure 6, we demonstrate the improved predictive power of the STRF when using a static output nonlinearity. We show a significant decrease ($p < 0.001$, Wilcoxon signed-rank) in both RMS error and variance of error when using the linear predictor (STRF) and an output nonlinearity, as opposed to the linear prediction alone.

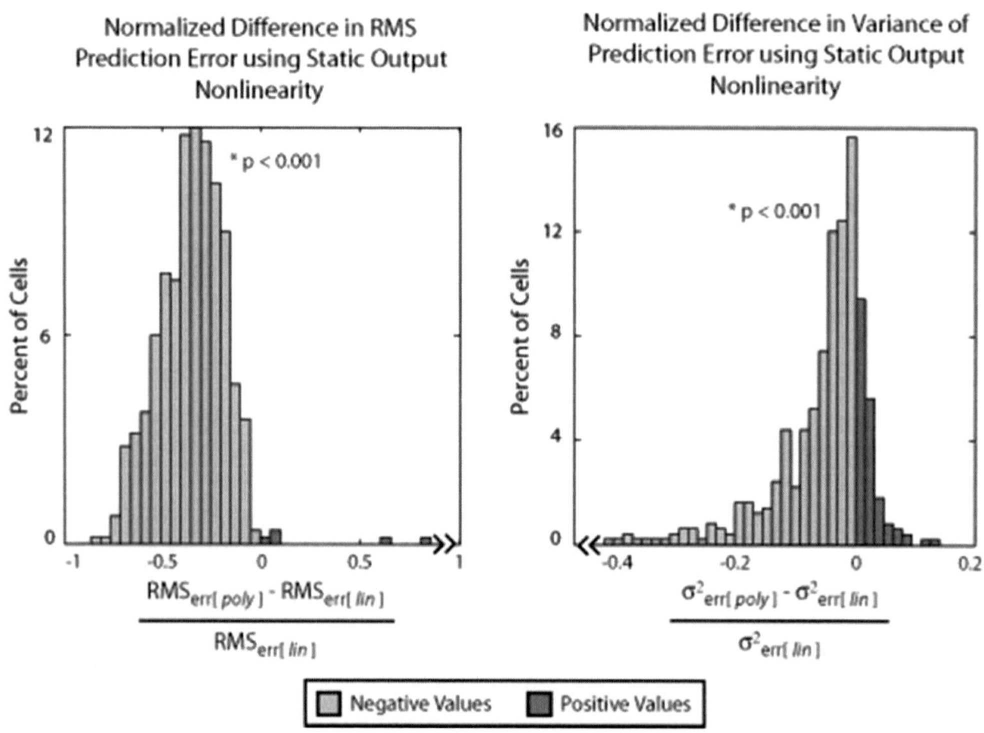

Figure 6. Reduction of Prediction Error with Static Output Nonlinearity. Distributions of the RMS prediction error (left) and variance of error (right) show a significant improvement in predictive power when using a static output nonlinearity, as opposed to the STRF alone ($p<0.001$, Wilcoxon signed-rank). The graphs show the difference in prediction errors (with respect to the actual response) normalized to the linear prediction error.

Discussion

The first extension of the STRF model is an STRF followed by an instantaneous non-linearity, first explored (as far as we know) in the early 1980s by Eggermont et al. (1983). This simplest of extensions already uncovers some interesting aspects of neural coding. This nonlinearity—a squaring nonlinearity in the main—is not solely a result of response rate saturation and half-wave rectification.

Significance of Squaring Nonlinearities

That in primary auditory cortex has interesting implications. The mean value of 2 is not so high that the output nonlinearity is just an over-rectification, with extreme sensitivity to small changes in input. Such a nonlinearity would have a high firing threshold and high gain, effectively reducing the dynamic range cells can encode. Given the overall reduction in firing rate as one moves up the auditory pathway, these nontrivial nonlinearities suggest cortical neurons are using an encoding scheme which enhances specific features. A squared output can encode a phase-specific component of Fourier energy in a local region of the stimulus. This may be an ideal way of preserving both local amplitude and phase information (Pollen and Ronner 1982). Second, squaring enhances stimulus selectivity: tuning of cells for stimulus parameters becomes narrower, and its edges steeper (see Predictions). Third, and probably most relevant, the squared outputs of linear filters are the building blocks for an energy model: combining the squared output of neighboring cells, all encoding the same region of the tonotopic axis and tuned to the same range of spectral densities and temporal periodicities, but differing in phase, results in responses whose characteristics are the auditory equivalent of the complex cell responses of visual cortex.

Exponential vs. Polynomial Output Nonlinearity

The exponent provides a compact way of characterizing the degree of linearity present in the neural response. The simplicity in using a single number allows for an efficient cross-cell comparison of the entire population of responses. Nevertheless, the complexity of the input-output nonlinearity is not fully characterized by a single number. The exponential is highly restrictive in the range of functions it can approximate. Therefore, after performing an overall characterization, we quantified the specific nonlinearity for each cell with a 3rd order polynomial function. The use of polynomials allows a broad range of nonlinear functions to be captured, while also providing an efficient parameterization using a small number of coefficients. Given that no responses showed spike rate saturation, the static output nonlinearities were well fit by a polynomial.

Overall Static Output Nonlinearity vs. a Per Channel Nonlinearity

The introduction of the static output nonlinearity is to a first approximation a global measure of the output characteristics of a cortical neuron: the simplest nonlinearity is a half-wave rectifier, as dictated by the physical limitations of neurons. Our model consists in a linear model (the STRF) followed by an instantaneous non-linearity. The STRF models the computations carried out by the auditory pathway up to and including the neuron. This information is then conveyed as firing output in a manner modeled to a large extent by the static output nonlinearity. In our model of a linear system followed by an instantaneous nonlinearity, the physiological properties of the cortical neuron result in the nonlinearity, and become an *explicit* feature of the neural computation. This is not to imply that in the physical instantiation of our model, the STRF is a representation of *all the neural processes* up until that point, nor that the static output nonlinearity has to do *exclusively* with the physical properties of the neuron producing a spike. However, in determining the algorithms used by the auditory pathway, the output nonlinearity is essential to the neural computation and its associated properties of noise-robustness and efficiency, which we believe are typical of cortical representations.

Each neuron we recorded from was actually receiving inputs from neurons with a range of best frequencies. The contribution from each of its spectrally distributed inputs should not necessarily be assumed linear in modulation. Ahrens et al. (2008) propose an overall input nonlinearity which conditions the input to the STRF based on stimulus level. One could extend the concept of input nonlinearity further to condition the input to the cortical model in a way that accounts for the subcortical processing—not just limited stimulus level. Perhaps, a more realistic extension of our model would entail the neuron integrating each spectral band nonlinearly before contributing the overall firing output. That is, instead of only a global static output nonlinearity, each frequency band should have its own local static nonlinearity. This more closely models the flow of information from downstream neurons and its subsequent integration for further processing. However, the main difficulty is that we have access only to the temporal output of the neurons, a one dimensional quantity. The use of our broadband sounds for spectro-temporal characterization is sufficient in the case of a global static output nonlinearity, but may not allow the disambiguation of many local nonlinearities.

Phase Locked vs. Phase Independent Nonlinearity

An established measure of complex (nonlinear) tuning is (Hubel and Wiesel 1965; Movshon, Thompson et al. 1978; Movshon, Thompson et al. 1978; Ahmed, Garcia-Lazaro et al. 2006). This ratio measures the degree to which a neuron is phase locked (f_1) to modulations in the stimulus relative to the degree to which the spike rate is elevated irrespective of modulation phase (f_0). This measure derives from the study of complex visual cortex neurons, which respond to a grating with an elevated firing rate throughout its presentation, but without specificity for any stimulus phase. Such a phase independent nonlinearity cannot be measured reliably in neurons which have low evoked firing rates and an appreciable response locked to stimulus modulations. Trivial output nonlinearities, namely rectification at 0 spikes/sec, are likely to interfere with the measurement of the evoked firing rate during stimulus presentation. Such rectification would be measured as an artificial elevation of the evoked rate and a decrease in the magnitude of the phase locked response. Despite the difficulty in measuring phase independent complexities in the response of AI neurons, it is plausible that such rate encodings of the sound environment co-exist with spike timing based schemes and may serve to extract distinct components from the sound envelope (Malone, Scott et al. 2007; Zheng and Escabi 2008).

Inherent Response Variability

The predictive power of a polynomial static output nonlinearity used in conjunction with the linear receptive field was demonstrated by an overall reduction in the prediction error.

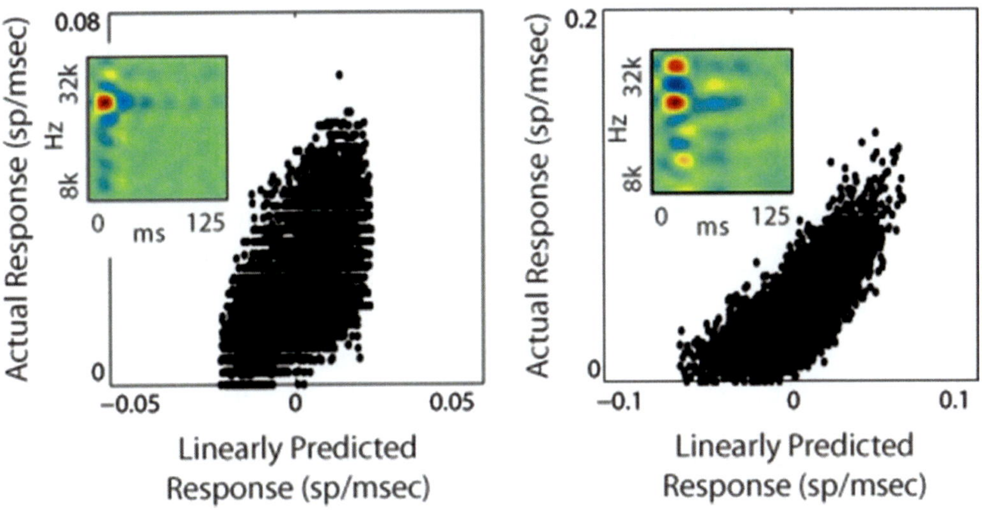

Figure 8. Inherently Variable Responses. The responses of two recorded neurons are depicted whose outputs were highly variable. Each point represents a point in time at which the actual response rate was sampled and a predicted response rate was computed. While an overall trend can still be seen, for any linearly predicted response value, there is a wide range of actual responses. For these neurons, while a static output nonlinearity will improve prediction errors, they will inevitably be high. The STRF of each neuron is inset.

Despite this improvement, the response characterization remains deterministic, in which a specific stimulus spectro-temporal envelope is predicted to evoke a unique response. However, in multiple presentations of a single stimulus, the responses of single neurons are highly variable from one trial to the next. The responses from two such neurons are displayed in Figure 8. Throughout stimulus presentation, even when the same response is predicted, the actual response takes on multiple values. A static output nonlinearity, such as is described in this paper, is ill equipped to account for these statistics. Only a formulation which takes other state variables into account and is probabilistic in nature can robustly characterize the response and its inherent variability.

Dynamic Tuning/Adaptive Tuning

The analysis in this study was conducted only after responses were allowed to reach a steady state regime. However, there is ample evidence that tuning at the level of primary auditory cortex evolves dynamically during stimulus presentation (Shechter, Dobbins et al. 2009). If the input-output properties of auditory neurons continuously evolve, the current static methods of characterization would be inadequate. The STRF method utilizes a short window of stimulus history to predict an instantaneous response, but its features (used to make that prediction) are *independent* of the stimulus and its history.

In conclusion, the majority of cells found in AI of the awake ferret responded nonlinearly with respect to the stimuli used to evoke them. This nonlinearity was nontrivial in that it had a squaring effect ($\alpha \approx 2$). Yet, despite the utility of static output nonlinearities (as measured by the improvement in predictive power), such a framework is insufficient to fully account for the measured nonlinearity in cortical responses.

Encoding of Spectro-Temporal Contrast: Phase Dependence

Introduction

The methods of the previous section allow one to demonstrate how processing of sound can be nontrivially nonlinear. However, we want to go further. For instance, the intelligibility of speech in a noisy environment is dependent on an enhancement of contrast between the spectral peaks of the speech signal and the background noise, thereby increasing the *effective* signal-to-noise (SNR) of the auditory stream (Chi, Gao et al. 1999). Formally, let us define "contrast" as a positive or negative deviation from an otherwise flat or constant auditory spectrum. We therefore define spectro-temporal contrast of a broadband sound as its squared spectro-temporal modulation envelope. Thus, equal positive and negative modulations of the spectrum away from its mean level have an equal measure of contrast, with larger deviations representing a higher degree of contrast.

Understanding the nature of non-linear processing with respect to the spectro-temporal contrast of sound is essential to understanding the robust processing of steady-state sounds, such as vowels in speech (Wang and Shamma 1994; Barbour and Wang 2002; Barbour and Wang 2003).

Smearing the spectral profiles or temporal profile of sound—thereby reducing auditory contrast—leads to deficits in discrimination of primarily vowel or consonant sounds, respectively (ter Keurs, Festen et al. 1992). However, contrast enhancement may lead to a partial recovery of deficits (Miller, Calhoun et al. 1999).

Since contrast is an important feature of sound which is essential for perception and discrimination, knowledge of how it is encoded and how it affects the encoding of other features is necessary for understanding how complex sounds are analyzed by the brain. Not only can we find a response to contrast, we can show the neural preference for contrast features can be orthogonal to those features represented by the linear STRF.

Methods

Computation of the Spectro-Temporal Contrast Receptive Field

Contrast is measured by the squared modulation amplitude of the spectro-temporal envelope. This value is high for extreme amplitudes (both positive and negative), and therefore is a measure of deviations of the stimulus from its overall level *L*. (Figure 7). We measure the neural preference to features in the stimulus contrast in much the same way that we measure the linear STRF from the responses to auditory gratings.

By reverse correlating the spike train output with the square of the spectro-temporal envelope of the stimulus immediately preceding each spike, we obtain the spectro-temporal contrast receptive field (CRF). For a spike train with spikes at times t_i, the CRF can be estimated as:

$$\overline{CRF}(x,\tau)=\frac{1}{N}\sum_{i=1}^{N}S^2(x,t_i-\tau) \tag{6}$$

where the bar above CRF implies a raw measurement (explained below).

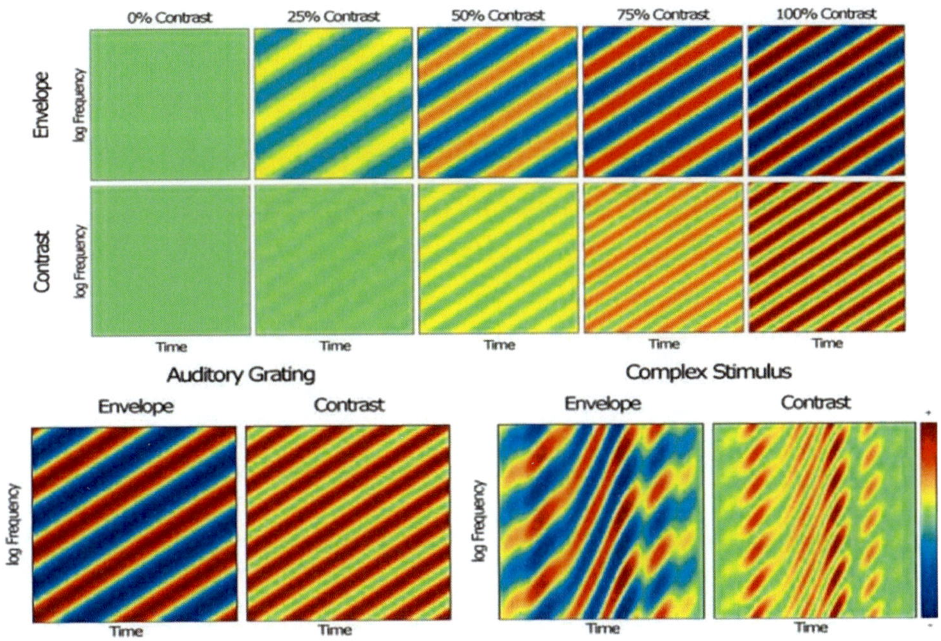

Figure 7. Spectro-Temporal Contrast: Contrast is defined as a degree of deviation from a background. We define spectro-temporal contrast as the squared spectro-temporal envelope of a sound. It is therefore a measure of (absolute) deviation, either positive or negative, from the mean level of that sound. We show in this figure spectro-temporal envelopes and their corresponding contrast. Note how the spectro-temporal contrast is high for both very positive and very negative values in the envelope.

The grating stimulus used for CRF estimation is optimal in that the set as a whole spans the range of spectral densities and temporal angular frequencies of interest. However, it is important to note also that the statistics of the stimulus are optimal for estimating the CRF given the nonlinear operation used on the spectro-temporal envelope (squaring, see previous section). With other stimuli, such as temporally orthogonal ripple combinations, the squaring operation would give rise to 'cross-terms' (because, for example, $(a+b)^2 \neq a^2+b^2$) making it difficult to account for the stimulus ensemble statistics and disambiguate between linear and quadratic responses. For example, a grating stimulus with a temporal periodicity of 4Hz will have a linear response at 4Hz and a contrast response at 8Hz. Similarly, an 8Hz stimulus will have a linear response at 8Hz and a contrast response at 16Hz. However, a composite stimulus modulated at both 4Hz and 8Hz will have a linear response at 4Hz and 8Hz, but a contrast response at 4Hz, 8Hz, 12Hz, and 16Hz. Disambiguating the linear and contrast responses is not straightforward, since they overlap in frequency content. Single auditory gratings—occupying a single point in the Fourier domain of spectral density and temporal periodicity—do not suffer from this drawback and their statistics are therefore easily accounted for.

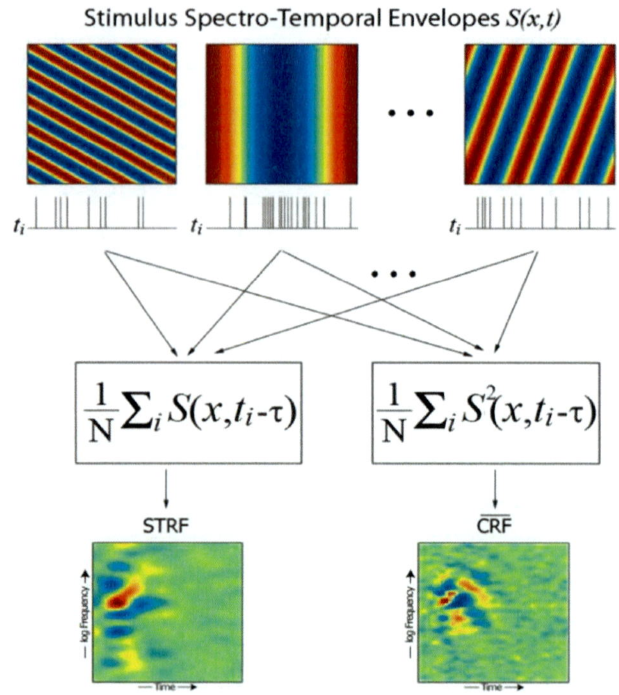

Figure 8. Computing the Raw CRF ($\overline{CRF}$): it is computed by reverse correlation similar to that used in computing the STRF. Instead of reverse correlating the neural response with stimulus spectro-temporal envelopes, we reverse correlate with the squared spectro-temporal envelopes, defined as a measure of spectro-temporal contrast. For every spike recorded, we average a time window of the stimulus spectro-temporal contrast history. In this example, spikes (represented by the tick marks under each spectro-temporal envelope) occur at times t_i . at frequency and time delay is computed by averaging the stimulus contrast value at the same frequency and at times $t_i - \tau$. The must then be disambiguated from second order contributions arising from partial wave rectification of the linear (STRF) response.

Disambiguation of the Contrast Receptive Field (CRF)

There still exists some ambiguity when measuring the CRF: we measure all quadratic sources in the response, whether from a linear response with a quadratic output nonlinearity or a response to spectro-temporal contrast. This is due to the fact that we only have access to the neural response. The latter source of squared statistics is exactly what we are trying to measure— the neural response to contrast. In addition, the linear response (predicted from the STRF) in conjunction with a squared static output nonlinearity will also contribute second order stimulus statistics to the neural response. Given that we reverse correlate with the squared stimulus envelope, both contributions are measured.

We account for this contribution by estimating the square of the contribution from the STRF. This ensures that there are no other confounding contributions to the squared statistics in the response, because the squared stimulus does not contain any cross terms. We measure, up to an overall scaling factor, the linear contribution to the squared statistics by squaring the 2-dimensional Fourier transform of the STRF, and then taking its 2-dime inverse Fourier transform:

$$L_2 = FFT^{-1}\left[FFT[STRF]^2\right] \tag{7}$$

The disambiguated CRF is obtained by subtracting from the measured CRF the projection of onto the measured CRF:

$$CRF = \overline{CRF} - L_2 \cdot \frac{\left\| L_2 \bullet \overline{CRF} \right\|}{\left\| L_2 \bullet L_2 \right\|} \tag{8}$$

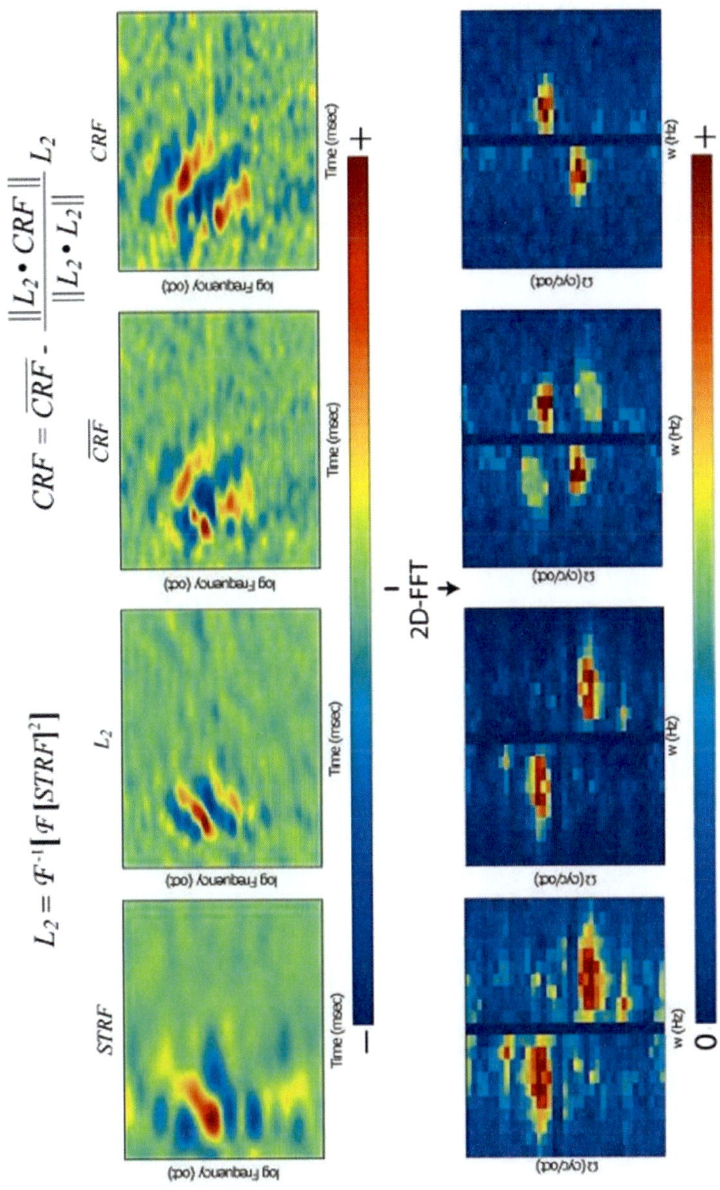

Figure 9. Disambiguation of the CRF: see next paragraph.

The is measured by reverse correlating the neural response with the stimulus spectro-temporal contrast. However, given any partial wave rectification (which has a strong second order component), any linear output will also have second order contributions to the response. This would be measured as part of the contrast response in the $\overline{CRF}$. We therefore remove any second order contributions present in the which are correlated with squared STRF output. Given that we present single auditory gratings, there are no stimulus "cross-terms" in the partially rectified linear response. We can therefore compute the squared STRF output (up to an overall scaling factor) by squaring each of its Fourier components independently. The squared STRF output is then projected onto the and subtracted out in order to obtain the CRF. In the bottom row, we plot the absolute values of the two-dimensional Fourier transforms of the measures in the top row. This is an equivalent representation of the same quantities, where each point in the Fourier domain corresponds to the response to a single auditory grating of spectral density and temporal periodicity w.

The CRF can be used to predict responses to the contrast of spectro-temporal envelopes in a similar manner as the STRF is used to predict responses to the envelopes. This is achieved by convolving in time the contrast of the spectro-temporal envelope with the CRF, and summing across all frequency bands, computed as:

$$r_{contrast}(t) = \int\int CRF(x,\tau) \cdot S^2(x,t-\tau)\, d\tau dx \, . \tag{9}$$

By comparing the actual neural response with predicted responses to the spectro-temporal envelope (by the STRF) and to its contrast (by the CRF), we can build a 2-dimensional output nonlinearity (which depends on the linear and contrast stimulus values), such that

$$r_{actual}(t) = NL_{2-D}(r_{lin}, r_{contrast}) \, . \tag{10}$$

Examples of such 2-dimensional output nonlinearities are shown in Figure 4.5.

SNR Computation

SNR is computed for the disambiguated CRF using roughly the same method as was described for the STRF above. We use the same bootstrap method to compute multiple estimates of the CRF and its Fourier space analog. The SNR at each point is taken as before to be the average power across the multiple bootstrapped estimates divided by their variance. The SNR of the CRF is then computed as the power-weighted mean of the SNR at each point.

Orthogonality, Spectro-Temporal Localization, and Direction Selectivity

We compare the features extracted by the STRF and the features extracted by the CRF by computing the point-wise correlation between the two measures. The correlation value is computed as in the one-dimensional case, where STRF and CRF are multiplied point-wise, where the product is summed across both dimensions and normalized accordingly. Correlation values of zero indicate orthogonality between STRF and CRF, whereas values near 1 or -1 indicate correlation or anticorrelation, respectively. We also determined the relative localization of features in the STRF and CRF by computing the correlation of their absolute values. Large correlation values indicate the STRF and CRF features co-localize to the same regions of spectro-temporal space, whereas smaller values indicate features of one occur when the other vanishes. Direction selectivity for spectro-temporal content arises when a neuron responds preferentially to spectro-temporal content which moves either up or down with time. Furthermore, a neuron may also respond preferentially to spectro-temporal contrast moving in a given direction—with either the same or differing directional selectivity present in the STRF and the CRF. We extracted the direction selectivity of STRF and CRF by fitting to a 2-dimensional Gabor function and computing the arctan of the ratio of preferred temporal periodicity and spectral density. The ratio of temporal periodicity and spectral density ranges from to ∞: the use of arctan maps this range onto the finite range of orientation angles from to $\pi/2$.

Examples:

In Figure 10 below, we depict the STRF and CRF characterization and their associated 2-dimenional nonlinearity for 4 different exemplar cells. We show the different response predictions in comparison to the actual response to a number of auditory grating stimuli and the improvement in predictive power (measured by correlation with the actual response) by analyzing the spectro-temporal envelope contrast. Qualitatively, the STRF and CRF localize to the same general region of spectro-temporal space, but closer inspection reveals that the two measures do not necessarily overlap. Furthermore, the STRF and CRF can have the same direction selectivity; however, this is not necessarily the case as they can be orthogonal as well.

STRF and CRF Output Nonlinearity

In order to assess the interdependence between linear and contrast responses of the cell, we need to analyze the two dimensional output nonlinearity in terms of its separability into a linear component and a contrast component. Empirically, the output nonlinearity had a typical inverted "J" shape, such that for high response values predicted by the STRF, the actual response is also high, but for low values of the STRF prediction, the actual response depends on the magnitude of the CRF prediction. We can distinguish between either a single output nonlinearity which acts on the sum of STRF and CRF output, or multiple output nonlinearities for the linear and contrast components of the response, corresponding to situations E and F in Figure 1 at the beginning of this chapter:

$$NL_{2-D}\left(r_{lin}, r_{contrast}\right) \overset{?}{=} \begin{cases} NL(r_{lin} + r_{contrast}) \\ NL_{STRF}(r_{lin}) + NL_{CRF}(r_{contrast}) \end{cases} \tag{11}$$

We first test the single output nonlinearity: we compute a relationship between actual response and predicted response when a) $r_{lin} = 0$, and b) $r_{contrast} = 0$: the specific values of and do not matter, but rather their summed value determines the neural response. The two nonlinearities constructed by setting and to 0, respectively, would therefore be equal.

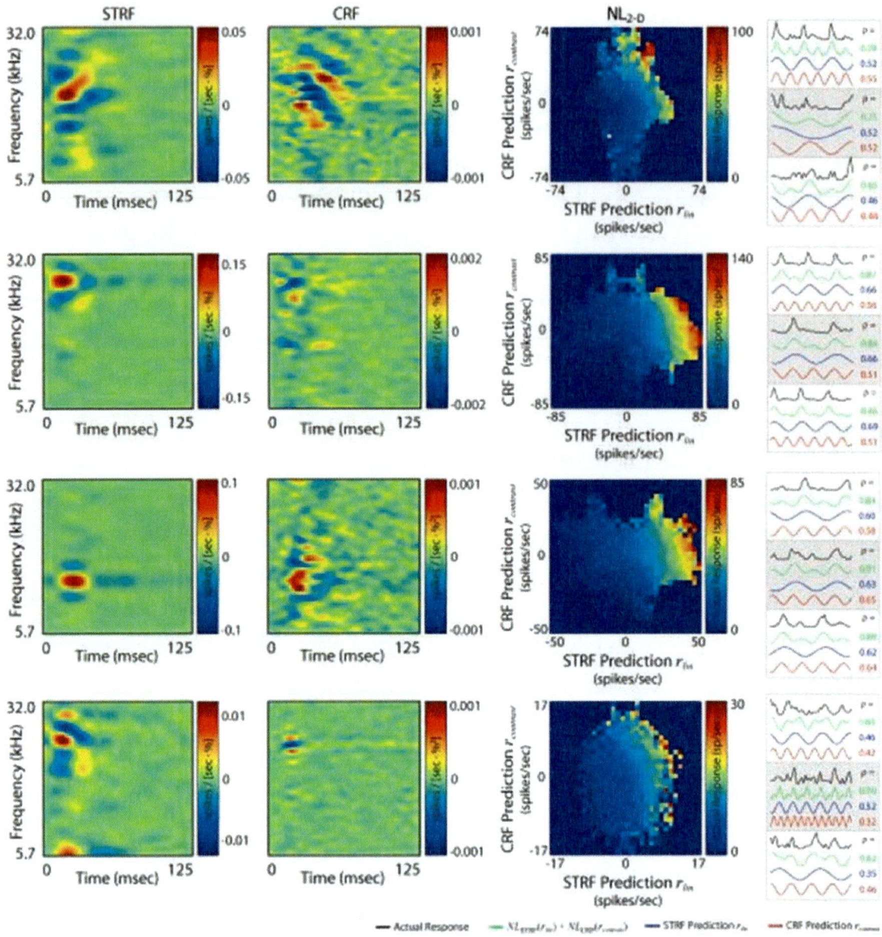

Figure 10. STRF and CRF for 4 cells (rows). For each cell, STRF (1st column), CRF (2nd column), two dimensional output nonlinearity (3rd column), and three example responses to single stimuli (4th column). The CRF measures the response to the stimulus spectro-temporal contrast. Using the STRF and CRF to predict the neural output, we compare the predicted to actual neural response (depicted in NL_{2-D}). With respect to single auditory grating stimuli, we show the actual response (black), the STRF prediction (blue), the CRF prediction (red), and the additive model (green). The correlation of actual response and prediction are shown in the corresponding colors. Note that the orientation of STRF and CRF features can be independent. Note the curved shape of the two dimensional output nonlinearity NL_{2-D}. The effect of contrast is most pronounced when the linear prediction is near zero. Values of the STRF and CRF are normalized to spike rate (spikes/sec) per percent stimulus modulation depth.

In our hands, this was never supported by the data as the two marginal output nonlinearities were not equivalent for most cells—indicating the independence of output nonlinearities for linear and contrast responses.

In order to reconstruct and from NL_{2-D}, we thus compute the partial derivatives of with respect to and and then integrated the resulting functions. This allows us to determine individual nonlinearities up to constant additive terms.

$$\frac{\partial NL_{2-D}}{\partial r_{lin}} = \frac{\partial NL_{STRF}(r_{lin})}{\partial r_{lin}} + \frac{\partial NL_{CRF}(r_{contrast})}{\partial r_{lin}} = \frac{\partial NL_{STRF}(r_{lin})}{\partial r_{lin}} + 0 = \frac{\partial NL_{STRF}(r_{lin})}{\partial r_{lin}} \tag{12}$$

and

$$\frac{\partial NL_{2-D}}{\partial r_{contrast}} = \cdots = \frac{\partial NL_{CRF}(r_{contrast})}{\partial r_{contrast}} \tag{13}$$

By computing and in this manner, we can reconstruct an estimate of which correlates well with the original 2-dimensional output nonlinearity (see (Shechter and Depireux 2012) for examples). In that paper, we then computed predicted responses as:

$$r_{pred} = NL_{STRF}(r_{lin}) + NL_{CRF}(r_{contrast}) \tag{14}$$

We measured a correlation coefficient between and for every stimulus. For a given cell, we then averaged these multiple values of for stimuli in which the variance of the response ($\sigma^2_{r_{actual}}$) exceeded 1.5 standard deviations of the distribution of all response variances. Using this method, we found an increase in predictive power of 9% (Figure 4.6B, $p < 0.001$, t-test) when using the CRF with an additive 2-dimensional output nonlinearity.

Orthogonality, Spectro-Temporal Localization, and Direction Selectivity

In order to determine if the STRF and CRF are encoding different features or co-encoding the same features, we measure a correlation of STRF and CRF. Practically, in AI we found that the two measures were generally uncorrelated with a trend towards anti-correlation (mean: $\rho = -0.02 \pm 0.1$, see (Shechter and Depireux 2012)). However, this might be cortical field-dependent.

Given the lack of correlation between STRF and CRF features, we should assess the localization of those features. While the STRF and CRF encode the same general region of spectro-temporal space, we measure the degree to which these features overlap by computing the correlation of the absolute values of the STRF and CRF.

By observation, their features generally overlapped only slightly, with CRF features localized in between excitatory and inhibitory features of the STRF (i.e., where the STRF was zero). This is reminiscent of an extra-classical receptive field described for the visual system: the CRF predicts a response where classically the STRF does not predict any induced response (Hubel and Wiesel 1965; De Valois, Thorell et al. 1985; DeAngelis, Robson et al. 1992)

In AI, we also compared the direction selectivity of STRF and CRF features. Direction selectivity arises when the neuron responds preferentially to spectro-temporal envelopes with content which moves up in time (or down) with respect to the spectral axis (Depireux, Simon et al. 2001). We fit the STRF and CRF to a 2-dimensional Gabor function

$$g(x,\tau) = e^{-\frac{(x-\mu_x)^2}{2\sigma_x^2} - \frac{(\tau-\mu_\tau)^2}{2\sigma_\tau^2}} \cdot \cos\left(2\pi\left(\Omega_g x + w_g \tau\right) + \phi_g\right) \quad (15)$$

and measured the directional preference as the arctan of the ratio of the Gabor temporal periodicity and Gabor spectral density (Daugman 1980). This was motivated by the existence of cells for which the orientation selectivity of the STRF and CRF were orthogonal (Figure 4.7C). We found no significant correlation between directional preferences of the STRF and the CRF ($\rho = -0.01$) and the two distributions were statistically indistinguishable ($p > 0.96$, t-test).

Discussion

We presented one aspect of contrast tuning as used by us in primary auditory cortex. Contrast is the deviations of the stimulus from a mean level, irrespective of sign, so we defined contrast as the squared spectro-temporal modulation envelope. We showed significant responses to the spectro-temporal contrast for about half of the cells we recorded from. This contrast receptive field was not an artifactual measurement resulting from a linear response processed by an output nonlinearity (such as partial wave rectification), since we were able to disambiguate such contributions from the STRF. This disambiguation was accomplished by computing the expected second order response which would result from a linear output (based on the STRF) compounded by a squaring output nonlinearity.

Contrast: Phase Dependent Response

As another aspect of contrast tuning, we can analyze the response to overall contrast as opposed to the local, time-varying, phase-dependent contrast tuning we have explored with the CRF. Such an overall response would not have fast temporal dynamics, but rather be represented in the baseline firing rate as a rate encoding of contrast. This phase-independent contrast tuning is analogous to complex visual neural responses, in which responses to a grating stimulus do not depend on its spatial phase (Hubel and Wiesel 1965; Movshon, Thompson et al. 1978). In the next section, we explore the phase-independent encoding of spectro-temporal contrast.

Encoding of Spectro-Temporal Contrast: Phase Independence

Introduction

One underlying assumptions in the measure of the STRF and CRF is that the mean firing rate remains constant across all stimulus conditions (Marmarelis and Marmarelis 1978). In other words, the overall rate does not depend on the spectro-temporal modulations, but rather on other parameters such as the mean level of the stimulus, the sound density, and temporal fine structure (Kowalski, Depireux et al. 1996; Elhilali, Fritz et al. 2004; Norena, Gourevitch et al. 2008). However, by analysis of the auditory environment over long timescale (with respect to modulations), the auditory system could make use of a rate code. Since it wouldn't follow the temporal dynamics of the stimulus, such a response would be independent of the specific phase of the stimulus.

This phase-independent contrast tuning is analogous to complex cell visual responses, in which the response to a grating stimulus does not depend on its spatial phase (Hubel and Wiesel 1965). Complex cells cannot be characterized by conventional reverse correlation techniques because they respond to (visual) gratings in any given spatial phase. Instead, they must be characterized by the mean changes in firing rate in response to the different spatial gratings (Movshon, Thompson et al. 1978). Similarly for the auditory system, a neuron which has a phase-independent tuning responds to the mere presence of specific features, irrespective of location along the spectral axis. Such feature extraction would be useful for generalization of a spectro-temporal structure (e..g, a formant ratio) from different sources or in varying conditions (e.g., different pitch). Alternatively, when analyzed in conjunction with the phase-locked response, a shift in baseline firing rate could be used to enhance transmission of information contained in the phase-locked component of the response.

A sometimes used measure of complex tuning is f_1/f_0 , where and respectively refer to the first harmonic and DC components of the Fourier transform of the response. This ratio measures the degree to which a neuron is phase locked to modulations relative to the degree to which the spiking rate is elevated irrespective of phase (Movshon, Thompson et al. 1978; Movshon, Thompson et al. 1978). In order to use this metric to classify cells as simple or complex, their response must be either primarily phase-locked or primarily phase-independent. However, a phase independent nonlinearity cannot be measured reliably by in neurons which have low evoked firing rates and a significant locked response to modulations. The use of strongly biases results (see Figures 5.1, 5.2), which should be taken into account when interpreting their results. Trivial output nonlinearities, namely rectification at 0 spikes/sec, interfere with the measurement of the evoked firing rate (taken as the mean number of spikes per stimulus duration) during stimulus presentation. Any rectification would induce an artificial elevation of the measured evoked rate and a decrease in the magnitude of the phase locked response (Figure 11). Despite the difficulty in measuring phase independent complexities in the response of AI neurons, it is plausible that such rate encodings of the sound environment co-exist with spike timing based schemes (Movshon, Thompson et al. 1978). We demonstrate phase-independent contrast tuning for cells in AI which also have reliable phase-locking responses.

Methods

Measuring the Phase-Independent Contrast Response

The STRF measures modulations of the response away from a mean firing rate. Under ideal conditions, the phase-independent contrast response (r_0) can be measured by computing the mean firing rate (f_0) for the duration of the stimulus.

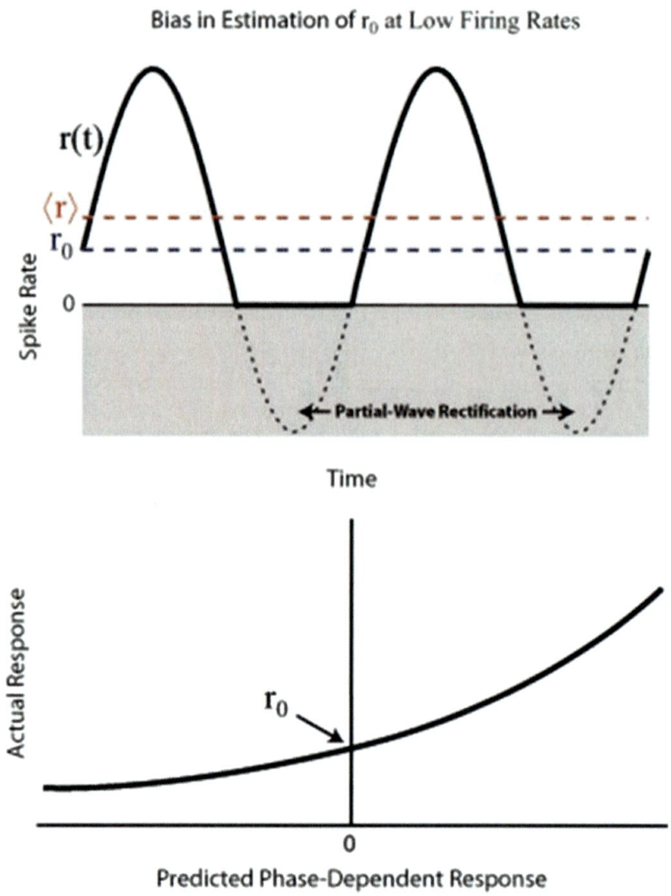

Figure 11. Measuring Phase Independent Response: Given a neural response consisting of a baseline firing rate (r_0) which is modulated sinusoidally, the baseline rate can be computed as the mean amplitude. Top. However, with partial wave rectification, the mean amplitude (red) over-estimates the true baseline firing rate (blue). Bottom. Using a linear model, we can predict modulations in the response away from its baseline rate and compare it to the actual response. We then measure a baseline rate as the neural response which occurs when the linear model predicts no modulation of the response.

However, when the response rates are relatively low (as is often the case in AI), the response is subject to partial wave rectification. This will cause an over-estimation of ($f_0 > r_0$). A more robust estimate of can be obtained by determining the firing rate of the neuron when the phase-dependent component of the response is zero (Figures11, 12): Using the STRF, we predict the response to each stimulus. We find a 3rd order polynomial fit between predicted and actual response for every spectral density and temporal periodicity. In the previous section, we used the same method to compute an overall output nonlinearity for the entire stimulus set, *as opposed* to computing an output nonlinearity for each stimulus independently as we do here. The zeroth order coefficient, where the fit intersects the ordinate, is the sustained firing rate of the neuron in response to a grating of the same spatial density and temporal periodicity (i.e., r_0): we measure distinct output nonlinearities which depend on the spectro-temporal statistics of the stimulus.

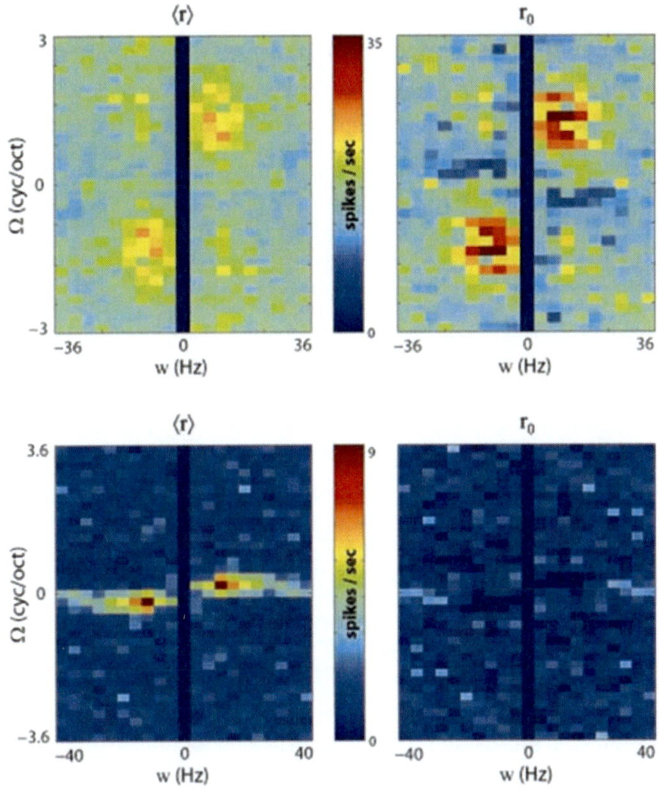

Figure 1. Estimation Errors in r_0 : Right: we measure the baseline firing rate r_0 in response to a set of gratings spanning a range of spectral densities and temporal periodicities using the method outlined in Fig.11. Left: Measuring the baseline firing rate as the mean firing rate $\langle r \rangle$ results in estimation errors in baseline firing rate. In some cases, the mean firing rate underestimates the magnitude of r_0 (top), while in others, the mean firing rate measures features which don't exist in r_0 (bottom).

Significance of r_0

We define significance of the phase independent contrast tuning based on whether is modulated by changes in spectral density and temporal periodicity. For a given cell, we measure mean and standard deviation of all values of r_0 . Of the points in which are at least 1 standard deviation away from its mean, we determine the fraction of points which are adjacent to other points that are also at least 1 standard deviation away from the mean.

$$\alpha_{r_0} = \frac{\#\ \text{adjacent significant points}}{\#\ \text{significant points}} \tag{16}$$

Values of near 1 imply significant phase independent responses, whereas values near 0 imply non-significant phase independent responses. An example is given in Figure 14, for two example cells with low and high values of α_{r_0} , resp.

Spectro-Temporal Distribution of Responses

In order to determine the relative localization of phase-independent and phase-dependent responses, we computed the correlation coefficient between a template function (T) corresponding to a high-pass, distributed response and two measures of the neural response: the absolute value of MTF (the Fourier transform of the STRF) and r_0.

$$T(\Omega, w) = \left|\frac{\Omega}{\Omega_{\max}}\right| + \left|\frac{w}{w_{\max}}\right| \tag{17}$$

The template has higher values for high spectral density and temporal periodicity. Positive correlation values between and the MTF or between and indicate stronger responses at high spatial densities and temporal periodicities. Conversely, negative correlation values indicate stronger responses at low spatial densities and temporal periodicities.

Results

Measuring the Phase-Independent Contrast Response

We measure the phase-independent contrast response by measuring the evoked firing rate during the presentation of a sinusoidal grating stimulus. The phase-independent component of the response can be measured as the mean firing rate. However, due to the partial-wave rectification of firing rates (since cells cannot fire less than 0 spikes/sec), the mean firing rate over-estimates the phase-independent tuning (Figures 5.1, 5.2). Instead, we use the STRF to predict the response for each stimulus, and fit that prediction to the actual response with a 3rd order polynomial.

We then take to be the phase-independent contrast response. In Figure 5.5, we show the individual nonlinearities for two different cells. Note that for cells without a reliable STRF, this measure of becomes equivalent to taking the mean rate during the entire stimulus presentation.

In Figure 15, we show the detailed complex response for 2 typical AI cells. The phase-independent contrast response is measured for each spectral density and temporal periodicity. We compute an output nonlinearity for *each* grating by comparing STRF predicted response to actual response.

r_0 is taken as the ordinate intersect, see Figure 11. Individual output nonlinearities are shown for 6 gratings, with the top 18 overlaid top right.

Phase independent and -dependent responses can be compared directly between and the MTF, respectively. For some cells, is inhibited for those stimuli to which the cell phase-locks (top). In other cells, is enhanced for stimuli with strong phase-locking (bottom).

Since each point in r_0 corresponds to a specific spectral density and temporal periodicity w, it follows that we should compare the r_0 tuning to the MTF tuning, since its dimensions are also in spectral density and temporal periodicity. Figure 16 shows how the STRF and its Fourier equivalent, the MTF , compare to the r_0 tuning for 4 cells.

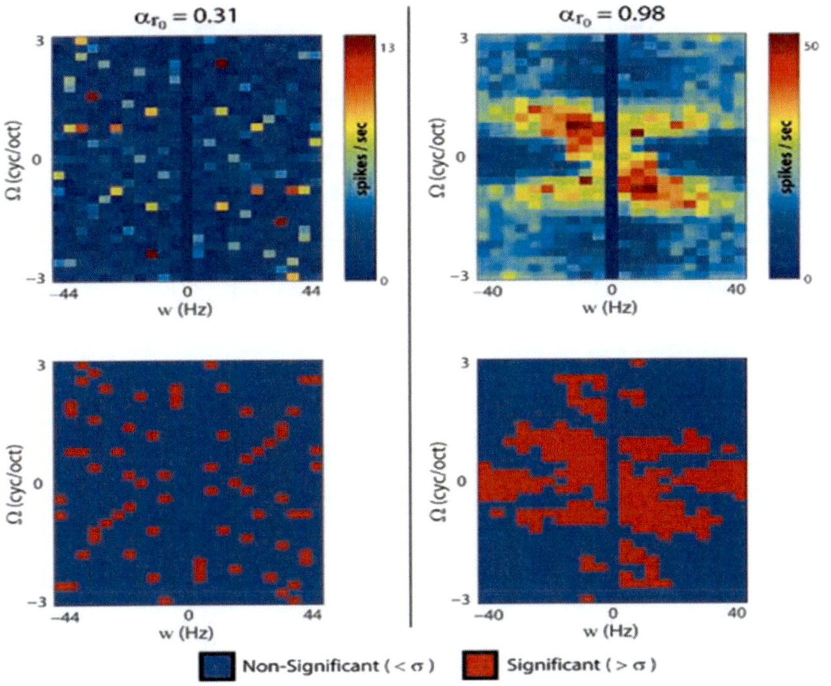

Figure 13. Measure of significance: for two cells in AI. A significant phase independent response was defined by (see text) i.e. the fraction of points adjacent to other points also at least 1 σ from the mean (in red) below each phase independent response. Left: A non-significant phase independent response will have points 1 σ from the mean response, but scattered randomly throughout stimulus space. Right: a significant phase independent response has clusters of significant points: is close to 1, and the phase independent response is deemed significant.

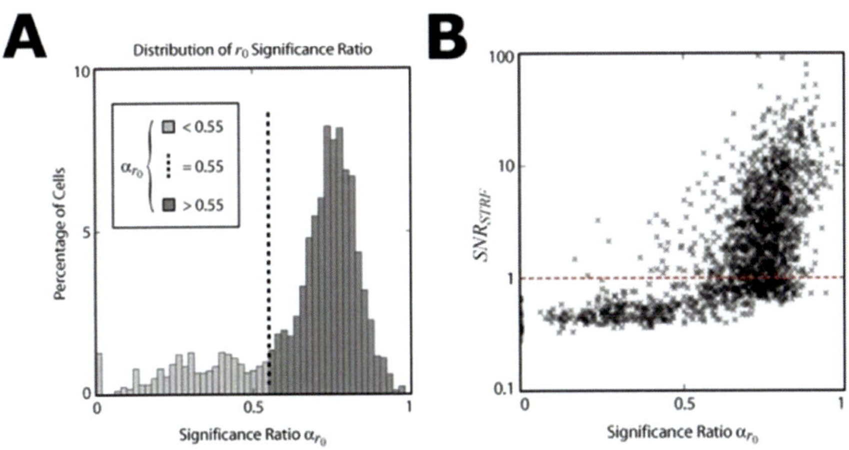

Figure 14. Significance of Phase Independent Response A. Distribution of α_{r_0} in AI. From this distribution, we determined a critical value of by visual inspection. In our hands, about 80% had significant phase independent response determined by $\alpha_{r_0} > 0.55$. B. as a function of α_{r_0}. Of the 1298 cells with significant tuning, 997 (77%) also had significant STRF determined by $SNR_{STRF} > 1$.

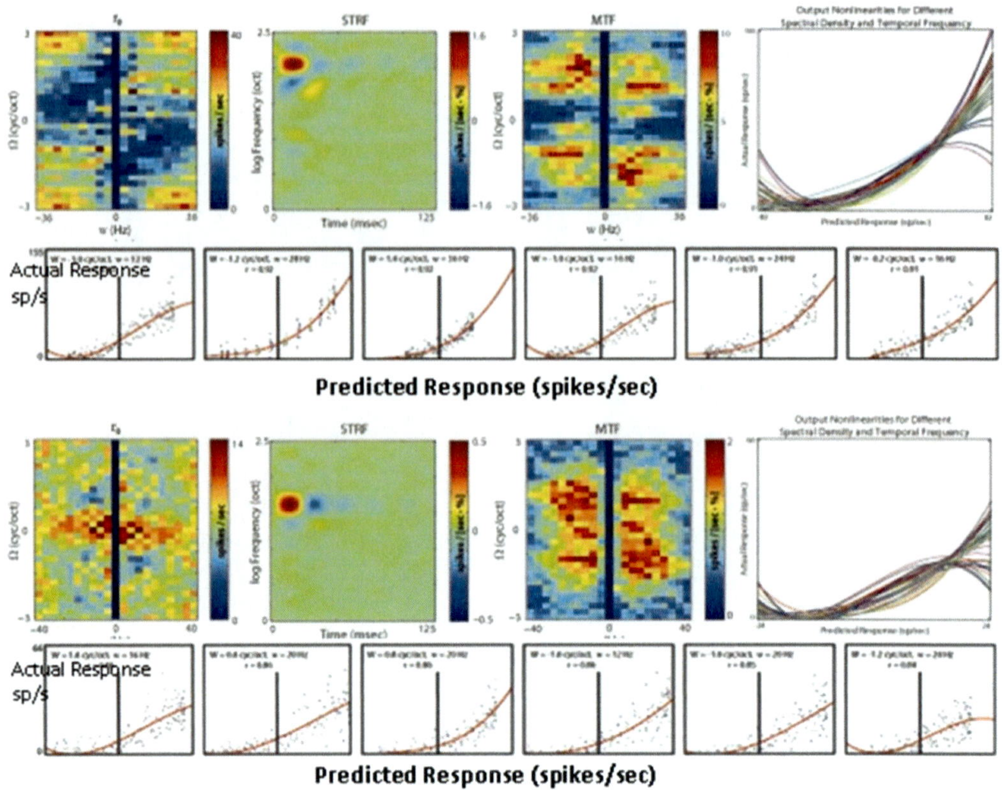

Figure 15. Individual Output Nonlinearities. See text below for details.

From empirical observation, we found STRFs in AI to generally be either low-pass or band-pass with a higher response power at low spectral densities and temporal periodicities. However, many cells demonstrate an opposite effect in r_0: These responses are generally high-pass in that they display a reduced for low spectral densities and temporal periodicities and a relatively higher overall firing rate for high spectral densities and temporal periodicities. In order to compare localization of response power in the phase-dependent (MTF) tuning and the phase-independent (r_0) tuning, we compute a correlation coefficient of both these values with a high-pass, decentralized template T, see Fig 17. Correlation values greater than 0 indicate an increases response for high spectral densities and high temporal periodicities (either as or increased phase-locking for the MTF). Conversely, correlation values less than 0 indicate an increase in the response for low spectral densities and low temporal periodicities.

Figure 17 shows the joint distribution of template correlation values for phase-dependent and phase-independent tuning and their marginals. The mean correlation value for the phase-independent tuning was and the mean correlation value for the phase-dependent tuning was -0.16 ± 0.11. These two distributions were significantly different ($p < 0.001$, t-test). These results match our initial observations that MTF power is generally centered on low spectral densities and temporal periodicities, whereas the response was generally distributed to higher spectral densities and temporal periodicities. In AI, about 75% cells showed this mismatched distribution of the response. The remaining cells showed the opposite effect where the MTF and were either both centralized or both distributed.

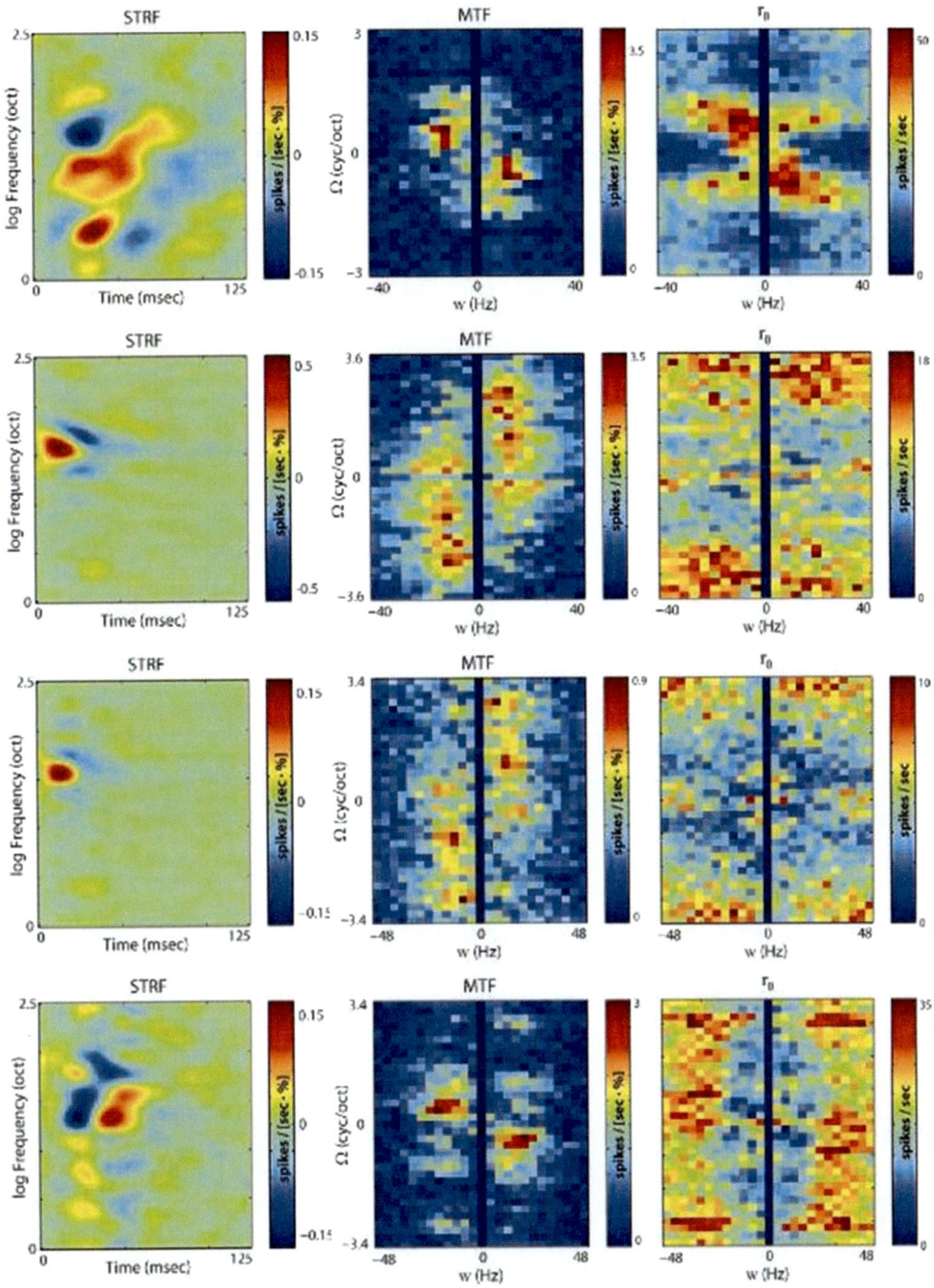

Figure 16. Example Phase Independent Tunings: characterization for 4 cells (rows). 1st column: STRF, 2nd column MTF, 3rd column r_0 . Phase independent and phase dependent responses can be compared directly between and the MTF, respectively.

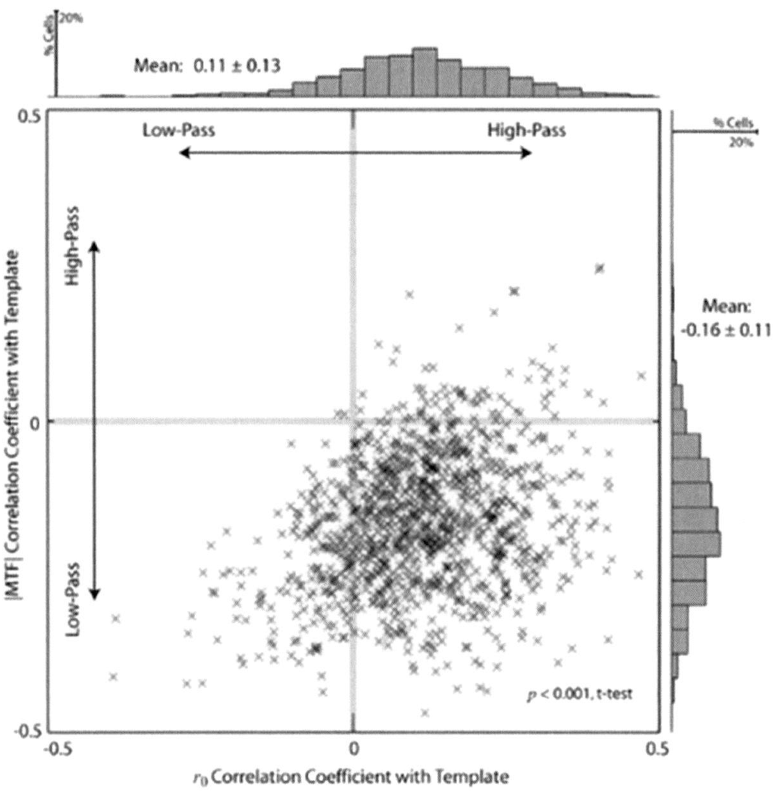

Figure 17. Relative localization of the phase dependent and -independent response: The marginal distributions of correlation coefficients are shown on their respective axes. The two distributions are significantly different. In AI, this reveals that the majority of cells (75%) respond with increased baseline firing rates for high spectral densities and temporal periodicities, and increased phase locking for low spectral densities and temporal periodicities.

Discussion

By applying a novel method for analyzing the response to spectro-temporal contrast, we uncover that AI neurons respond in a phase-independent to contrast, often simultaneously with a phase-dependent response. This response may be a reduction or an increase in the overall firing rate for regions of spectro-temporal space for which the STRF has energy.

Stationarity of the Mean Response in the STRF Model

Our stimuli are constructed as a noise carrier, modulated in spectrum and time according to spectral density and temporal periodicity. The STRF, by construction, attributes the baseline firing rate as a response to this underlying noise carrier; modulations in the firing rate away from that baseline rate are attributed to the modulations in the stimulus spectro-temporal envelope (Marmarelis and Marmarelis 1978; Kowalski, Depireux et al. 1996; Elhilali, Fritz et al. 2004). In other words, in the linear model, the baseline firing rate is assumed constant with respect to changing statistics *in the envelope*. While this is good as a first approximation, extending the STRF model as done in this and the previous section show that *is* influenced by the spectro-temporal statistics of the modulation envelope. Furthermore, even for a single measurement of r_0, taking the mean firing rate during stimulus presentation will typically overestimate the true evoked firing rate, particularly because of partial wave rectification.

The different classes of tuning for (with respect to phase-locked tuning) may effectively serve to enhance the signal-to-noise in the neural output. The reduced baseline firing rate for well phase-locked modulations might suppress uncorrelated neural activity which does not convey information about the stimulus (modulations). Alternatively, an increase in baseline firing for well phase-locked stimulus modulations may raise the set point of neural firing in order to ensure transmission of information regarding the stimulus.

Relation to f_1/f_0

A sometimes used metric for distinguishing simple and complex type responses is f_1/f_0 —a ratio of phase-locked to average response. While it has been applied in the auditory system, the results were inconclusive, with a finding of a unimodal distribution of this ratio. This is in stark contrast to the bimodal distribution found in visual cortex. That cells typically have tuning which has both phase-locked and sustained components is a strong predictor that the conventional metric will not be sufficient to classify the cells into simple and complex sub-populations. Furthermore, due to the fact that most cells have both phase-locked and sustained response components, the effects of partial wave rectification must be taken into consideration when computing r_0. With the method presented in this chapter, one can achieve a fuller characterization of the phase-independent contrast response and its relation to the linear, phase-locked response by comparison across different spectral densities and temporal periodicities both within and across response modality.

General Discussion

Neural processing in sensory systems is measured by quantifying the preference of neurons to features along specific stimulus dimensions. Linear methods are widely used in modeling the function of sensory processing, since they provide a good first approximation of stimulus-response relationships and are good predictors of neural responses to novel stimuli (Marmarelis and Marmarelis 1978; Eggermont, Johannesma et al. 1983; de Ruyter van Steveninck and Bialek 1988; Rieke, Warland et al. 1997; Jones, Depireux et al. 2004). However, cortical responses are inherently nonlinear. These nonlinearities cannot -by definition- be characterized by linear methods.

The auditory system is an ideal model system for investigating non-linear coding. The stimulus is well defined, and easily parameterized and controlled, thus the exact nature of input-output relationships can be methodically explored. In our work, and in this chapter, we showed

- Neurons in AI employ nontrivial squaring nonlinearities: We hypothesized that the encoding of complex spectro-temporal content in primary auditory cortex employs non-trivial squaring nonlinearities, ideal to extract stimulus contrast. To test this hypothesis, we compared neural responses to responses predicted from a linear characterization of the same neuron and determined the slope of a linear regression between the logarithms of predicted and actual responses.

- Contrast is encoded in AI in a phase dependent manner. We explored the representation of spectro-temporal contrast in primary auditory cortex. Contrast is a measure of deviation away from a mean or background, defined as the squared spectro-temporal modulation envelope. We hypothesized that the firing rate of neurons in AI would be significantly modulated by stimulus contrast in a phase-dependent manner. To test this hypothesis, we computed the linear and contrast receptive fields as measures of the correlation between neural responses and stimulus spectro-temporal modulations and spectro-temporal contrast, respectively. We compared these two characterizations and measured the degree to which taking stimulus contrast into account improved our ability to predict neural responses.
- Contrast is concurrently encoded through rate and temporal codes. We explored an alternate encoding scheme for contrast in primary auditory cortex. One of the underlying assumptions of the linear model is that the mean firing rate is constant with respect to changing spectro-temporal modulations. However, by using multiple timescales and encoding schemes, the auditory system could encode both short timescale modulation features and long timescale contrast statistics. Such a response would be independent of the stimulus phase, and thus independent of stimulus placement along the spectral axis. We hypothesized that AI neurons encode the overall stimulus spectro-temporal contrast by changing their baseline firing rate for different stimulus statistics. To test our hypothesis, we measured the baseline firing rate during the presentation of each stimulus taken from a set of auditory gratings with different spectro-temporal content. We accounted for any partial wave rectification in the response by measuring the firing rate at times when the linear characterization predicted no phase dependent modulation of the firing rate. We compared the phase-independent response to the phase dependent response across stimulus conditions.

Implications for Studies of Neural Systems and Future Directions

The methods presented here allowed us to address a long standing question regarding the existence of complex responses in AI. While we did not find a clear dichotomy between phase locked and phase invariant tuning, our results strongly suggest the emergence of complex cell type responses already in AI. The implications of such responses with regards to speech represent a higher level of abstraction, which allows sensory processing systems to generalize objects across different input conditions. The cooperative role between phase dependent and phase independent tuning is also an important aspect of tuning. Do these modes of information transfer act in tandem to ensure faithful transmission of information? Or rather, are they independent streams conveying different aspects of the same input?

Even by itself, the analysis of phase dependent contrast tuning can be extended in a very specific way. We noted that contrast responses are generally weak compared to the linear response. This is directly seen in the characteristic shape of the 2 dimensional nonlinearities. There is a strong modulation of the response by phase dependent contrast tuning when the linear response is predicted to be zero. To access this aspect of phase dependent contrast tuning, we can enhance the response to contrast by presenting *counter-phase modulation grating* stimuli (CPMG) (Heeger 1993). Such gratings are built by adding two identical gratings but with temporal angular frequencies of opposite sign (Figure 6.1). The result is a spectral profile which is stationary on the spectral axis, but amplitude modulated in time by positive and negative modulation values. By varying the relative phase of the two gratings, CPMGs allow us to minimize the linear response (since in most cells, there is a level of symmetry with respect to the direction of the envelope) and measure directly the contribution of contrast. This systematic change in relative phase effectively moves the CPMG spectral envelope along the tonotopic axis, probing different parts of the receptive fields of neurons for their relative response to contrast vs. linear features.

The ability to probe different parts of the receptive field by changing the relative phase of the CPMG components would allow us to study the effect of the presence of contrast in different parts of the receptive field, by manipulating density, periodicity, and relative phase. The quantity of interest is the ratio of phase locking to contrast relative to phase locking to linear features. If we present a CPMG of 4 Hz to a cell that encodes the presence of contrast, we will have a response to the 4 Hz, and the 8 Hz *contrast* periodicity, the relative magnitudes of the two responses being determined by the phase difference of the two gratings added to create the CPMG. For some optimal phase difference, the ratio of the 8Hz of the response to the 4Hz will increase, corresponding to when modulations are present in the part of the receptive field that modulates overall firing rate in response to contrast. In other words, the 8Hz /4Hz ratio will display complex spectral enhancement as a function of relative phase.

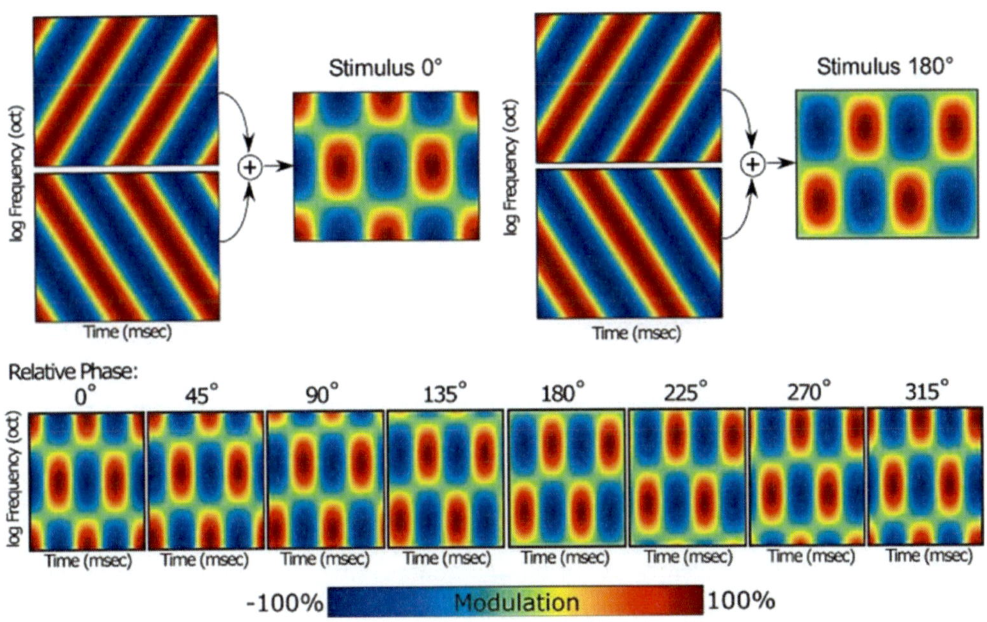

Figure 18. Construction of Counter-Phase Modulation Gratings The stimuli are created by adding two gratings of equal spectral density, but opposite temporal periodicity and varying phases. The contrast response is enhanced when the two component gratings have an optimal phase difference, such that the contrast response (the second Fourier component) is enhanced and the linear response (first Fourier component) is reduced.

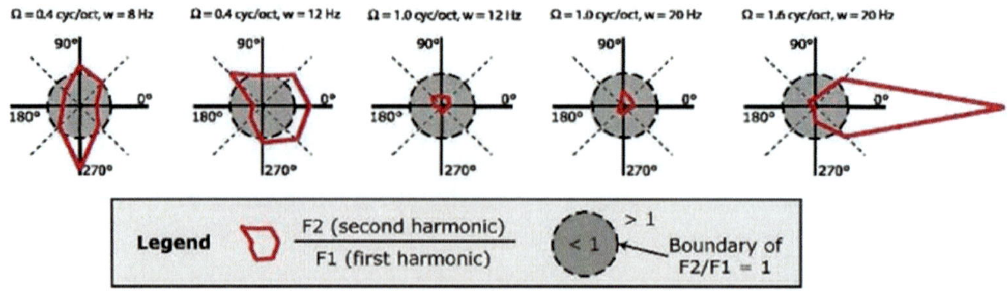

Figure 19. Response to the CPMG of Figure 18 is measured by the ratio of the second harmonic (F2) in the Fourier transform of the response relative to the first harmonic (F1). The region inside the gray circle indicates values where (small contrast response), whereas points outside this circle indicate (complex spectral enhancement). This neuron showed appreciable contrast responses for specific spectral densities and temporal periodicities, but not for others.

The result of Figure 19 is shown to underline the necessity of adapting any methodology to the experimental question. Another possibility, not shown here, is to use "band-limited stimuli for which "the modulation of the spectro-temporal envelope is non-zero only over a restricted range of frequencies (say, an octave) while the bandwidth of the stimulus remains constant (say, 6 octaves). Integral to our approach is an incorporation of both biological and computational methodology. We have found that neurons encode multiple aspects of the auditory environment concurrently using different modes of information transmission. Analysis of neural output on different timescales and with respect to different stimulus features reveals the multifaceted nature of neural coding.

Acknowledgments

Most of the work here was done with the help of Yadong "KK" Ji, who provided extensive help in animal care and data acquisition, as well as Peter Marvit and Heather Dobbins who contributed to the discussion of ideas presented here. This research was funded by NIH/NIDCD RO1 DC005937 awarded to DAD.

References

Ahmed, B., J. A. Garcia-Lazaro, et al. (2006). "Response linearity in primary auditory cortex of the ferret." *J. Physiol.* 572(Pt 3): 763-73.

Ahrens, M. B., J. F. Linden, et al. (2008). "Nonlinearities and contextual influences in auditory cortical responses modeled with multilinear spectrotemporal methods." *J. Neurosci.* 28(8): 1929-42.

Barbour, D. L. and X. Wang (2002). "Temporal coherence sensitivity in auditory cortex." *Journal of Neurophysiology*. 88(5): 2684-99.

Barbour, D. L. and X. Wang (2003). "Auditory cortical responses elicited in awake primates by random spectrum stimuli." *Journal of Neuroscience*. 23(18): 7194-206.

Calhoun, B. M. and C. E. Schreiner (1998). "Spectral envelope coding in cat primary auditory cortex: linear and non-linear effects of stimulus characteristics." *European Journal of Neuroscience* 10(3): 926-40.

Chi, T., Y. Gao, et al. (1999). "Spectro-temporal modulation transfer functions and speech intelligibility." *Journal of the Acoustical Society of America* 106(5): 2719-32.

Daugman, J. G. (1980). "Two-dimensional spectral analysis of cortical receptive field profiles." *Vision Res.* 20(10): 847-56.

de Boer, A. E. and H. R. De Jongh (1975). "On cochlear encoding: Potentialities and limitations of the reverse-correlation technique." *Acoust. Soc. Am.* 63: 115-135.

de Boer, E. (1967). "Correlation studies applied to the frequency resolution of the cochlea." *J. Auditory Res.* 7: 209-217.

de Ruyter van Steveninck, R. and W. Bialek (1988). "Real-Time Performance of a Movement-Sensitive Neuron in the Blowfly Visual System: Coding and Information Transfer in Short Spike Sequences." *Proceedings of the Royal Society of London Series B* 234(1277): 379-414.

De Valois, R. L., L. G. Thorell, et al. (1985). "Periodicity of striate-cortex-cell receptive fields." *J Opt Soc Am A* 2(7): 1115-23.

DeAngelis, G. C., J. G. Robson, et al. (1992). "Organization of suppression in receptive fields of neurons in cat visual cortex." *J. Neurophysiol.* 68(1): 144-63.

Deller JR., J. R., J. H. L. Hansen, et al. (2000). Discrete-Time Processing of Speech Signals. Hoboken, NJ.

Depireux, D. A., J. Z. Simon, et al. (2001). "Spectro-temporal response field characterization with dynamic ripples in ferret primary auditory cortex." *J. Neurophys.* 85(3): 1220-34.

Dobbins, H. D., P. Marvit, et al. (2007). "Chronically Recording with a Multi-Electrode Array Device in the Auditory Cortex of an Awake Ferret." *J. Neurosci. Meth.* 159(1).

Drullman, R., J. M. Festen, et al. (1994). "Effect of temporal envelope smearing on speech reception." *Journal of the Acoustical Society of America* 95(2): 1053-64.

Eggermont, J. J., A. M. Aertsen, et al. (1983). "Prediction of the responses of auditory neurons in the midbrain of the grass frog based on the spectro-temporal receptive field." *Hearing Research* 10(2): 191-202.

Eggermont, J. J., P. M. Johannesma, et al. (1983). "Reverse-correlation methods in auditory research." *Q Rev Biophys* 16(3): 341-414.

Elhilali, M., J. B. Fritz, et al. (2004). "Dynamics of precise spike timing in primary auditory cortex." *Journal of Neuroscience* 24(5): 1159-72.

Fishbach, A., Y. Yeshurun, et al. (2003). "Neural model for physiological responses to frequency and amplitude transitions uncovers topographical order in the auditory cortex." *J. Neurophysiol.* 90(6): 3663-78.

Fritz, J. B., M. Elhilali, et al. (2007). "Adaptive changes in cortical receptive fields induced by attention to complex sounds." *J. Neurophysiol.* 98(4): 2337-46.

Heeger, D. J. (1993). "Modeling simple-cell direction selectivity with normalized, half-squared, linear operators." *J. Neurophysiol.* 70(5): 1885-98.

Heil, P. (1997). "Auditory cortical onset responses revisited. II. Response strength." *J. Neurophysiol.* 77(5): 2642-60.

Hubel, D. H. and T. N. Wiesel (1965). "Receptive Fields and Functional Architecture in Two Nonstriate Visual Areas (18 and 19) of the Cat." *J. Neurophysiol.* 28: 229-89.

Jones, L. M., D. A. Depireux, et al. (2004). "Robust temporal coding in the trigeminal system." *Science* 304(5679): 1986-9.

Klein, D. J., D. A. Depireux, et al. (2000). "Robust spectrotemporal reverse correlation for the auditory system: optimizing stimulus design." *Journal of Computational Neuroscience.* 9(1): 85-111.

Knight, R. T., W. R. Staines, et al. (1999). "Prefrontal cortex regulates inhibition and excitation in distributed neural networks." *Acta Psychol.* (Amst) 101(2-3): 159-78.

Kowalski, N., D. A. Depireux, et al. (1996). "Analysis of dynamic spectra in ferret primary auditory cortex. I. Characteristics of single-unit responses to moving ripple spectra." *Journal of Neurophysiology.* 76(5): 3503-23.

Kowalski, N., D. A. Depireux, et al. (1996). "Analysis of dynamic spectra in ferret primary auditory cortex. II. Prediction of unit responses to arbitrary dynamic spectra." *Journal of Neurophysiology.* 76(5): 3524-34.

Lee, Y. W. and M. Schetzen (1965). "Measurement of the Wiener kernels of a nonlinear system by cross-correlation." *Int. J. Control* 2: 237-254.

Linden, J. F., R. C. Liu, et al. (2003). "Spectrotemporal structure of receptive fields in areas AI and AAF of mouse auditory cortex." *Journal of Neurophysiology* 90(4): 2660-75.

Machens, C. K., M. S. Wehr, et al. (2004). "Linearity of cortical receptive fields measured with natural sounds." *Journal of Neuroscience* 24(5): 1089-100.

Malone, B. J., B. H. Scott, et al. (2007). "Dynamic amplitude coding in the auditory cortex of awake rhesus macaques." *J. Neurophysiol.* 98(3): 1451-74.

Marmarelis, P. Z. and V. Z. Marmarelis (1978). Analysis of physiological systems: The white-noise approach. New York, Plenum Press.

Marmarelis, V. (1993). Nonlinear dynamic modeling of physiological systems, Wiley-IEEE Press.

Miller, R. L., B. M. Calhoun, et al. (1999). "Contrast enhancement improves the representation of /epsilon/-like vowels in the hearing-impaired auditory nerve." *J. Acoust Soc. Am.* 106(5): 2693-708.

Moller, A. R. (1983). "Frequency selectivity of phase-locking of complex sounds in the auditory nerve of the rat." *Hear Res* 11(3): 267-84.

Movshon, J. A., I. D. Thompson, et al. (1978). "Receptive field organization of complex cells in the cat's striate cortex." *J. Physiol.* 283: 79-99.

Movshon, J. A., I. D. Thompson, et al. (1978). "Spatial summation in the receptive fields of simple cells in the cat's striate cortex." *J. Physiol.* 283: 53-77.

Norena, A. J., B. Gourevitch, et al. (2008). "Increasing spectrotemporal sound density reveals an octave-based organization in cat primary auditory cortex." *J. Neurosci.* 28(36): 8885-96.

Ohzawa, I., G. C. DeAngelis, et al. (1990). "Stereoscopic depth discrimination in the visual cortex: neurons ideally suited as disparity detectors." *Science* 249: 1037-41.

Pollen, D. A. and S. F. Ronner (1982). "Spatial computation performed by simple and complex cells in the visual cortex of the cat." *Vision Res.* 22: 101-118.

Rieke, F., D. Warland, et al. (1997). Spikes: Exploring the Neural Code. Cambridge, MIT Press.

Rust, N. C., O. Schwartz, et al. (2005). "Spatiotemporal elements of macaque v1 receptive fields." *Neuron* 46(6): 945-56.

Sahani, M. and J. Linden (2002). How linear are auditory cortical responses? Advances in Neural Information Processing Systems, Vancouver, MIT press, MA.

Schnupp, J. W., T. D. Mrsic-Flogel, et al. (2001). "Linear processing of spatial cues in primary auditory cortex." *Nature* 414(6860): 200-4.

Schreiner, C. E. and B. M. Calhoun (1994). "Spectral envelope coding in cat primary auditory cortex:Properties of ripple transfer functions." *Aud. Neurosci.* 1: 39-61.

Sen, K., F. E. Theunissen, et al. (2001). "Feature analysis of natural sounds in the songbird auditory forebrain." *Journal of Neurophysiology* 86(3): 1445-58.

Shechter, B. and D. A. Depireux (2007). "Stability of spectro-temporal tuning over several seconds in primary auditory cortex of the awake ferret." *Neuroscience* 148(3): 806-14.

Shechter, B. and D. A. Depireux (2010). "Nonlinearity of coding in primary auditory cortex of the awake ferret." *Neuroscience* 165(2): 612-20.

Shechter, B. and D. A. Depireux (2012). "Contrast tuned responses in primary auditory cortex of the awake ferret." *Eur. J. Neurosci.* 35(4): 550-61.

Shechter, B., H. D. Dobbins, et al. (2009). "Dynamics of spectro-temporal tuning in primary auditory cortex of the awake ferret." *Hear Res.* 256(1-2): 118-30.

Tan, Q. and L. H. Carney (2003). "A phenomenological model for the responses of auditory-nerve fibers. II. Nonlinear tuning with a frequency glide." *J. Acoust Soc. Am.* 114(4 Pt 1): 2007-20.

ter Keurs, M., J. M. Festen, et al. (1992). "Effect of spectral envelope smearing on speech reception. I." *J. Acoust Soc. Am.* 91(5): 2872-80.

Theunissen, F. E., K. Sen, et al. (2000). "Spectral-temporal receptive fields of nonlinear auditory neurons obtained using natural sounds." *Journal of Neuroscience* 20(6): 2315-31.

Tramo, M. J., J. J. Bharucha, et al. (1990). "Music perception and cognition following bilateral lesions of auditory cortex." *Cognitive Neurosci.* 2: 195-212.

Tramo, M. J., G. D. Shah, et al. (2002). "Functional role of auditory cortex in frequency processing and pitch perception." *Journal of Neurophysiology* 87(1): 122-39.

Valentine, P. A. and J. J. Eggermont (2004). "Stimulus dependence of spectro-temporal receptive fields in cat primary auditory cortex." *Hear Res.* 196(1-2): 119-33.

Versnel, H., N. Kowalski, et al. (1995). "Ripple analysis in ferret primary auditory cortex: III. Topographic distribution of ripple response parameters." *Aud. Neurosci.* 1: 271-285.

Wang, K. and S. Shamma (1994). "Self normalization and noise-robustness in early auditory representations." *IEEE Transactions on Speech and audio* 2(3): 421-435.

Watson, A. B. and A. J. Ahumada, Jr. (1985). "Model of human visual-motion sensing." *Journal of the Optical Society of America A-Optics & Image Science* 2(2): 322-41.

Young, E. D. (2008). "Neural representation of spectral and temporal information in speech." *Philos Trans. R. Soc. Lond B Biol. Sci.* 363(1493): 923-45.

Zhang, X., M. G. Heinz, et al. (2001). "A phenomenological model for the responses of auditory-nerve fibers: I. Nonlinear tuning with compression and suppression." *J. Acoust Soc. Am.* 109(2): 648-70.

Zheng, Y. and M. A. Escabi (2008). "Distinct roles for onset and sustained activity in the neuronal code for temporal periodicity and acoustic envelope shape." *J. Neurosci.* 28(52): 14230-44.

In: Handbook of Modern Techniques in Auditory Cortex
Editors: Didier A. Depireux and Mounya Elhilali
ISBN: 978-1-62808-894-6

Chapter 5

Nonlinear Spectro-Temporal Modeling in the Auditory System

V. Z. Marmarelis
Department of Biomedical Engineering,
University of Southern California, Los Angeles, California, US

Introduction

Mathematical and computational modeling provides the quantitative means for understanding the function of physiological systems. Data-based models constitute efficient "summaries" of the scientific observations (data) of a given system. Hypothesis-based models represent our formal understanding of the mechanisms that subserve the function of a given system. Both data-based and hypothesis-based modeling approaches are useful (and probably necessary) in advancing our understanding of the function of a given system in a manner that is supported by experimental evidence. There are many possible mathematical and computational forms that these models may assume. They generally employ differential operators (differential equations describing the system dynamic states) and/or integral operators (convolution integrals or Volterra functionals describing the dynamic/causal relationships between "input-output" variables of interest). Of course, at the age of digital processing, these differential and integral operators assume their discretized forms.

These operators are placed either in linear or nonlinear mathematical/computational context, depending on the actual functional characteristics of the subject system. It has been found that most physiological systems exhibit nonlinearities, but many can be studied adequately with linear approximations of the actual nonlinear system dynamics. Nonlinear modeling presents still several practical and methodological challenges that are compounded by the occasional presence of multiple interacting variables, interference, noise and system nonstationarities (i.e. the change of the system functional characteristics over time). For this reason, linear time-invariant (i.e. stationary) methods have been used more extensively so far and in the context of only a few (typically two) variables. Nonetheless, the actual scientific and medical requirements in the realm of biomedical system modeling demand the gradual extension of our modeling capabilities in the direction of *nonlinear and multi-variable systems* (Marmarelis 2004).

This is especially true in the case of the auditory system which is the subject of the present book, because of its intrinsic nonlinearities and its fundamental multivariate nature, either in the form of multiple neural recordings or due to the required spectral processing of auditory signals (e.g. temporal flow of speech formants). This provides the motivation for the present chapter, which introduces a general modeling framework for the *nonlinear spectro-temporal processing* in the auditory system. The presented modeling methodology is data-based and generally applicable to arbitrary combinations of observable input-output variables in the manner selected by the investigator. This methodology seeks to extract mathematical/computational representations (models) of the *dynamic nonlinear input-output transformations* of interest with the ability to predict the system response to an arbitrary set of inputs within the power/bandwidth range of the data used for model estimation. Sophisticated efforts of spectro-temporal modeling of the auditory system have been made in the linear and nonlinear context (Atencio et al. 2008, 2009; Eggermont 1993, 2011; Elhilali et al. 2004, 2007, 2009; Lewis et al. 2000, 2002, 2003; Shamma et al. 2011; Theunissen et al. 2001) following the pioneering work of Aertsen and Johanesma on the spectro-temporal receptive field (1981). Particular mention is merited for the nonlinear analysis of the auditory system using the eigen-structure of 2nd-order kernel estimates by Lewis et al. (2002, 2003) and the spectro-temporal analysis of auditory receptive fields by Schreiner and Atencio using the concept of "maximally informative dimensions" (2012).

Modeling methodologies are broadly classified into "parametric" or "hypothesis-based", which utilize structural or compartmental models postulated on the basis of existing knowledge about the function of the subject system, and "nonparametric" or "data-based" (e.g. the Volterra approach), which seek mathematical/computational representations of the transformation of observable "input" signals into "output" signals. Since both classes of modeling approaches have their strengths and weaknesses, their synergistic use is advisable whenever this is feasible in each specific application context. With regard to nonlinear biomedical systems, the nonparametric approach appears to offer significant practical advantages when adequate data can be collected, because it does not require the a priori postulation of a model structure – a challenge that is often daunting in biomedical applications. Because the auditory system is no exception with regard to its intrinsic functional complexity, the nonparametric modeling approach is advocated for its study in this chapter. This general approach simplifies the model *specification* task and yields nonlinear dynamic models "true to the data". It also yields *robust* model estimates in the presence of ambient data noise or systemic interference and it is extendable to systems with *multiple* inputs and outputs, including spectro-temporal data relevant to the auditory system. However, this approach also requires appropriate (broadband) input-output experimental or natural data and needs proper attention to maintain model compactness. Further research is also needed to be able to ascribe meaningful physiological interpretation to the obtained model.

The proposed methodology is rooted in the general Volterra modeling approach and, specifically, utilizes a recent variant that employs the concept of *Principal Dynamic Modes* (PDMs) for the efficient computational representation of the multi-input/multi-output (spectro-temporal in this case) dynamic characteristics of the system (Marmarelis 2004). The study of the auditory system requires the frequency-domain representation of the signals and their transformations. For this reason, the presented spectro-temporal variant of the PDM-based Volterra modeling employs a filter-bank of band-pass filters to pre-process the data and study the dynamic transformations of the auditory signal content over time within each frequency band of interest, which is viewed as a distinct "input" signal (spectro-temporal modeling). This general methodology and the requisite background are summarized in the following section.

Methodology

Nonparametric modeling employs the mathematical concept of a *functional* that represents formally the input-output transformation performed by the subject *system*. For causal physical and physiological systems, a functional F defines the mapping of the past and present values of the *input* signal onto the present value of the *output* signal $y(t)$:

$$y(t) = F\left[x(t'), t' \leq t\right] \tag{1}$$

Nonparametric modeling methods seek a mathematical/computational representation of this functional F using input-output data. This formulation implies that the effects of an instantaneous change in the input upon the output spread over time. This makes suitable for the study of *dynamic* systems, although the latter are usually associated with differential equation models (parametric models). This conceptual/mathematical framework can be extended to the case of nonlinear dynamic systems, as well as systems with multiple inputs and multiple outputs. The advocated general approach of nonparametric modeling of nonlinear dynamic biomedical systems from input-output data is rooted on the Volterra functional expansion (or Volterra series) and its many elaborations or variants (Marmarelis 2004). The Volterra functional series expansion (Volterra, 1930) is applicable to all analytic functionals (extension of the Taylor series expansion) and can approximate to any desired degree of accuracy all continuous and stable functional (extension of the Weierstrass theorem). Therefore, it represents a general model form for all nonlinear dynamic system with *finite memory* – a key fact recognized by Wiener in connection with the identification of nonlinear systems (Wiener 1958). The requirement of finite memory is necessary for the convergence of the Volterra functional series expansion (i.e., for the stability of the system) and excludes chaotic systems and non-dissipative nonlinear oscillators (Marmarelis 2004).

The Volterra series expresses the output signal in terms of the input signal by means of a hierarchy of multiple convolution integrals (the Volterra functional) as:

$$y(t) = k_0 + \int_0^\infty k_1(\tau)x(t-\tau)d\tau + \int_0^\infty\int k_2(\tau_1,\tau_2)x(t-\tau_1)x(t-\tau_2)d\tau_1 d\tau_2 + \ldots + \int_0^\infty \ldots \int k_r(\tau_1,\ldots,\tau_r)x(t-\tau_1)\ldots x(t-\tau_r)d\tau_1\ldots d\tau_r + \ldots \tag{2}$$

where the *r-th* order functional convolves a *kernel* function $k_r(\tau_1, \tau_2, \ldots, \tau_r)$ with r time-shifted versions of the input signal and represents the *r-th* order nonlinearity of the subject system. The Volterra kernels (viewed as weighting functions in these convolutional integrations) define the system functional characteristics for each order of nonlinearity r and constitute the objectives of estimation from input-output data in order to obtain a nonparametric model. The significant values of the kernels of a physical system practically extend over a finite time interval μ (the system "memory"), which represents the time-spread of the causal effects of an input change upon the output signal. Thus, the Volterra kernels are causal functions and symmetric with respect to their arguments (i.e., invariant to permutations of their arguments). They characterize completely the system dynamics and allow prediction of the output for any given input, when a complete Volterra model of the subject system is available. The first-order Volterra kernel, $k_1(\tau)$, is akin to the "impulse response function" of linear system theory, although it does not determine the response to an impulsive input in the nonlinear context which incorporates the diagonal values of the high-order kernels (Marmarelis & Marmarelis 1978, Marmarelis 2004). It should be viewed simply as the linear component of the nonlinear system. Its Fourier transform provides the frequency response characteristics of the system in a linear context (akin to the "transfer function" of linear system theory). Most biomedical systems exhibit linearized behavior for very small input signals.

The second-order kernel, $k_2(\tau_1, \tau_2)$, represents the lowest order nonlinear interactions between two values of the input past as they affect the output present value. It can be viewed as the two-dimensional pattern by which the system weighs all possible pair-product combinations of input past values in order to generate the second-order component of the Volterra model output. Higher order kernels represent the patterns of nonlinear interactions among *multiple* values of the input past equal in number to the order of the kernel. Only second-order kernels are usually estimated in practice, because the estimation of higher order kernels requires large datasets and extensive computational effort, while their interpretation is difficult due to their high dimensionality. For this reason, we have developed the alternate approach of modeling higher order nonlinearities using kernel expansion on properly selected bases that facilitate estimation and interpretation (Marmarelis 2004), as elaborated below.

Since inductive, data-based modeling of physiological systems is performed using sampled data, the mathematical expression of the Volterra model in Eq. (2) must be adapted to discrete-time:

$$y(n) = k_0 + T\sum_{m} k_1(m)x(n-m) + T^2 \sum_{m_1}\sum_{m_2} k_2(m_1, m_2)x(n-m_1)x(n-m_2) + \ldots \tag{3}$$

where n represents the discrete-time index $(n = t/T)$, denotes the discrete-time lag with denoting the sampling interval (sufficiently small relative to the bandwidth of the system). The discretized kernels are sampled versions of the unknown continuous-time Volterra kernels of the system, having significant values over M (the ratio of the effective kernel memory to the sampling interval *T)*. The values of the discretized kernels can be estimated from input-output via least-squares fitting of Eq. (3) according to the matrix equation:

$$\mathbf{y} = \mathbf{Xk} + \boldsymbol{\varepsilon} \tag{4}$$

where the input matrix **X** is properly constructed to conform with the discretized Volterra model of Eq. (3) and is the error vector of the model-prediction residuals. Note that the vector **k** of unknown discretized kernel values enters linearly in Eq. (4), although the model is nonlinear in terms of the input-output relation. The size P of the unknown kernel vector determines the computational burden of this estimation problem and depends on the system memory and on the nonlinear order of the system Q as:

$$P = (M+Q)(M+Q-1)...(M+1)/Q! \tag{5}$$

i.e. it is increasing roughly as M^Q. It is evident that the parameter *M* is critical for the estimation task because it determines the number of unknowns and the size of the key matrix that must be inverted in least-squares estimation, preventing the estimation of high-order kernels with large memory *M*. There are two confounding issues in practice: (a) the rapid increase of discrete kernel values *P* as the model order Q and/or the system memory M increase ("curse of dimensionality"); (b) the difficulty of interpreting high-dimensional kernels. This has motivated the introduction of kernel expansions on properly selected bases which mitigate the problem of dimensionality by compacting the kernel representation and, at the same time, facilitating interpretation. General bases were initially used (e.g. the Laguerre basis) but, subsequently, system-customized bases were developed leading to the concept of Principal Dynamic Modes (Marmarelis 2004).

Estimation of Volterra Models Using Kernel Expansions

The kernel expansion methodology employs a properly selected basis of *L* functions $\{b_j(\tau)\}$, defined over the kernel memory [0, *M*], to expand the kernels as (Marmarelis 1991, 1993, 1997):

$$k_r(\tau_1, \cdots, \tau_r) = \sum_{j_1=1}^{L} \cdots \sum_{j_r=1}^{L} a_r(j_1, \cdots, j_r)\, b_{j_1}(\tau_1) \cdots\, b_{j_r}(\tau_r) \tag{6}$$

The basis functions can be viewed as Impulse Response Functions of a linear filter-bank receiving the input signal x(t) and generating the outputs $\{v_j(t)\}$ of this filter-bank ($j = 1,...,L$) as convolutions of the input x(t) with the respective basis function $b_j(\tau)$. The system output y(t) can be expressed in terms of the signals $\{v_j(t)\}$ as:

$$y(t) = k_0 + \sum_{r=1}^{Q} \sum_{j_1=1}^{L} ... \sum_{j_r=1}^{L} a_r(j_1,...,j_r)\, v_{j_1}(t)...v_{j_r}(t) \tag{7}$$

where are the coefficients of the r th-order kernel expansion. This expression of the modified Volterra model (MVD) is isomorphic to the block-structured model shown in Figure 1 (also known as "Wiener-Bose" model in honor of Norbert Wiener and his student Amar Bose who first introduced it in the study of nonlinear system identification). The Wiener-Bose model is equivalent to the Volterra model if and only if the kernel expansions of Eq. (6) hold precisely for all r (i.e. the selected basis $\{b_j(\tau)\}$ must be complete for the expansion of the particular kernels). In practice, it is sufficient that the selected basis provide adequate approximations of the kernels. The kernel estimation problem thus reduces to the estimation of the unknown expansion coefficients $\{a_r\}$ using the expression (7). This leads to the *modified* input-output matrix equation:

$$\mathbf{y} = \mathbf{V}\mathbf{c} + \boldsymbol{\varepsilon} \tag{8}$$

where the matrix is constructed with the outputs of the filter-bank according to Eq. (7). Note that the symmetries of the kernels must be taken into account by requiring that in Eq. (7). The number of columns in matrix for a Qth-order MDV model is:

$$P = (L+Q)!/(L!Q!) \tag{9}$$

and the number of rows is equal to the number of output samples N. For estimation efficiency, the number of required basis functions L must be much smaller than the memory of the system. Thus, our efforts are aimed at minimizing L by judicious choice of the expansion basis.

The determination of the structural parameters and of the MDV model, which determine the size of matrix $\mathbf{V}$, is of particular practical importance. For this reason, we have developed a statistical criterion for model order selection that proceeds sequentially by considering a sequence of MVD models of increasing order " r ", where is a sequential index sweeping through the double loop of increasing and values. The model order is selected when a threshold criterion on the reduction of the Normalized Mean-Square Error (NMSE) of the model prediction is not met for two successive order increases. This threshold is (Marmarelis 2004):

$$\theta_r = \lambda \Omega_r \frac{(P_{r+1} - P_r)}{(N - P_r)} \tag{10}$$

where $E[\Omega_r] = E[\boldsymbol{\varepsilon}_r' \boldsymbol{\varepsilon}_r]$, and P_r is defined by Eq. (9) for the structural parameters and that correspond to model order r. The search for the putative "minimum set" of such basis functions may commence with the use of a general complete orthonormal basis (such as the Laguerre basis proposed originally by Wiener) and may advance with the notion of a system-customized basis, such as the "Principal Dynamic Modes" that are discussed below.

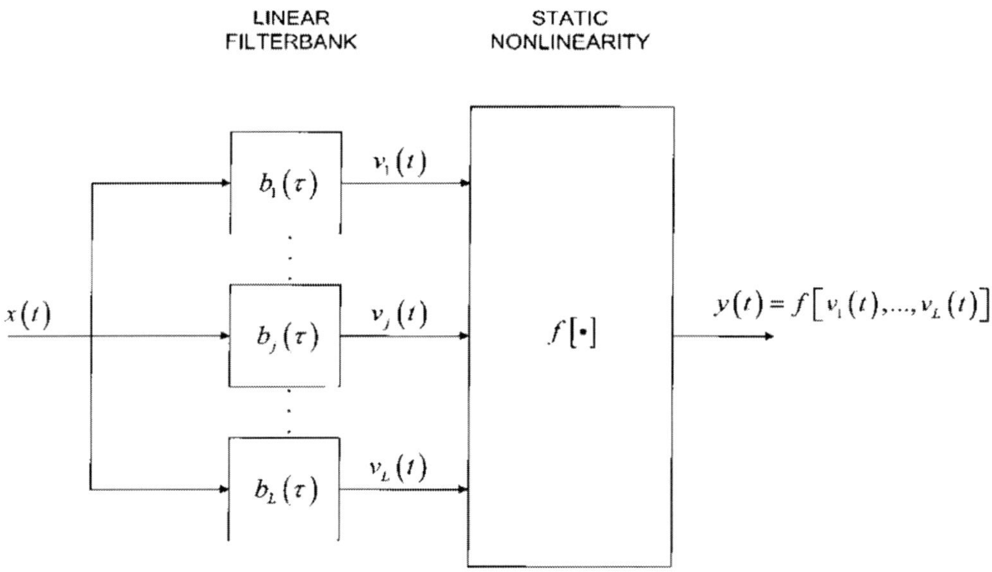

Figure 1. The Wiener-Bose model which is equivalent to the Volterra model when the Volterra kernels can be represented as expansions on the basis $\{b_j(m)\}$. This modular model is isomorphic to the modified Volterra model of Eq. (7), with the static nonlinearity f being a multinomial expansion.

Multi-Input/Multi-Output (MIMO) Formulation and Spectro-temporal Modeling

The presented single-input/single-output formulation of the nonlinear modeling problem can be extended formally to the Multi-Input/Multi-Output (MIMO) case by considering a separate set of Volterra kernels for each input and output pair-combination, as well as "cross-kernels" for the interactions between inputs as they affect each output (Marmarelis 2004). For example, the case of a 2nd-order system with two-inputs, *x(t)* and *p(t)*, and one output, *y(t)*, has the Volterra model:

$$
\begin{aligned}
y(t) = k_0 &+ \int_0^\infty k_p(\tau)\, p(t-\tau)\, d\tau + \int_0^\infty k_x(\tau)\, x(t-\tau)\, d\tau \\
&+ \iint_0^\infty k_{pp}(\tau_1,\tau_2)\, p(t-\tau_1)p(t-\tau_2)\, d\tau_1 d\tau_2 + \iint_0^\infty k_{xx}(\tau_1,\tau_2)\, x(t-\tau_1)x(t-\tau_2)\, d\tau_1 d\tau_2 \\
&+ \iint_0^\infty k_{px}(\tau_1,\tau_2)\, p(t-\tau_1)x(t-\tau_2)\, d\tau_1 d\tau_2 + \varepsilon(t)
\end{aligned}
\tag{11}
$$

where k_x and k_{xx} denote the kernels for input $x(t)$, k_p and k_{pp} denote the kernels for input $p(t)$, k_{px} denotes the cross-kernel between the two-inputs, and $\varepsilon(t)$ denotes the model-prediction residuals which includes possible measurement errors or modeling inaccuracies. The estimation of these kernels from sampled input-output data can be achieved via kernel expansion and least-squares fitting of an adjusted input-output equation, similar to Eqs. (7) and (8), that involves the convolutions of the two inputs with the respective kernel expansion bases (Marmarelis 2004).

This formulation can be extended to an arbitrary number of inputs and outputs, where each output has its own set of characteristic kernels. The kernels of this MIMO model formulation can be indexed with a pair of indices i and j that denote the corresponding causal relation between input i and output j. When the inputs and/or outputs have a specific spatial arrangement, then these indices denote spatial location and we refer to the respective kernels as "*spatio-temporal*". For instance, in the visual system, the kernels of a retina model describing the connection between many photoreceptors in the visual field and a ganglion cell or a cortical model of a "generalized receptive field" defining the dynamic nonlinear relation between the spatio-temporal visual field and a cortical neuron are spatio-temporal (Marmarelis 2004). Likewise, in the auditory system, the dynamic nonlinear relation between various frequency-bands of the stimulating acoustic signal (input index i) and the response of auditory neurons (output index j) can be described by "*spectro-temporal*" kernels, where the index i now denotes specific bands in the frequency spectrum of the acoustic stimulus and in the respective dynamics of the system. This particular formulation is of interest in the present chapter. The *MIMO spectro-temporal model* has considerable complexity but represents a rather complete description of the dynamic nonlinear transformations performed by the auditory system at any chosen level of processing (from the cochlea to the auditory cortex). Naturally, the complexity of the spectro-temporal model is commensurate with its extensive capabilities. The estimation of this general and powerful model can be achieved from input-output data that have sufficiently broadband content (such as natural sounds or broadband stimuli, but not contrived sinusoids or "clicks") following the proposed methodology.

Although the kernel expansion technique brings considerable model estimation efficiencies, it does not remove the “curse of dimensionality” associated with the multi-dimensional structure of high-order kernels. In order to mitigate this problem, we have introduced the concept of customized bases for each system, leading to the concept of *Principal Dynamic Modes* (PDM), which aims at identifying the minimum set of "basis" functions (distinct and characteristic for each system) that are capable of representing adequately the system dynamics (i.e. provide satisfactory expansions of the kernels) with minimum model complexity following the Wiener-Bose modular model form. To achieve this, we must also obtain the proper set of static nonlinear functions that transform the outputs of the filter-bank composed of the selected PDM basis in order to generate the system output in an efficient manner. This procedure is described below.

Customized Bases for Kernel Expansion and PDMs

As indicated above, the introduction of customized bases for kernel expansion is motivated by considerations of estimation efficiency and model compactness. We describe below a customized basis that we have found to provide considerable benefits in several applications to date (Marmarelis 2004, 2012). We propose a "near-optimal" basis for kernel expansion that is composed of the *Principal Dynamic Modes (PDMs)* of each given system, obtained via the following procedure. In applications to date, estimation of Volterra models has been limited to second-order by practical considerations of estimation accuracy and length of required data, as well as the difficulty of interpreting multi-dimensional high-order kernels. For the computation of the PDMs, we use the *eigen-structure of the 2nd-order kernel estimate and the 1st order kernel estimate* to compute the PDMs via Singular Value

Decomposition (SVD) of a rectangular matrix composed of the 1st order kernel (as a column vector) and the 2nd order kernel (as a block matrix) multiplied by the standard deviation of the input signal (to make the 1st and 2nd order kernels compatible in terms of input units). The significant singular vectors (typically corresponding to the singular values that are greater than 10% of the maximum singular value) are selected as the PDMs of the system. The selection threshold for the significant singular vectors may vary, depending on the signal-to-noise ratio in the data and the study requirements. Occasionally we seek the "global" PDMs of a class of systems of interest (e.g. a population of patients or control subjects) by fusing the obtained PDMs for each subject (also termed "subject PDMs") via SVD of a rectangular matrix containing all the subject PDMs from the ensemble of interest, weighted by the respective singular values.

The resulting PDMs form a filter-bank that receives input signals and generates (via convolution) the PDM output signals that are subsequently transformed by properly defined nonlinear functions to form additively the system output, as depicted schematically in Figure 2 for a two-input/one-output system with three PDMs for each input. These nonlinear functions define the static nonlinear transformation of each PDM output (which may be viewed as an "internal" or "state" variable of the system) and they are termed the "Associated Nonlinear Functions" (ANF). They are distinct for each PDM and represent the nonlinear characteristics of the system for the respective PDM dynamics. Thus, the PDM-based model is similar in modular structure to the Wiener-Bose model (as seen in Figure 2) in that it separates the dynamics (PDMs) from the nonlinearities (ANFs), but it is also distinct from the Wiener-Bose model in that it employs a (near-)minimal, system-customized set of basis functions in the filter-bank (the PDMs) and separates the multi-input static nonlinearity to PDM-associated single-input static nonlinearities (the ANFs). Since the "separability" of the system nonlinearity cannot be generally assumed or guaranteed, we include in the PDM-based model "cross-terms" involving various PDM outputs that are properly selected to capture the non-separable nonlinearities of the system in an efficient manner (see below).

This issue attains greater importance in the case of multiple inputs that give rise to many "cross-kernels" describing interactions among the various inputs. The use of the "significant cross-terms", representing the most significant interactions among the inputs as they impact the output, obviates the need for inclusion of cross-kernels with considerable practical benefits – especially when the number of model inputs is large. The validity of this practical approach for the effective representation of input interactions must be ultimately examined via the predictive capability of the resulting model. In actual applications to date with a relatively small number of inputs (<4), this approach was found to yield results comparable to the formal inclusion of cross-kernels, with improved model compactness. The selection of the significant cross-terms is based on a statistical test on the computed correlation coefficient between each cross-term (e.g. the pair product of PDM outputs) and the output signal. Each computed correlation coefficient is subsequently tested for statistical significance using the *w-statistic* (Marmarelis & Marmarelis 1978). The model output prediction is composed of the sum of all ANF outputs and cross-terms, along with an estimated constant baseline value (see Figure 2). Cubic ANFs and pair-product cross-terms have been used so far and shown to be adequate in applications to date. This, however, must be examined in each particular application as a trade-off between prediction accuracy and model compactness.

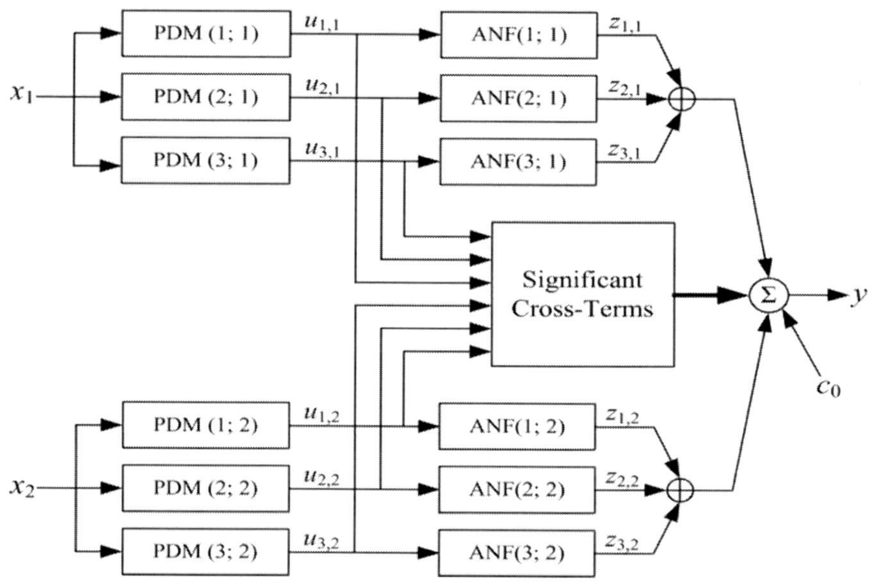

Figure 2. Schematic diagram of the PDM-based model for a two-input/one-output system with 3 PDMs for each input, x_1 and x_2. The output $u_{j,m}(n)$ of the j-th PDM, $p_{j,m}$, for the m-th input, x_m ,is the convolution of this PDM with the respective input: $u_{j,m}(n) = \text{conv}\{p_{j,m}, x_m\}$. The ANFs are usually cubic polynomials: $z_{j,m} = f_{j,m}(u_{j,m}) = a_{1,j,m}\, u_{j,m} + a_{2,j,m}\, u_{j,m}^2 + a_{3,j,m}\, u_{j,m}^3$. The selected cross-terms, $\{c_{i,j}\, u_{i,1}(n)\, u_{j,2}(n)\}$, have significant correlation with the output y, which is the sum of all ANF output components $\{z_{j,m}\}$, the selected significant cross-terms and a constant value c_0.

As an example, the output of the PDM-based model of a two-input system is expressed as:

$$y(t) = c_0 + \sum f_h[u_h(t)] + \sum f_m[w_m(t)] + \text{Cross-Terms} + \varepsilon(t) \tag{12}$$

where $\{u_h\}$ and $\{w_m\}$ are the PDM outputs corresponding to the two inputs (i.e. convolutions of each input with the respective PDMs), and $\{f_h\}$ and $\{f_m\}$ are the ANFs associated with each PDM. The ANFs may take any nonlinear form (with unknown parameters to be estimated from the data), but are typically given polynomial form (usually cubic). The "Cross-Terms" in Eq. (12) are composed of pair products of $\{u_h\}$ and $\{w_m\}$ that have significant correlation with the output, according to the w-statistic. The coefficients of the selected Cross-Terms are estimated, along with c_0 and the coefficients of the (cubic) ANFs via least-squares regression of Eq. (12).

This PDM formulation can be extended to multiple inputs and outputs with the use of corresponding sets of PDMs. It has been found extremely useful to employ "global PDMs" in these MIMO PDM-based models (instead of the PDMs of each input-output relation) that are common for all input-output relations of a given MIMO system. The intrinsic differences among the various input-output relations are captured by the respective ANFs. An example of this from an application to the pre-frontal cortex of non-human primates is presented in the following section.

Frequency-domain Representation of Volterra Models

Since frequency-domain analysis is important in the auditory system, the basic Volterra model of Eq. (2) can be represented in the frequency domain using multi-dimensional Fourier transforms of the kernels (Rugh 1981, Marmarelis 2004):

$$Y(\omega) = 2\pi k_0 \delta(\omega) + K_1(\omega)X(\omega) + \frac{1}{2\pi}\int_{-\infty}^{\infty} K_2(\omega, \omega - u)X(\omega)X(\omega - u)\,du + \ldots$$

$$\ldots + \frac{1}{(2\pi)^{r-1}}\iint\int_{-\infty}^{\infty} K_r(u_1, \ldots, u_{r-1}, \omega - u_1 \ldots - u_{r-1})X(u_1)\ldots X(u_{r-1})\ldots X(\omega - u_1 \ldots - u_{r-1})\,du_1 \ldots du_{r-1} + \ldots \quad (13)$$

Since stationary random signals do not have proper Fourier transforms, the expression of Eq. (13) is strictly mathematically valid only for deterministic inputs. Nonetheless, the use of finite data-records of sampled data in practice makes this mathematical issue moot, since Discrete or Fast Fourier Transforms of the finite data-records are used as approximations of the putative input-output stationary processes. Eq. (13) indicates that for a generalized sinusoidal input: $x(t) = Ae^{j\omega_0 t}$, the rth-order Volterra functional generates at the system output the harmonic:

$$Y_r(\omega) = 2\pi A^r K_r(\omega_0, \omega_0, \ldots, \omega_0, \omega_0)\delta(\omega - r\omega_0) \quad (14)$$

In practice, sinusoidal inputs are not complex analytic and the resulting output components include lower harmonics of the same parity (odd or even). This odd/even separation of the Volterra functionals and output harmonics can be used in practice to gain additional insight into the possible odd/even symmetries of the system nonlinearity. If we consider an input comprised of a pair of complex analytic sinusoids: $x_2(t) = Ae^{j\omega_1 t} + Be^{j\omega_2 t}$, then intermodulation terms are generated by the Volterra functionals due to nonlinear interactions. For instance, the 2nd-order functional contributes second harmonics at frequencies ($2\omega_1$) and ($2\omega_2$), as well as an intermodulation term at frequency ($\omega_1+\omega_2$), with amplitudes and phases determined by at the respective frequencies:

$$Y_2(\omega) = 2\pi A^2 K_2(\omega_1, \omega_1)\delta(\omega - 2\omega_1) + 2\pi B^2 K_2(\omega_2, \omega_2)\delta(\omega - 2\omega_2) + 4\pi AB K_2(\omega_1, \omega_2)\delta(\omega - \omega_1 - \omega_2) \quad (15)$$

This analytical example demonstrates the generality and potential of the Volterra representation in the frequency domain, which is critical for the auditory system. An illustrative example of an actual application of the proposed MIMO PDM-based modeling method in the pre-frontal cortex of non-human primates is presented below in order to demonstrate the potential of this approach in an actual application context (no such application to the auditory system is available yet).

Illustrative Example

For illustrative purposes, we present an example from an actual application of the PDM-based MIMO approach to a cognitive system: the prefrontal cortex of non-human primates during a behavioral task (DMS: Delayed-Match-to-Sample) that was recently published (Marmarelis et al. 2012). This model has 4 inputs (the activity of 4 neurons in Layer 2 of the prefrontal cortex) and 4 outputs (the activity of 4 neurons in Layer 5 of the prefrontal cortex). The structure of this PDM-based model for a single output neuron is shown in the schematic diagram of Figure 3. Four such models are combined for the full 4-input/4-output system of this study (Marmarelis et al. 2012).

The experimental methods used for data collection are described in (Hampson et al. 2012). We analyzed the collected data in two phases of the DMS task: (1) the "Match Presentation" phase between the icon presentation for matching and the NHP behavioral response, and (2) the "Sample Presentation" phase between the sample-icon presentation and the NHP ackonowledgement. We estimated the 1st and 2nd order Volterra kernels using Laguerre expansions with 5 Laguerre basis functions of the appropriate Laguerre parameter *alpha* determined through a search procedure. Since we are interested in a MIMO model that is valid during both phases of this behavioral task (Sample and Match), we obtained the "global" PDMs by "fusing" the respective PDMs for the two phases, following the procedure presented above. The obtained global PDMs are shown in Figure 4.

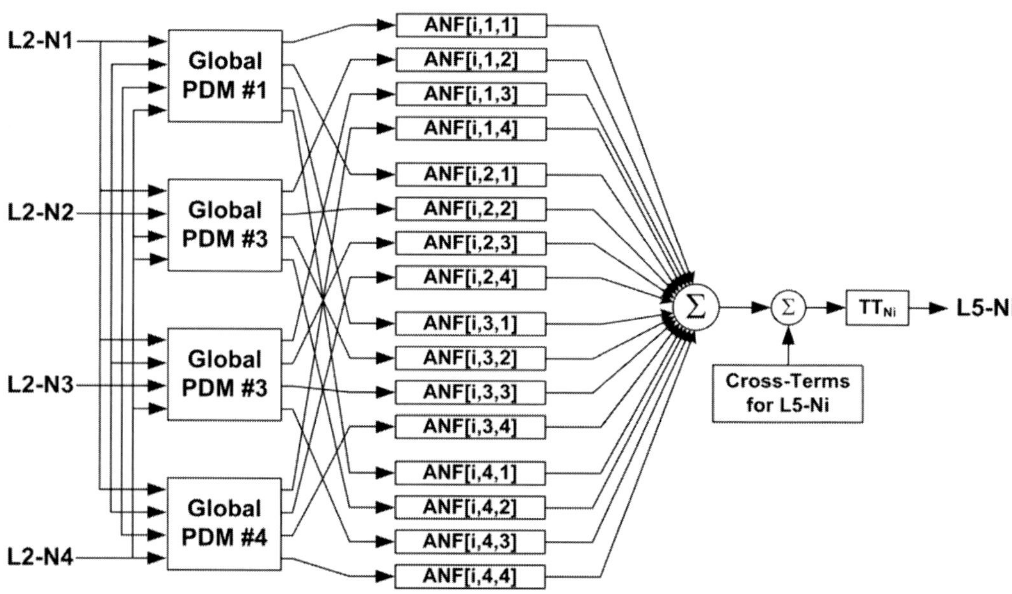

Figure 3. Schematic diagram of the PDM-based MIMO model employing 4 global PDMs with 4 PFC-L2 input neurons for a single PFC-L5 output neuron Ni (i=1,2,3,4) (N1: upper-left unit, N2: upper-right unit, N3: lower-left unit, N4: lower-right unit).). In the notation ANF[i, j, k), i=output #, j=input #, k=PDM #. The threshold-trigger (TT) operator includes an exponential refractory component (taken from Marmarelis et al. 2012).

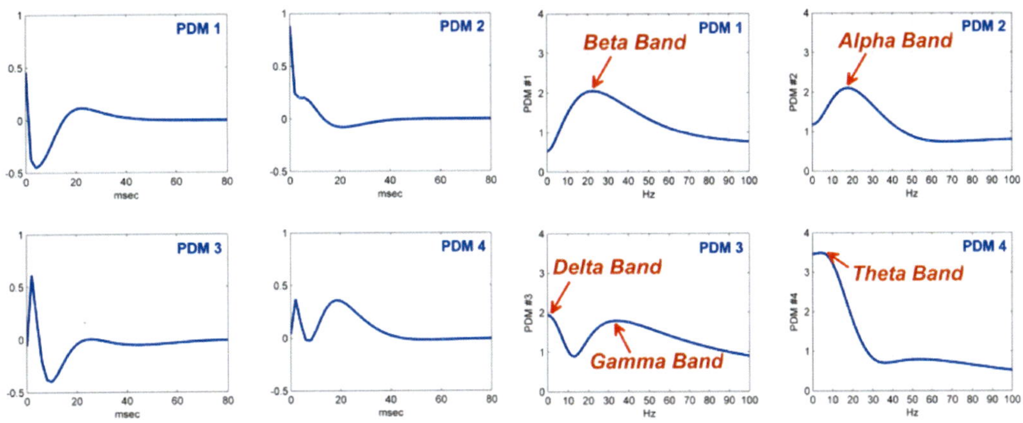

Figure 4. The four global PDMs of the MIMO model in the time domain (left) and in the frequency domain (right) that are obtained from the data of NHP1504 during the Sample Presentation and Match Presentation phases of 40 successful DMS trials of Session 0726. The annotated resonant peaks in the frequency-domain representation of these global PDMs correspond to well-known frequency-bands of neuronal ensemble activity (α, β, γ, δ, θ) that have been associated in previous EEG studies with specific cognitive functions (taken from Marmarelis et al. 2012).

The frequency-domain representations of the obtained global PDMs exhibit characteristics resonant peaks that correspond to celebrated bands of neural rhythms associated with various cognitive functions, as discussed in the following section. For instance, the 1st PDM (top left) exhibits a resonant peak ~25 Hz in the beta-band that has been associated in previous studies of the prefrontal cortex in non-human primates (using EEGs and local field potentials) with sensorimotor integration and preparation for motor action. Similar interpretation can be given to the other PDMs (see Discussion). This exemplifies the potential utility of the proposed approach.

The relative importance/contribution of these global PDMs to the output neuron activity during this specific task is quantified via the estimated ANFs which represent the amplitude nonlinearities of the system and are computed as the conditional probabilities of having a spike at the output neuron for given value of the respective PDM output. The computed ANFs for this system are shown in Figure 5. Note that the ANF abscissa is the amplitude of the respective PDM output and the ordinate is the relative contribution of the respective input-PDM "channel" to the probability of firing at the respective output neuron. The latter has arbitrary units and combines with the outputs of the other ANFs and the cross-terms to define the internal variable that generates the prediction of the output spike-train upon application of the TT operator. For each output neuron, the maximum number of ANFs is the product of inputs times PDMs (i.e. $4\times4=16$ ANFs in this case). Generally, some of these ANFs make insignificant contributions to the likelihood of firing at the output neurons, suggesting "pruning" of the ANFs using a statistical significance test. This pruning yielded the significant ANFs shown in Figure 5 with blue line, while the insignificant (pruned) ANFs are shown in green line. We observe that only 25 out of a total of 64 ANFs (39%) are found to be significant in this case, demonstrating considerable reduction of MIMO model complexity without degradation of model predictive performance. The latter point was examined and confirmed through the computation of Receiver Operating Characteristic (ROC) curves based on the actual data. The ROC curves are the most commonly used evaluation tools when true-positive predictions must be balanced against false-positive predictions (the numbers of normalized true-positive and false-positive predictions are plotted against each other for each putative threshold value of the threshold-trigger operator TT, which incorporates an exponential refractory component).

The ANFs provide quantitative guidance about which input-PDM channels are affecting the firing of each output neuron, affording a level of functional insight in terms of information processing by this neural network that has been heretofore unavailable. This important point is further discussed in the following section. We note thata the significant cross-terms were generally found to be a small proportion of all pair-product combinations (less than 10%) and seem to have only small impact on the MIMO model prediction performance -- primarily in terms of reducing the number of false-positives. For instance, the total number of significant cross-terms in this model was 26, representing only 5.4 % of the total 480 pair-products.

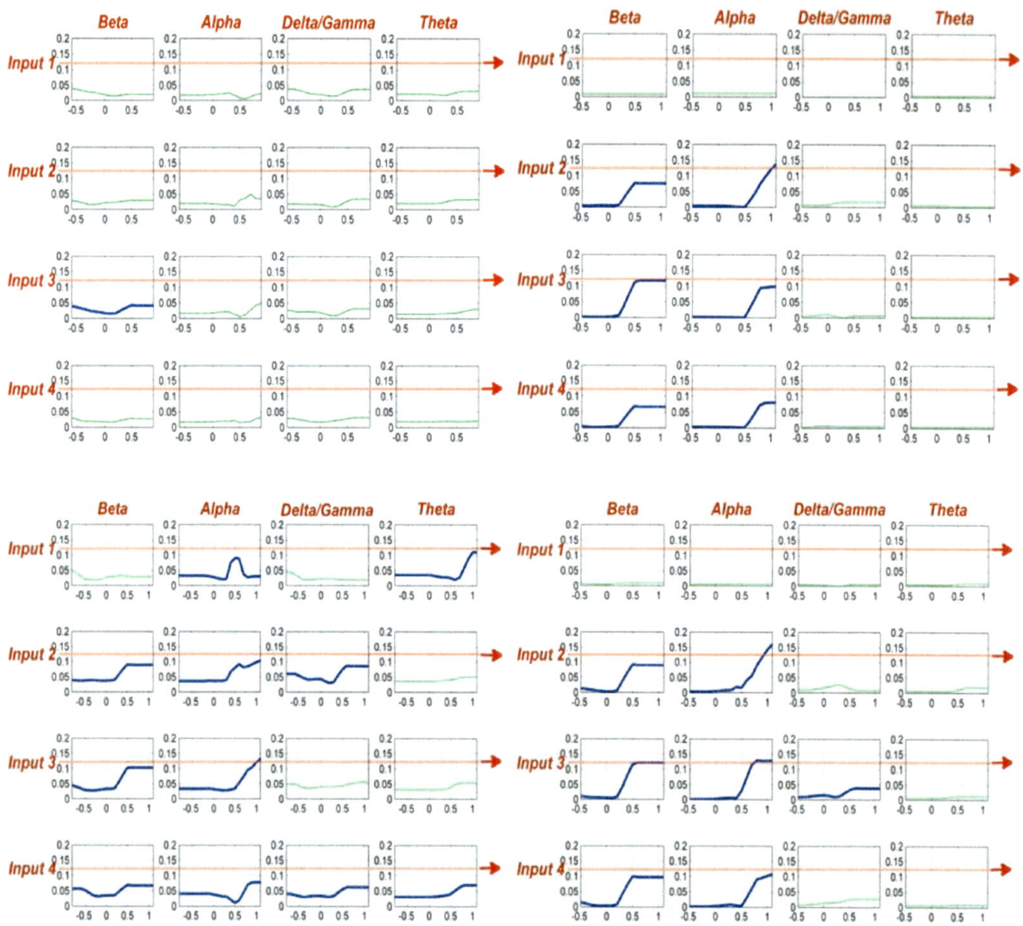

Figure 5. The 64 ANFs for the four output neurons in Layer-5 of the prefrontal cortex of NHP 1504. The ANFs for each output are plotted as 4×4 sets of panels where the 4 inputs correspond to 4 rows and the 4 PDMs to 4 columns. The significant ANFs are plotted in blue and the ones that make insignificant contributions to output firing (47 out of 64) are pruned and shown in green (taken from Marmarelis et al. 2012).

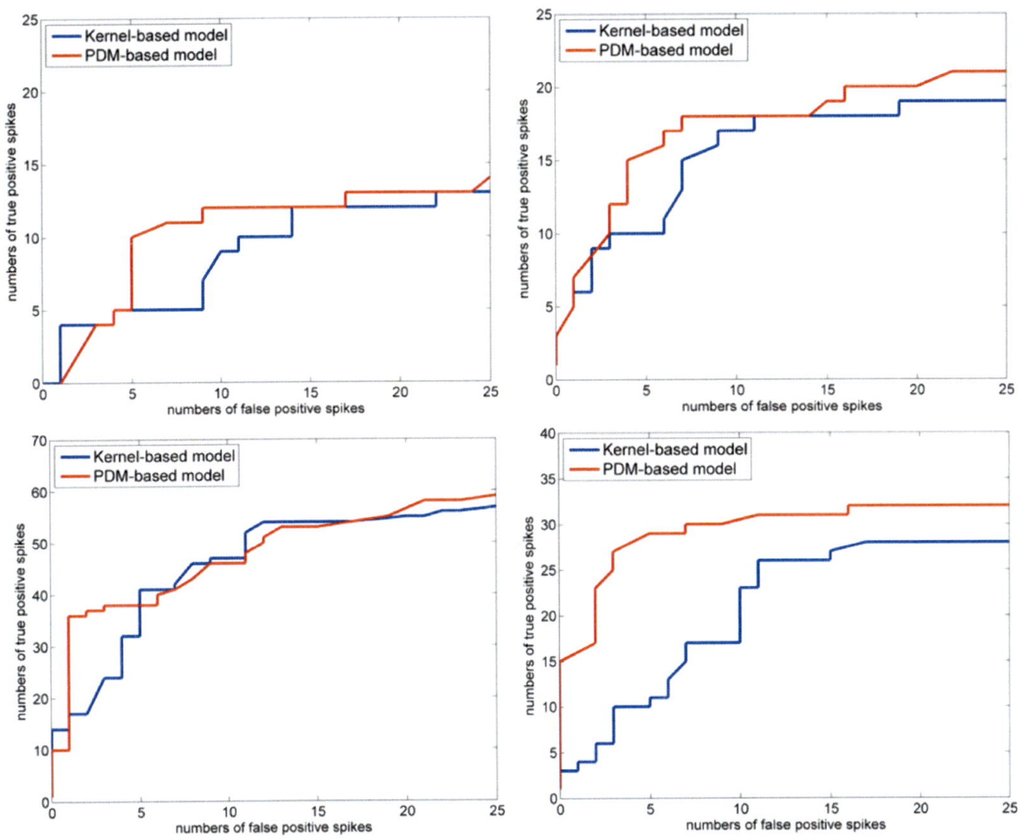

Figure 6. The ROC curves obtained for the PDM-based MIMO model with the pruned ANFs of Figure 5 (red line) and for the kernel-based MIMO model (blue line) for each of the four output neurons. Overall, the two types of MIMO models exhibit comparable performance (with a slight advantage for the PDM model), although the complexity of the PDM-based model is significantly reduced. The axes show the numbers of the true-positives (ordinate) and false-positives (abscissa).

The predictive performance of this PDM-based MIMO model was evaluated through the computation of ROC curves which are shown in Figure 6. We believe that the ROC curve should be viewed as a metric of model performance only for low probability of false-positive predictions (e.g. < 0.003 for mean firing rates up to 15 spikes per second in this study). The ROC curves of the full kernel-based MIMO model are also shown in Figure 6 (blue lines) and are comparable in performance, with a slight advantage exhibited by the PDM-based model (red lines). Note that the kernel-based MIMO model has many more free parameters (greater model complexity). This supports the proposition that the PDM modeling approach may indeed offer a more parsimonious alternative for practical MIMO modeling of neuronal ensembles.

Discussion

This chapter presents a variant of a general nonlinear modeling methodology that utilizes the novel concept of Principal Dynamic Modes (PDMs) (Marmarelis 2004) to obtain efficient dynamic nonlinear models of the input-output relation between multi-dimensional sets of signals, including complex interactions between neuronal ensembles. The proposed methodology is deemed suitable for advanced spectro-temporal modeling of the auditory system which is the focus of this book.

The main strengths of the proposed approach are its general applicability and its ability to provide unique insights and reveal rich information about the complex functional characteristics of the system under study. This may be of particular importance for the advanced study of the auditory system, as well as other sensory systems (e.g. visual, somatosensory, sensorimotor etc.) or brain regions (e.g. the hippocampus, the prefrontal cortex etc.). An illustrative example of the actual application of the proposed PDM-based modeling approach to the prefrontal cortex of non-human primates is presented as an initial demonstration of the potential capabilities of this approach (see specific discussion points below).

The main weaknesses of the proposed approach are the fundamental requirement of appropriate data (broadband and of adequate quantity) on the variables of interest and the considerable effort required for the proper methodological implementation of this sophisticated approach and the interpretation of the resulting models. It is the labored view of the author that these "apparent weaknesses" are *sine qua non* for the advanced analysis of complex systems. It is fundamentally unreasonable to expect that complex systems can be effectively studied and understood without adequate data or sophisticated analysis.

The adequacy of the required data need be emphasized. In addition to sufficient quality and quantity of measurements/data on all variables of interest, an effective input ensemble ought to include broadband natural data under the operating conditions that are relevant to the objectives of the study. This sounds obvious, and yet it is rather common that experimental investigations constrain significantly the operation of the system under study (for practical convenience or ostensible "clarity of observation") but draw conclusions from the analysis of these constrained data that extend beyond the imposed experimental conditions.

Some of the key benefits of the proposed approach that were illustrated in the presented example are the following (Marmarelis et al. 2012):

(1) The obtained global PDMs revealed unique information about the functional characteristics of the prefrontal cortex. Specifically, the 1st PDM (top left of Figure 4) exhibits a resonant peak ~25 Hz in the beta-band that has been associated in previous EEG studies of the prefrontal cortex in non-human primates with sensorimotor integration and preparation for motor action. The 2nd PDM (top right of Figure 4) exhibits a resonant peak ~15 Hz in the high end of the alpha-band (10-15 Hz) associated in previous EEG studies with internalized attention and memory load, as well as processing of internal mental content. The 3rd PDM (bottom left of Figure 4) exhibits a resonant peak ~35 Hz in the low end of the gamma-band associated in previous EEG studies with sensory and working memory tasks. The 3rd PDM also has high values in the delta-band (<4 Hz) that has been associated in previous studies with short-term plasticity, anticipation of reaction, hormonal secretion, general neuropsycological performance and deep sleep. The 4th PDM (bottom right of Figure 4) exhibits a theta-band resonant peak ~7 Hz that has been associated in previous studies with memory tasks, such as memory formation, delineation of memory-encoding from memory-retrieval, and cortical synchronization. It is not possible to

acquire this type of detailed information with existing methods – note, in this regard, that the PDMs reveal characteristics of the functional *connections* between Layer 2 and Layer 5 of the prefrontal cortex and they do not refer simply to *spectral characteristics* of the EEG signals (or field potentials). This is a fundamental distinction that must be emphasized *between the system and the signals* which is often blurred.

(2) The obtained ANFs provide unique quantitative information about which input-PDM channels are affecting the firing of each output neuron and to what degree, affording a level of functional insight in terms of information processing by this neural network that has been heretofore unavailable. For example, we see in Figure 5 that one output neuron (top left) is inactive during this task, but the other three output neurons are active in the alpha and beta bands. Furthermore, the third neuron in the output Layer 5 (bottom left) is also active in the theta band (in connection with the 1st and 4th neurons in the input Layer 2) and in the gamma/delta bands (in connection with the 2nd and 4th neurons in the input Layer 2). This type of information, if confirmed and validated with extensive future studies, is rather unique and offers novel insights into the function of the prefrontal cortex.

It is posited that this type of analysis can be performed in the auditory system as well, where the various inputs can be distinct neurons or ensembles or acoustic stimuli at various frequency bands of interest (spectro-temporal modeling). The information in specific frequency bands of auditory interest is defined via pre-processing of the data through a band-pass filter-bank. The PDMs and ANFs of the resulting model will then describe the detailed dynamic interactions among the observed "inputs" of interest with reference to the "outputs" of interest. For instance, possible resonant peaks of the obtained PDMs will reveal the presence of possible amplitude modulation of the respective input-output causal connection. It is hoped that this chapter will help inseminate such future efforts for the advanced study of the auditory system.

Acknowledgment

This work was supported in part by the Biomedical Simulations Resource at the University of Southern California under NIH/NIBIB grant P41-EB001978.

References

Aertsen A. M. amd P. I. Johannesma (1981). The spectro-temporal receptive field: a functional characteristic of auditory neurons. *Biological Cybernetics* 69:407-414.

Atencio C. A, T. O. Sharpee and C. E. Schreiner (2008). Cooperative nonlinearities in auditory cortical neurons. *Neuron* 58:956-966.

Atencio C. A., T. O. Sharpee and C. E. Schreiner (2009). Hierarchical computation in the canonical auditory cortical circuit. *Proc. Nat. Acad. Sci. U.S.A* 106:21894-21899.

Atencio C. A, T. O. Sharpee and C. E. Schreiner (2012). Receptive field dimensionality increases from the auditory midbrain to cortex. *J. Neurophysiol.* 107: 2594–2603.

Eggermont J. J. (1993). Wiener and Volterra analyses applied to the auditory system. *Hearing Research* 66:177-201.

Eggermont J. J. and X. Wang (2011). Temporal Coding in Auditory Cortex. In: *The Auditory Cortex*, pp. 309-328.

Elhilali M., Fritz J. B., Klein D. J., Simon J. Z., Shamma S. A. (2004). Dynamics of precise spike timing in primary auditory cortex. *Journal of Neuroscience* 24:1159-1172.

Elhilali M., Fritz J. B., Chi T., Shamma S. A. (2007). Auditory Cortical Receptive Fields: stable entities with plastic abilities. *Journal of Neuroscience* 27:10372-82.

Elhilali M., Ma L, Micheyl C, Oxenham A and Shamma SA (2009). Temporal coherence in the organization and representation of auditory scenes. *Neuron* 61:317–329.

Hampson R. E., Gerhardt G. A., Marmarelis V. Z., Song D., Opris I., Santos L., Berger T. W. and Deadwyler S. A. (2012). Facilitation and restoration of cognitive function in primate prefrontal cortex by a neuroprosthesis that utilizes minicolumn-specific neural firing. *J. Neural Eng.* 9 056012.

Lewis E. R., K. R. Henry and W. M. Yamada (2000). Essential roles of noise in neural coding. *Biosystems* 58:109-115.

Lewis E.R., K.R. Henry and W.M. Yamada (2002). Tuning and timing in the gerbil ear: Wiener kernel analysis. *Hearing Research* 174:206-221.

Lewis E. R. and P. van Dijk (2003). New variations on the derivation of spectrotemporal receptive fields for primary auditory nerve fibers. *Hearing Research* 186:30-46.

Marmarelis PZ & Marmarelis VZ (1978). *Analysis of Physiological Systems: The White-Noise Approach*. Plenum, New York. *Russian translation*: Mir Press, Moscow, 1981. *Chinese Translation*: Academy of Sciences Press, Beijing, 1990.

Marmarelis VZ (1991). Signal transformation and coding in neural systems. *IEEE Transactions on Biomedical Engineering* 36:15-24, 1989.

Marmarelis VZ (1993). Identification of nonlinear biological systems using Laguerre expansions of kernels. *Annals of Biomedical Engineering* 21:573-589, 1993.

Marmarelis VZ (1997). Modeling methodology for nonlinear physiological systems. *Annals of Biomedical Eng*ineering 25:239-251, 1997.

Marmarelis VZ (2004). *Nonlinear Dynamic Modeling of Physiological Systems*. Wiley Interscience & IEEE Press, New Jersey, 2004.

Marmarelis V. Z., D. C. Shin, D. Song, R. E. Hampson, S. A. Deadwyler and T. W. Berger (2012). Nonlinear modeling of dynamic interactions within neuronal ensembles using Principal Dynamic Modes. *Journal of Computational Neuroscience* (*in press*).

Rugh W. J. (1981). Nonlinear System Theory: The Volterra-Wiener Approach. Johns Hopkins University Press, Baltimore, Maryland.

Shamma SA, Elhilali M, Micheyl C (2011). Temporal coherence and attention in auditory scene analysis. *Trends in Neurosciences* 34:114-123.

Theunissen FE, David SV, Singh NC, Hsu A, Vinje WE and Gallant JL (2001). Estimating spatio-temporal receptive fields of auditory and visual neurons from their responses to natural stimuli. *Neural Networks & Comp. Neural Syst.* 12:289-316.

In: Handbook of Modern Techniques in Auditory Cortex ISBN: 978-1-62808-894-6
Editors: Didier A. Depireux and Mounya Elhilali

Chapter 6

Spectro-Temporal Receptive Fields and High-Order Stimulus-Response Functions: Methods, Validation and Physiological Mechanisms

Stephen V. David[1], Michael Oliver[2], Jack L. Gallant[2] and Frédéric E. Theunissen[2]
[1]Oregon Hearing Research Center,
Oregon Health and Science University, Oregon, US
[2]Helen Wills Neuroscience Institute,
University of California, Berkeley, California,US

Introduction

The estimation of stimulus-response functions (SR-functions) continues to play a central role in neurophysiological research in all sensory systems. The description of these SR-functions can be traced back the classical concept of the receptive field (RF) of a visual neuron (Hartline 1940): the region of stimulus space that elicits a response. Because sensory stimuli vary in time and neural systems have memory, receptive fields must also include a temporal component. When these dynamical relationships are described by a linear filter operating on a multi-dimensional stimulus, they are referred to as spatio-temporal RFs in vision (Hida and Naka 1983), spectro-temporal RFs in audition (Aertsen and Johannesma 1981), or simply STRFs. Since the initial implementations using linear filters, researchers have used the term STRF more generally to describe a dynamical model that operates on any transformation of the stimulus. The STRF can include nonlinear transformations of the stimulus providing filter input, static nonlinearities applied to filter output, and filters that are themselves nonlinear, such as the second order Volterra filter or its variant, the spike-triggered covariance (Brenner, Bialek et al. 2000; Nemenman, Bialek et al. 2004). In this chapter we review analytical tools for estimating STRFs defined in this broad sense and how this approach has been used to study auditory representations in the brain.

Section I of this chapter reviews analytical methods used for STRF estimation (see also the chapter by Atencio and Schreiner in this volume), with an emphasis on numerical approaches that can be used for high dimensional representations. Section II reviews three general approaches to testing hypotheses about auditory coding based on these analytical methods: comparing two alternative STRF models estimated from the same dataset, varying the statistical properties of stimuli used for STRF estimation, and controlling the behavioral state of awake animals during stimulus presentation. Finally, section III reviews recent studies that have used these approaches to test specific hypotheses about the functional properties of neural networks involved in auditory processing.

I. STRF Estimation

This section reviews methods that have been developed to estimate the STRF, defined in the broad sense of SR-functions. Ultimately, this problem is equivalent to the complete specification of joint stimulus-response probability distribution, $p(\vec{S}, R)$, for a stimulus, S, and response, R. The stimulus influencing the response at any moment can have a large number of dimensions in both space and time, the latter reflecting the stimulus history that influences neural representations. In practice, experimental data are usually insufficient to estimate all the moments of this very high-dimensional joint probability distribution. Some simplifying assumptions are required to reduce the distribution to lower dimensionality and make the problem tractable.

Classically, the problem of estimating has been simplified by considering only the low-order moments of the probability distribution, using a Volterra series expansion. The linear, first-order Volterra model captures the first moment of $p(\vec{S}, R)$, that is, the correlation between stimulus and response. The second order Volterra model captures the second moment, and so forth. Although theoretically well-motivated, expansion into higher-order moments is not guaranteed to converge rapidly and can often require unrealistically large data sets for model estimation. Thus more recent attempts to model nonlinear SR functions have sought to project the stimulus and/or response into a new subspace where the first moment captures more of the stimulus-response distribution. In the auditory system, these projections have typically included representing the stimulus with its spectrogram or cochleogram. In this framework, the SR-function can be thought of as a NLN cascade model: a representation of the stimulus using a general nonlinear (N) basis set, a linear projection into a subspace (L), and a nonlinear SR- function (N) from that stimulus subspace to the space of neural response.

This first section of the chapter is organized around approaches used to estimate SR-functions using this framework. We begin with methods used to estimate the linear filter: the projection of the stimulus space into a single dimension. These methods include both analytical and numerical solutions to the regularized linear regression problem. We show how the numerical solution can be particularly useful when the stimulus is first represented using a high dimensional over-complete basis set. We then describe methods that have been used to fit the output nonlinearity, i.e. the nonlinear relationship between the output of the linear filter and the neural response. Finally, we review higher-order models where the stimulus is projected into subspaces with dimensions greater than one. These methods include spike-triggered covariance, where the subspace is determined by the second order moment of $p(\vec{S},R)$, and more general approaches that use information theoretic measures (Sharpee, Rust et al. 2004; Fitzgerald, Sincich et al. 2011).

I.1. The Linear Filter and Ridge Regression Algorithm

The simplest formulation of the function that describes the transformation between a stimulus and a neural response is the linear filter (Kay 1993). This basic linear filtering algorithm has played a significant role in the study of auditory coding and is the foundation of the more complex STRF models that will be described in the following sections.

In the continuous formulation, the predicted response, $\hat{r}(t)$, is the convolution of the stimulus with a linear filter that extends back in time to include the memory of the neural system and spans spatial dimensions that make up its receptive field. In most cases in the auditory system, spatial dimensions correspond to frequency-tuned cochlear channels, and this spatial dimension can be described by the center frequency of each frequency band, *f*. However, in order to allow for alternative stimulus representations, as in examples that follow, we will refer to this dimension more generally as the stimulus space, *x*. The linear filter is then written as:

$$\hat{r}(t) = F_{lin}\{s(t,x)\} = r_o + \iint h(t-\tau,x)s(\tau,x)\,d\tau\,dx$$

In practice, both time and space are discretized, and for notational simplicity the filter can be collapsed into a single time-space vector,

$$\hat{r}_i = r_0 + \vec{h}\cdot\vec{S}_i$$

where the stimulus is designated by the vector $s(t,x) = \vec{S}_i$. The filter, $\vec{h}$, and stimulus, $\vec{S}$, have a dimensionality *M*, which is equal to the number of time delays times the number of spatial dimensions. The vector notation also facilitates the geometric interpretation of the linear model: the stimulus, $\vec{S}$, is projected along a single stimulus dimension defined by $\vec{h}$. Moreover, without any additional modification of the model, the relationship between the projected stimulus and the predicted response is simply linear.

The least mean square error (LMSE) solution to this linear regression problem is well known and is given by:

$$\hat{\vec{h}} = C_{ss}^{-1}\vec{C}_{sr}, \tag{1}$$

where C_{ss} is the stimulus auto-covariance matrix and C_{sr} is the stimulus-response cross-covariance vector. These covariances are estimated by averaging across all stimulus-response data pairs in the data set for $i \in \{1, N\}$, where N is the number of stimulus response pairs in the data set. The notation can be simplified once more by writing $\{\vec{S}_i\}$ as an NxM matrix, **S**. In addition to representing the number of spatial and temporal dimensions of the filter, M is also the number of parameters in the linear regression problem. The LMSE solution to the linear regression problem shown in (1) can then be rewritten (assuming zero mean stimulus and response values) as:

$$\hat{\vec{h}} = \left(\mathbf{S}^{\mathbf{T}}\mathbf{S}\right)^{-1}\mathbf{S}^{\mathbf{T}}\vec{r} \quad (2)$$

Equations (1) and (2) are known as the normal equations. When the stimulus auto-covariance matrix is diagonal, as it is the case for Gaussian white noise, the solution for the linear filter reduces to $(\mathbf{S}^T\vec{r})/N$. Thus for spiking neurons and a white noise stimulus, the optimal linear filter can simply be obtained by averaging the stimulus preceding each spike. This solution is called the spike-triggered average (STA) (de Boer 1967; de Boer and Kuyper 1968) and has been used extensively to characterize the receptive fields of neurons at various stages in the auditory processing stream (Aertsen and Johannesma 1981; Hermes, Aertsen et al. 1981; Clopton and Backoff 1991; Richard, Leppelsack et al. 1995).

In general, however, one would like to estimate the stimulus-response function when the neural system is processing behaviorally relevant natural stimuli such as environmental sounds, speech sounds, etc. In those cases, we have shown that one can use the analytical solution shown in (2) while paying particular attention to the inversion of the stimulus covariance matrix. We implement a regularized solution where the stimulus covariance matrix is decomposed into its eigenvectors. We then obtain a pseudo-inverse by solving the problem in the subspace spanned by the eigenvectors with the largest eigenvalues (Theunissen, Sen et al. 2000; Theunissen, David et al. 2001). Equation (1) is rewritten as:

$$\hat{\vec{h}} = Q_{SS}\Lambda^{-1}Q_{SS}^{T}C_{SR} \quad (3)$$

where Q_{ss} is the eigenvector matrix of C_{ss} and Λ is the diagonal matrix of its eigenvalues. In subspace regression (also called Principal Component regression), the inverse of these eigenvalues is set to zero for all dimensions where the eigenvalue is smaller than a threshold fraction of the largest eigenvalue. This equation can also be solved in the Fourier domain when the stimulus second order statistics are stationary (Theunissen, Sen et al. 2000; Theunissen, David et al. 2001). The solution in the Fourier domain allows for substantial savings in computational resources and greater estimation accuracy.

Subspace regression is mathematically very similar to ridge regression (Hoerl and Kennard 2000). In ridge regression, the term (also called L2 penalty) is added to the mean square error function to "penalize" regression weights that deviate from zero. It can then be shown that the analytical solution for h becomes:

$$\hat{\vec{h}} = Q_{SS}\left(\frac{1}{\Lambda+\lambda}\right)Q_{SS}^{T}C_{SR} \tag{4}$$

Eigendimensions that have small eigenvalues relative to λ will effectively be projected out in a manner that is similar to subspace regression. Thus λ behaves as a threshold parameter and as λ approaches zero, equation (4) becomes equivalent to equation (3).

Finally, it is also well known that the LMSE solution for the linear filter is equivalent to the maximum likelihood solution when it is assumed that the neural system can be modeled as a linear filter plus Gaussian noise:

$$p(r \mid \mathbf{S}, \vec{h}) = N(\vec{S}\cdot\vec{h}, \sigma^2)$$

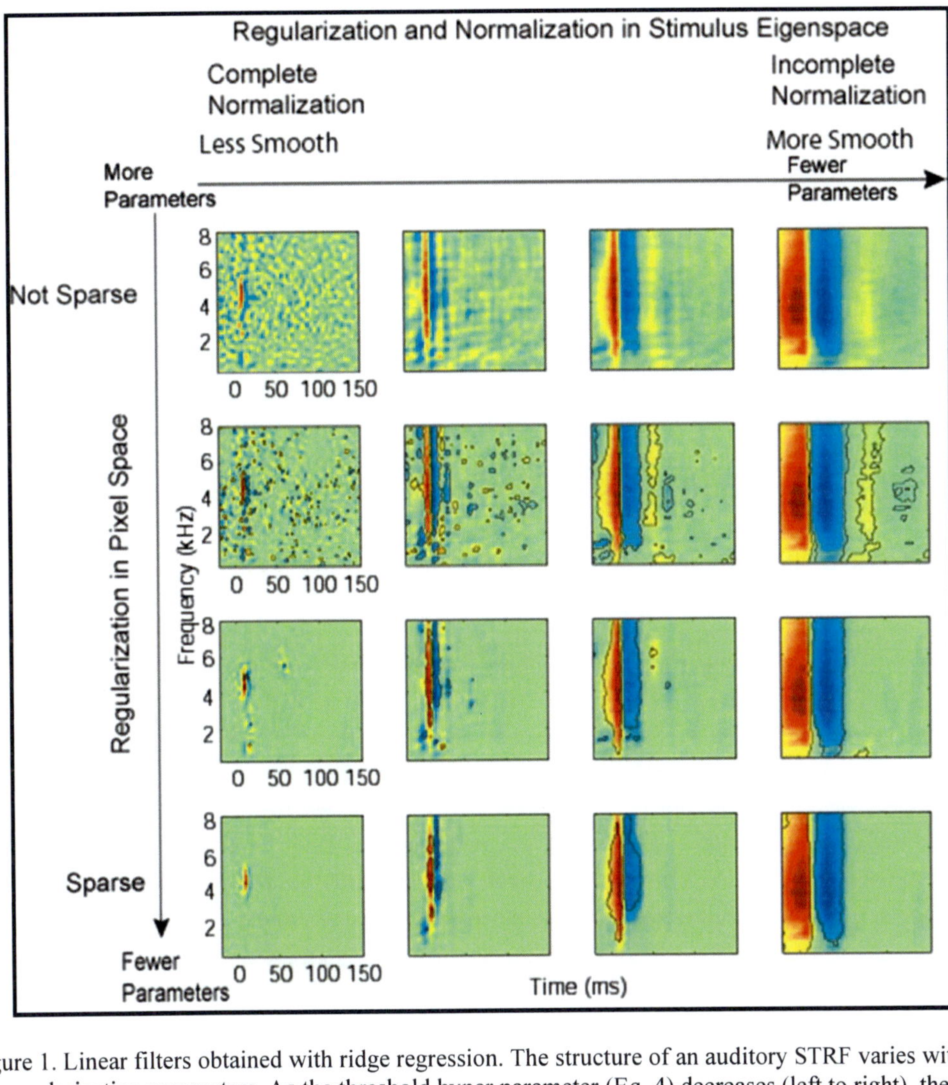

Figure 1. Linear filters obtained with ridge regression. The structure of an auditory STRF varies with the regularization parameters. As the threshold hyper parameter (Eq. 4) decreases (left to right), the STRF becomes smoother. The regularization in the pixel space (top to bottom) creates a sparser STRF.

It can also be shown that the ridge regression penalty can be reformulated in terms of a Gaussian prior on the filter coefficients:

$$p(\vec{h}) = N(0, \lambda^{-1} I).$$

The maximum *a posteriori* (MAP) solution then leads to the minimum least square solution with the ridge regression penalty (Wu, David et al. 2006).

When using subspace or ridge regression, one can implement additional regularization of the STRF estimate, for example, by thresholding filter parameters, h, based on the estimation of their standard error. With this double regularization procedure one obtains a family of linear filters for various values of the two hyper parameters (i.e., parameters guiding the fit procedure that reflect prior assumptions about the system and influence the final model fit parameters), the subspace threshold and standard error threshold. Figure 1 illustrates the effect of these two hyper parameters on the estimates of a STRF of an avian auditory neuron. A "best" solution out of this family of STRFs can be determined using cross-validation.

Since the second order statistics of natural sounds obey power law relationships (Singh and Theunissen 2003), the lower spatial and temporal Fourier dimensions have the largest eigenvalues. Thus, the ridge regression hyper parameter effectively acts as a smoothness parameter for the STRF estimation. In contrast, the hyper parameter based on the standard error of the coefficients acts as a sparseness parameter. Similar "smoothness" and "relevance" regularization has been used to estimate the STRF of auditory neurons in mice (Sahani and Linden 2003).

1.2. Gradient Descent Method Algorithms

The analytical solution for the linear filter in equation (4) yields fast and robust solutions. However, this approach suffers from two significant limitations. First, it requires computing the eigenvalue decomposition of the stimulus auto-correlation matrix. Although this computation is efficient when S has a small number of dimensions, it quickly becomes computationally expensive as well as underspecified by the data for large dimensional spaces. This problem of dimensionality is a particularly serious limitation when regression techniques are used for fitting STRF models that use a high dimensional stimulus representation to capture input nonlinearities (see subsequent sections). Second, an analytical solution can incorporate only a limited number of priors (such as the Gaussian prior in ridge regression). Using numerical gradient approaches allows one to circumvent these limitations.

Gradient descent uses the fact that the mean square error is a convex function of the linear filter parameters. The convexity property of the error function extends to a larger class of models, the generalized linear models, as we will elaborate below. For a particular value of the filter parameters, $\hat{h}^m$, the mean square error function is given by:

$$MSE^m = \frac{1}{N}\sum_{i=1}^{N}\left(\vec{S}_i.\hat{\vec{h}}^m - r_i\right)^2 \tag{5}$$

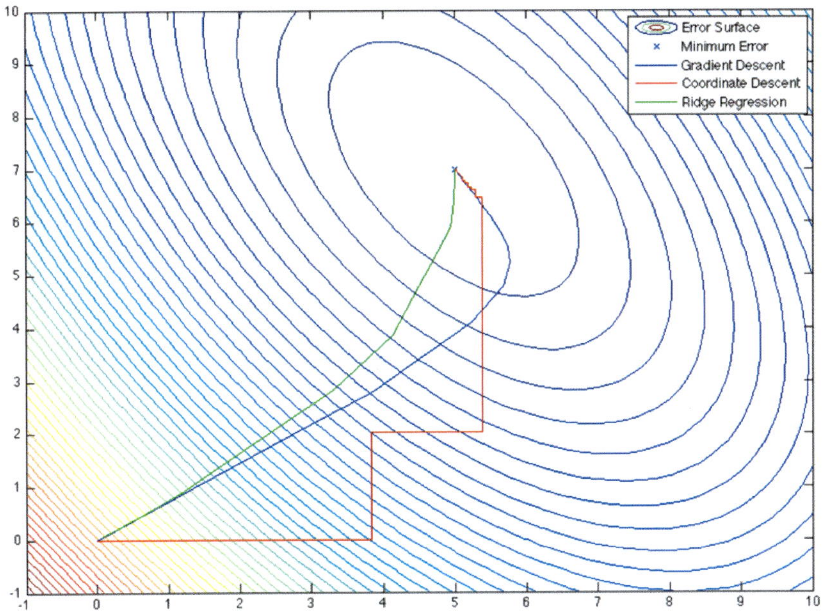

Figure 2. Solution paths for ridge regression (green), gradient descent (blue) and coordinate descent (red).

The gradient at any point of this error function is a slope that points in a direction of decreasing error. To find the minimum error, the gradient descent algorithm chooses a starting point, calculates the gradient of the error function at that point and takes a small step in the direction opposite of the gradient until the error function stops decreasing. The gradient for the MSE, using the matrix notation defined above is given by:

$$\vec{g}^m = S^T \left((\hat{\vec{h}}^m \cdot S) - \vec{r} \right) \tag{6}$$

One can see from the above equation that gradient descent methods circumvent the need to invert the stimulus auto-covariance matrix.

Several variants of the gradient descent algorithm exist. In coordinate descent the update is only performed in the dimension of with largest slope. Threshold gradient descent performs a compromise between gradient and coordinate descent by updating all dimensions for which the gradient exceeds a particular threshold. Scaled conjugate descent (SCG) takes advantage of the fact that the stimulus covariance matrix is symmetric and positive definite to optimize the direction and size of the steps. Scaled conjugate descent is very fast and this advantage can be exploited for very high dimensional cases.

In many gradient descent methods, regularization is achieved by initializing at zero and using early stopping to prevent over-fitting. In early stopping, the parameter updates are stopped before one reaches the minimum of the error function, as estimated from the fitting data set. Although this might seem counterintuitive, this early stopping point is the minimum of the error function given certain prior probabilities of the filter parameters. Thus early stopping can provide solutions that are more accurate when generalized to other data sets.

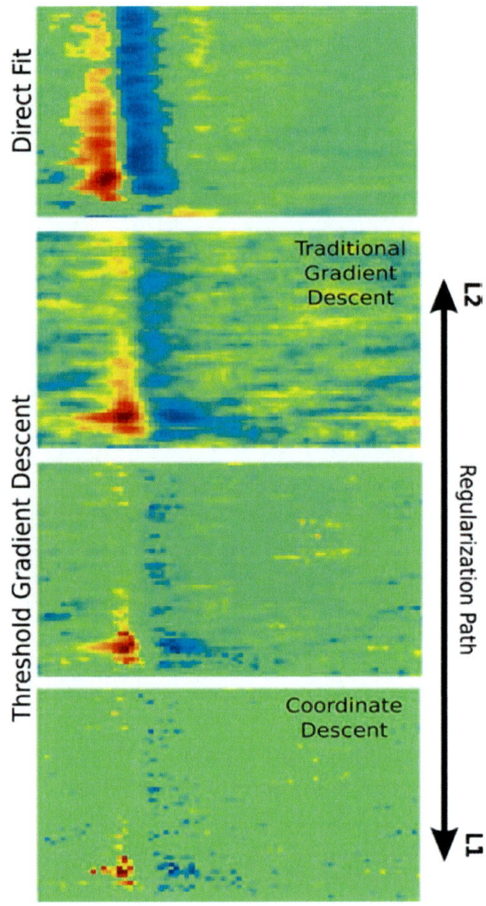

Figure 3. STRFs obtained for the same data with the direct fit (Top) and with threshold gradient descent with threshold values of 0 (ordinary gradient descent), 0.5 (combination), and 1 (coordinate descent).

Mathematically, it can be shown that early stopping corresponds to specific prior assumptions about filter parameter values (Friedman and Popescu (submitted)), and in this sense gradient descent with early stopping is an efficient implementation of MAP estimates. For example, traditional gradient descent approximates the Gaussian prior (or L2 regularization) used in ridge regression, while the coordinate descent approximates the Laplace prior (or L1 regularization also called LASSO). In Figure 3, we show examples of STRFs obtained for an avian auditory neuron using Ridge Regression, gradient descent, coordinate descent and the solution that corresponds to a combination of these two priors. As illustrated on the figure, STRFs obtained using coordinate descent are sparser and it has been shown that, in certain situations, they can yield higher predictions in cross-validation data (David, Mesgarani et al. 2007).

1.3. Input Nonlinearity and Large Basis Set Algorithms

Neurons and neuronal circuits are composed of many nonlinear biophysical elements (Aguera y Arcas, Fairhall et al. 2003; Abbott and Regehr 2004) and it is known that many of these nonlinearities perform key computations (Egelhaaf and Reichardt 1987; Karklin and Lewicki 2003; Gabbiani, Krapp et al. 2004; Pena and Konishi 2004). It is therefore essential to include nonlinear elements in STRF estimation. In this section, we will describe an approach to model the input nonlinearity by using an over complete basis set to represent the stimulus. In section I. 4 we will describe methods for fitting a one-dimensional output nonlinearity after projection onto the linear filter, and in section I. 5 we will describe approaches that involve projections of the stimulus into a subspace of 2 or more dimensions and nonlinear mappings between this stimulus subspace and the response. In all three sections, the methodology involves a linearization step that allows us to use some of the fitting methods described above for the linear filter.

It is well known that applying the linear filter framework directly to capture the stimulus-response functions of high-level sensory neurons can fail dramatically. For example auditory neurons above the cochlear nucleus do not phase-lock to the sound pressure waveform and thus cannot be described by a linear filtering operation on this signal. However, in this case, a simple solution exists. For high-level auditory neurons, the sound pressure waveform can be decomposed into a time-frequency representation using the sound spectrogram. Sounds can be represented as spectrograms with either linear or log amplitude transformations or even more realistic models of the peripheral auditory filter bank (Gill, Zhang et al. 2006). In these new basis sets the relationship between the stimulus and the neural response can once again be described by a linear filtering operation. Note, however, that the novel stimulus representation included a nonlinear step: the estimation of the amplitude of a Fourier component.

More recently, it has been shown that this form of stimulus pre-processing can be generalized by using very large and over-complete representations (Kay, Naselaris et al. 2008; Willmore, Prenger et al. 2010). In mathematical notation, the procedure can be summarized as:

$$\hat{r}_i = F_{non-linear}\{\vec{S}_i\} \cong \vec{h} \cdot f(\vec{S}_i), \text{ where } f : \vec{S} \in \Re^M \to \vec{S}' \in \Re^L \text{ with L>M.}$$

These over-complete basis sets are designed to either capture known properties of the biological system or linearize specific nonlinearities, such as full rectification. This higher dimensional stimulus representation can then be used as input to a linear encoding filter. This procedure can only work 1) if the linear regression methods are regularized and 2) if the dimensionality remains tractable. Gradient descent methods can be used both for regularization and to solve the problem when the stimulus dimensions become very large.

I.4. Output Nonlinearities and Generalized Linear Model (GLM) Algorithms

Some nonlinearities in the system can also be caused by output nonlinearities such as those that could be expected from the rectification and compression observed in spiking neurons. The output nonlinearity can be written in mathematical notation as:

$$\hat{r}_i = F_{non-linear}\{\vec{S}_i\} \cong f(\vec{h} \cdot \vec{S}_i).$$

For static nonlinearities and one-dimensional responses (e.g. single neurons or single voxels), f is a function of real numbers $f : \Re \rightarrow \Re$.

It can be shown that for Gaussian white noise, f and $\vec{h}$ can be solved separately and successively (Marmarelis and Marmarelis 1978): $\vec{h}$ can still be obtained from the stimulus-response cross-correlation (or the STA for spiking neurons) and f can be solved sequentially using many available nonlinear fitting routines such as spline approximations (Pillow, Paninski et al. 2005) or other approaches that also take into account the probability distributions of the response (Kouh and Sharpee 2009). Unfortunately this simple approach fails for non-Gaussian stimuli and in those cases f and must be solved simultaneously. Moreover the values of and their interpretation might be erroneous if the nonlinearity is not taken into account (Christianson, Sahani et al. 2008; Sharpee, Miller et al. 2008).

There are two related solutions to this problem. The first is to use an iterative procedure for invertible f functions as proposed by Hunter and Korenberg (Hunter and Korenberg 1986). In brief, is initially obtained from equation (1) above and a first estimate for f is fitted sequentially. Then, the inverse of f is used to transform responses r into the estimate of the linear output of the system (e.g r' could be the membrane potential that causes the spiking behavior, r). A new linear filter is then estimated between and r' and the procedure is repeated until convergence. The primary difficulty in the application of this algorithm is that the inversion of the nonlinear function can produce extreme and noisy estimates for r' which could lead to poor convergence behavior. An alternative algorithm that avoids the use of the inverse has been suggested to alleviate this problem (Korenberg and Hunter 1999).

The second method is to use the very powerful framework of the generalized linear model (GLM). Using the GLM one can obtain solutions for the linear filter not only for particular static output nonlinearities but also for the entire exponential family of response distributions.

In the linear model: $\mu_i = \hat{r}_i = \hat{\vec{h}} \cdot \vec{S}_i$ and $R_i \sim N(\hat{r}_i, \sigma^2)$, where R_i is the random variable describing the responses given the stimulus, $\vec{S}_i$. R_i is assumed to have a Gaussian distribution with mean given by the linear prediction.

In the GLM: $g(\mu_i) = g(\hat{r}_i) = \hat{\vec{h}} \cdot \vec{S}_i$ and $R_i \sim \Im(r, \theta_i) = \exp\left[rb(\theta_i) + c(\theta_i) + d(r)\right]$

The function g is a monotone, differentiable function called the link function that describes the nonlinear transformation between the linear estimator $\eta_i = \hat{\vec{h}} \cdot \vec{S}_i$ and the predicted response (note that the inverse of the link function, g^{-1}, is the equivalent of the f function in the first part of this section). $\mu_i = \hat{r}_i$ is the expectation value (or mean) of the distribution of responses given $\vec{S}_i$. This distribution belongs to the exponential family and has the form given by $\Im(r, \theta_i)$. Some of the distributions that belong to this class are the Gaussian, the Binomial, and the Poisson. If g is the identity function and $\Im(r, \theta_i)$ is Gaussian, the GLM is identical to the classical linear model. The Poisson distribution is particularly relevant since it is a better description of the distribution of counts (spike rates) that one obtains from spiking neurons than the Gaussian distribution.

Similar to the linear model, the linear filter in the GLM can be estimated by maximizing the likelihood function, or as is usually convenient the log of the likelihood function. And because the likelihood function is convex with respect to $\vec{h}$, gradient descent methods can be used to find the unique solution. The gradient of the log likelihood (L) along dimension j of ($j \in \{1, M\}$; see Section I. 1) is (Dobson 2002):

$$\frac{\partial L}{\partial h_j} = \sum_{i=1}^{N} s_{ij} \frac{(r_i - g^{-1}(\vec{h} \cdot \vec{S}_i))}{\text{var}(R_i)} \left(\frac{\partial g^{-1}(\eta_i)}{\partial \eta_i} \right) \tag{7}$$

One can therefore use the gradient descent methods described above to fit the GLM. Also when the derivative of the inverse link function is equal to the variance of the response distribution, the gradient in the GLM (Equation 7) is identical to the gradient obtained from the LMSE in the linear case (Equation 6) and thus identical algorithms can be used in both cases. The link functions that have this property are called canonical link functions and are shown in Table 1.

The GLM approach with canonical link functions and Poisson distributions has been applied to model neural responses with relative success (Paninski, Pillow et al. 2004; Pillow 2005). In the auditory system, GLM models have also been shown to yield better predictions than models that did not include a nonlinear output function (Calabrese, Schumacher et al. 2011). However, the full flexibility of the algorithm has not yet been exploited in that the effect of modeling different noise distributions and link functions has not been systematically investigated or exploited to its full potential.

I.5. Dynamical Nonlinearities and the Spike-triggered Covariance (STC) Algorithm

The previous two sections have focused on methods to estimate a static input or output nonlinearity and therefore to model the neural system with what is called a nonlinear-linear-nonlinear (NLN) cascade model, where the linear filter (L) is a projection from an high dimensional nonlinear stimulus representation (the first N) into a 1 dimensional subspace that is followed by a nonlinear output function (the second N).

Table 1.

Type of Regression	Link Function	Noise Distribution
Linear	$g(\mu) = \mu = \vec{h} \cdot \vec{S}$	Gaussian
Logistic	$g(\mu) = \ln(\frac{\mu}{1-\mu}) = \vec{h} \cdot \vec{S}$	Binomial
Poisson	$g(\mu) = \ln(\mu) = \vec{h} \cdot \vec{S}$	Poisson

Although this approach can be very powerful, it does not capture all possible SR-functions. The alternative is to project the stimulus into a subspace with dimensions greater than 1 and fit multi-dimensional output function from that stimulus subspace to the response. In this section, we will describe how the second order terms of the Volterra expansion (Marmarelis and Marmarelis 1978) can be described in this framework and how it can derived using methods that are similar to those described above. We will also show how this approach relates to the method of spike-triggered covariance.

The extension of the linear filter to the second order is given by:

$$\hat{r}(t) = F_{2nd}\{s(t,x)\} = r_o + \iint h_1(t-\tau,x)s(\tau,x)\,d\tau\,dx$$
$$+\iint\iint h_2(t-\tau_1,t-\tau_2,x_1,x_2)s(\tau_1,x_1)s(\tau_2,x_2)\,dx_1\,dx_2\,d\tau_1\,d\tau_2$$

or in discrete form:

$$\hat{r}(t) = r^0 + \sum_{i=1}^{M} h_i^1 s_i + \sum_{i=1}^{M}\sum_{j=1}^{M} h_{ij}^2 s_i s_j$$

(note that the superscripts 1 and 2 on h denote the first and second order terms and not the power operation). The previous equation can be expressed in linearized vector form as:

$$\hat{r} = r^0 + \vec{h}^1 \cdot \vec{S}^1 + \vec{h}^2 \cdot \vec{S}^2, \tag{8}$$

where and $\vec{S}^2 = \begin{pmatrix} s_1 s_1 \\ s_1 s_2 \\ \vdots \\ s_2 s_1 \\ \vdots \end{pmatrix}$ are M^2x1 vectors. In this linearized formulation, the second order terms could in theory be found using the normal equation and ridge regression (as long as r^0 and h^1 are zero). However, in this case the stimulus auto-covariance matrix that corresponds to S^2 has size M^2xM^2, which, in most applications, will be too large for eigenvalue decomposition. For example, a 10x10 image patch with 10 delays in time yields M=1000 and therefore a second order stimulus covariance matrix of size 10^6 by 10^6.

One solution is to use Gaussian white noise as a stimulus, in which case the second order stimulus auto-covariance can be written as a scalar times an identity matrix and can therefore be considered a simple scaling. In this case, one could just compute the cross-covariance to obtain the h^2 filter. This is the underlying principle of the method known as spike triggered covariance (STC) (Brenner, Bialek et al. 2000; Nemenman, Bialek et al. 2004). This method has been used to recover the components of the receptive fields of complex visual cells (Touryan, Felsen et al. 2005). However, one is still able to obtain a solution using gradient descent methods since these methods only require the computation of vector dot products of size 1xM^2. Moreover, the gradient descent approaches incorporate regularization, which becomes crucial given the high number of filter parameters that are being fitted. In addition, with the advance of fast gradient descent algorithms (such as SCG), solutions can be found in time that grows linearly with size (M^2 in this case).

The second order filter is difficult to interpret and visualize without further processing. One of the very useful insights of the STC framework has been to examine the eigenvectors of the spike-triggered stimulus-response cross covariance matrix to find the subspace of the original stimulus space that is sampled (or explored) when response events occur (Brenner, Bialek et al. 2000). The same principle can be applied to the normalized second order filter h^2. First, we rewrite the second order filter as a matrix instead of a vector:

$$\vec{h}^2 = \begin{pmatrix} h_{1,1}^2 \\ h_{1,2}^2 \\ \vdots \\ h_{2,1}^2 \\ \vdots \\ h_{M,M}^2 \end{pmatrix} = \begin{pmatrix} h_{1,1}^2 & h_{1,2}^2 & \cdots & h_{1,M}^2 \\ h_{2,1}^2 & h_{2,2}^2 & & \vdots \\ \vdots & & \ddots & \\ h_{M,1}^2 & \cdots & & h_{M,M}^2 \end{pmatrix} = \mathbf{H}^2 \qquad (9)$$

The second order term can then be rewritten as $\vec{S}_i^T \mathbf{H}^2 \vec{S}_i$. Then we compute the eigenvalue decomposition of $\mathbf{H^2}$ to write it as: $\mathbf{H}^2 = \mathbf{S}_e \Lambda \mathbf{S}_e^T$, where S_e is the matrix of eigenvectors of $\mathbf{H}^2$ and Λ is the diagonal matrix of its eigenvalues. A stimulus can then be expressed in the basis set spanned by the eigenvectors of S_e: $\vec{S}_i = k_{i1}\vec{S}_{e1} + k_{i2}\vec{S}_{e2} + \cdots + k_{iM}\vec{S}_{eM}$. The second order term can then be rewritten as: $\vec{S}_i^T \mathbf{H}^2 \vec{S}_i = k_{i1}^2 \lambda_1 + k_{i2}^2 \lambda_2 + \cdots + k_{iM}^2 \lambda_M$, where λ_i are the eigenvalues composing Λ.

We can draw some useful conclusions from this representation. First, one can clearly see that the second order term can be visualized and interpreted by examining the eigenvectors corresponding to the largest eigenvalues. Each of these eigenvectors can be interpreted in a fashion that is similar to the linear filter in the sense that the predicted response depends on the dot product between the stimulus and these eigenvectors. Second, one can explicitly observe that the nonlinearity that is fitted in the second order term is quadratic.

In addition to helping visualize the model parameters, this representation also suggests a novel approach to obtain a more general fit of this dynamical nonlinearity. Since the subspace spanned by the first few vectors of $\mathbf{S_e}$ corresponds to the stimulus space that is conditioned on the response, we can attempt to use the projection to fit a more general nonlinear function. More explicitly, one can write:

$$\hat{r}_i = F(k_{i1}, k_{i2}, \cdots, k_{iL}) \text{ where } L<M. \qquad (10)$$

Here, F is a multivariate general nonlinear function and it would be fitted sequentially. This approach has not yet been used extensively in the auditory system.

1.6. Multicomponent STRFs Based on Information Theoretic Measures

In the previous sections, we described classical methods for STRF estimation (linear filter, GLMs, Volterra series) that obtain an estimate of the STRF solution by minimizing a cost function based on the likelihood of particular noise distributions (normal or exponential in the case of GLMs), particular nonlinearities (specified by the link function in GLMs or the quadratic relationship implied in STC) and priors used for regularization.

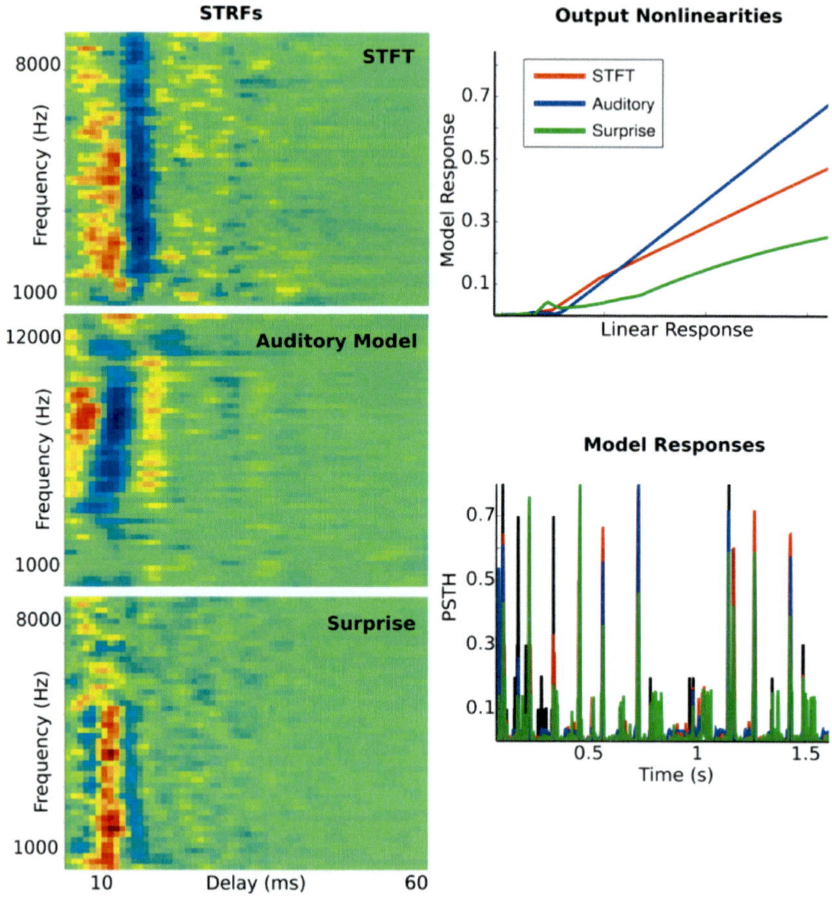

Figure 4. The NLN cascade model applied to the same auditory neuron for different choices of stimulus representations. The left column shows STRFs obtained with the STFT (spectrogram), the Lyon's Cochlear model (Auditory Model), and the surprise model for the input nonlinearity. The upper right plot shows static output nonlinearities fit for each of these STRFs, using a non-parameteric cubic spline fit. The bottom right plot shows the real PSTH (peri stimulus time histogram, black) and model responses for a particular stimulus. It is clear from this example that the choice of stimulus preprocessing can change the shape of the linear filter, the output nonlinearity and the predicted responses.

Information theoretic approaches allow the relaxation of some of these assumptions by allowing the nonlinearites or noise distribution to be inferred directly from the data. In a technique known as Maximally Informative Dimensions (MID) multicomponent STRFs such as those obtained with the STC method but without assuming a particular link function as in the GLM or a quadratic form as in STC (Sharpee, Rust et al. 2004). The MID approach has been used in audition to describe and quantify the emergence of higher order representations as one moves up the auditory processing chain (Atencio, Sharpee et al. 2012). More recently, Fitzgerald et al. have proposed another multi-component STRF technique in which mutual information is minimized under a set of constraints (Fitzgerald, Sincich et al. 2011). This second approach yields the model that satisfies particular observed stimulus-responses correlations while making minimal assumptions about non-observed statistics. In this manner it provides a data driven approach to the joint estimation of the noise distribution and the multi-component STRF.

I.7. Software Implementation

Although many of the regression routines described above exist as high-level functions in programming languages such as R, Python or Matlab, we have written a comprehensive toolbox in Matlab that implements most of the algorithms above. This toolbox is called strfLab and is available at http://strflab.berkeley.edu. The code in *strfLab* is organized in a three-layer framework: the fitting layer, the resampling layer and the wrapper layer. The layers are organized hierarchically, such that functions of one layer call functions in the layer below. The bottommost layer is composed of the model fitting routines (e.g. ridge regression, gradient descent). The resampling layer allows the data to be reformatted in the most efficient manner for the fitting routines as well as for validation. The topmost layer consists of general-purpose wrapper functions that call the various lower level functions. This architecture is advantageous both from the user's perspective and from the developer's perspective.

Box 1. Sample strfLab code to obtain a linear STRF for an auditory neuron

```
% Initialize a GLM by specifying the size of the spatial and temporal dimensions of the
    filter and the identity as the link function.
    strfAud = linInit(size(stimAud,2), [0:60], 'linear');
    % Store the stimulus response data pairs in strfLab global structures
    strfData(stimAud,respAud);
    % Choose Coordinate Descent as the fitting algorithm for the linear model
    options.optimOpt=trnGradDesc;
    options.optimOpt.coordDesc = 1;
    options.optimOpt.earlyStop = 1;
% Fit model. Here we are using 90% of the data for fitting and 10% for early stopping
    (regularization)
    fittingIdx=1:floor(.9*globDat.nSample);
    stoppingIdx =floor(.9*globDat.nSample)+1:globDat.nSample);
    strfTrainedAud=strfOpt(strfAud,fittingIdx,optionsAud,stoppingIdx);
```

From a user's perspective, all interface with the toolbox occurs through high-level function provided by the topmost level. These high-level functions called without arguments return an *Options* structure with default values. The user can thus quickly perform data analysis with the default values but can also change them effortlessly. Thus, with this framework, relatively sophisticated analyses can be performed with a few lines of code (See Box 1). Moreover, the user can rapidly test a range of model parameters or model architectures by writing simple wrapper loops.

From a developer's perspective, the layer architecture and the use of Options structure that can incorporate variable number of arguments allows for rapid and robust development. For example, a programmer can write a low level new model fitting routine that can be easily incorporated in the program. Similarly, new options (and thus new features) can be added to existing routines without any issues of compatibility with previous code.

II. STRF Validation and Hypothesis Testing

The central idea driving hypothesis tests based on STRF comparisons is that the model better describing the underlying system should do a better job predicting the neural response to an arbitrary novel stimulus (Theunissen, Sen et al. 2000; David and Gallant 2005; Wu, David et al. 2006). From this perspective, the analytical structure of the model (i.e., the representation of the stimulus inputs, any nonlinearities applied to the stimulus by the model, and the fit procedure) represents a hypothesis about the underlying neural system that produces the observed response. If some element of the model structure captures an important functional property of the system, then that model should do a better job predicting responses than a model lacking the critical feature. Prediction accuracy provides an objective, quantitative measure for comparison of two or more models.

In the same way that a variety of error metrics can be used for model estimation, the same variety of metrics can also be used for evaluating prediction accuracy, including correlation coefficient (Theunissen, David et al. 2001; Paninski 2004), mean-squared error (Linden, Liu et al. 2003), coherence (Hsu, Borst et al. 2004), maximum likelihood (Theunissen, David et al. 2001; Paninski 2004), or mutual information (Sharpee, Rust et al. 2004). If neural noise distributions were well known and characterized, then one could argue that measures based on maximum likelihood, maximum posterior or mutual information are the most appropriate from a theoretical standpoint (Wu, David et al. 2006). In practice, however, it is not clear if there is a single "best" error metric, as each suffers from its own potential bias because of data limitations (Hsu, Borst et al. 2004; Wu, David et al. 2006). In most cases where multiple metrics have been tested, they have largely agreed on how they rank the relative performance of different models (e.g., see Schinkel-Bielefeld, David et al. 2012).

Because of the complexity of regression methods used for STRF fitting, especially for nonlinear models, there is a danger that one model might appear to perform better simply because it does a better job of fitting experimental noise. This potential bias is largely avoided by a simple cross-validation procedure (Theunissen, Sen et al. 2000; David and Gallant 2005; Wu, David et al. 2006) in which the neural dataset is broken into two parts. The STRF is fit with the larger part, the *estimation dataset*, (typically 80-90% of the data). Predictions are then tested using the smaller remaining part, the *validation dataset*, which was not used at any previous stage of model fitting. When this approach is used, models cannot be "over-fit" to noise present in the validation dataset and measured prediction accuracy must instead reflect a characterization of the true stimulus-response relationship.

Before discussing specific examples, we provide a brief overview of general experimental approaches used for hypothesis testing in this STRF prediction framework.

II.1. Model Comparison: Two Models, One Dataset

In its most common application, prediction analysis provides a tool for comparing how well two different models describe auditory tuning observed in dataset in which a large variety of stimuli were presented while recording neural activity (David and Gallant 2005; Gill, Zhang et al. 2006; Wu, David et al. 2006; David, Mesgarani et al. 2007). This method of model comparison represents a classical method for characterizing any complex nonlinear system, including auditory neurons, and exemplifies the majority of methods described elsewhere in this volume.

We illustrate this approach with a very simple simulation representative of the output nonlinearities described in Section I. 4 (Figure 5). Here, the neural output response (e.g., spike rate) is modulated at a single time lag by a single scalar input (e.g., stimulus intensity). As is observed in many neurons, larger inputs produce larger outputs. However, as is also typical for neurons, the relationship is not linear, with a threshold preventing small inputs from having any effect on output and saturation of outputs for large inputs. Gaussian additive noise introduces variability that might be observed in the response averaged over a finite number of trials so that the sampled data do not exactly match the underlying tuning of the neuron.

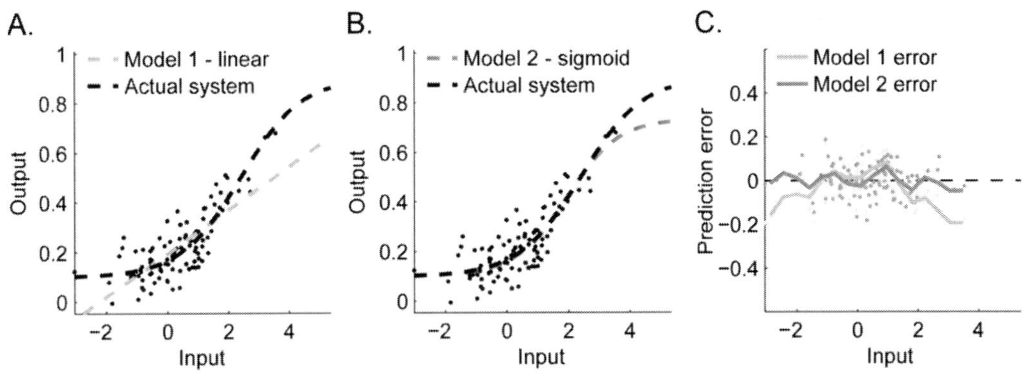

Figure 5. STRF model comparison. A. Black dots represent noisy data sampled from a system with a simple one-dimensional input-output relationship (black dashed curve). A. Linear fit to the data (gray line) captures the tendency of larger inputs to produce larger outputs. B. However, a fit that accounts for a nonlinear sigmoidal relationship between input and output describes the system much more accurately. C. Model accuracy can be quanitified by prediction error. The nonlinear model from B has much smaller error (dark gray) than the linear fit (light gray), especially for very large and small inputs. Because of its more accurate predictions, one can conclude that the nonlinear model more accurately describes the underlying system.

Because the input-output relationship is largely monotonic, one might initially attempt to describe the data using a linear model (Section I. 1, Figure 5A). For this reduced system, the linear fit requires finding a single weight that scales the input to match the output. Predictions by this model are then described by a straight line. The linear model explains some variance in the test dataset that was not used for fitting, but systematic errors appear very small and large inputs, where the effects of nonlinear thresholding and saturation are the strongest (Figure 2C).

Based on prior knowledge of threshold and saturation nonlinearities in neural systems, one might instead describe the same dataset with a more complex GLM in which the output of the linear filter is scaled by a sigmoid function (Section I. 4, Figure 5B). Fitting the nonlinear sigmoid model requires more parameters, but it does a better job predicting the same validation dataset than the linear model (Figure 5C). Because the second model more accurately predicts neural responses in the validation data set, one can conclude that it represents the better model for describing this data.

II.2. Stimulus Space Comparison: One Model, Two Datasets

An alternative form of hypothesis testing with STRFs has grown increasingly popular in recent years. Rather than comparing the predictive power of two different models, one can fit a single model using two separate datasets, distinguished by stimuli with different statistical properties. If the model captures all the important nonlinear features of the system, then the fits should be comparable. If however, the two stimulus sets activate unmodeled nonlinearities differentially, then the models fit to the two datasets will not agree.

This approach has been used to test for circuitry specialized for processing natural stimuli, by comparing STRFs fit to a commonly used synthetic noise stimulus and to an ethologically relevant natural or naturalistic stimulus (Aertsen and Johannesma 1981; Theunissen, Sen et al. 2000; David, Mesgarani et al. 2009; Schneider and Woolley 2010). In general, however, this approach is not limited to the comparison of natural and synthetic stimuli. One can compare two different types of synthetic stimuli, e.g., modulated noise that differs in spectral density (Norena, Gourevitch et al. 2008; Schneider and Woolley 2010), or two different sets of natural stimuli, e.g., vocalizations at different sounds levels (Nagel and Doupe 2008).

As in the case of model comparison (Section II. 1), stimulus-dependent model differences can be quantified by comparing predictive power for stimuli belonging to the same category as the estimation set to predictive power for stimuli from the other category. (It is important to emphasize that in both cases, the test stimuli should be validation datasets that were reserved from estimation. To reduce noise, it is also helpful to use the same validation datasets for testing both models.) If STRF predictive power does not generalize across stimulus categories then some additional, unmodeled nonlinearity must be activated differentially between those conditions.

Figure 6 illustrates this approach using the same simple system as in the previous example. In addition to the first dataset, in which inputs were centered on a mean of 0 (close to threshold), a second dataset was collected with inputs around a mean of 3 (well above threshold). Linear models fit separately to these datasets each describe the input-output relationship in that dataset reasonably accurately (Figures 7A-B). However, the fits are different, with a steeper slope (i.e., higher gain) in the fit to the second, above-threshold dataset. While each model may predict responses better in their own stimulus domain, they fail dramatically to predict responses in the other domain (Figure 6C).

This initial analysis establishes that some nonlinearity must exist in the system that is not captured by the current model. If the analysis stops here, one can conclude simply that the current model is not adequate for describing the system in its entirety. In the case of a natural versus synthetic stimulus comparison, one can also conclude that the fit to the natural stimulus dataset provides a more accurate characterization of filter properties engaged under normal behavioral conditions. Studies using this approach have also been described in detail in a previous chapter (see chapter by Schreiner and Atencio)..

However, stimulus-dependent differences in model fits can also provide new insights into important nonlinearities at work in the system. Consider the hypothetical situation in which the idea for the sigmoid nonlinearity did not previously exist for the system in Figure 6. The separate fits represent piece-wise linear approximations to the underlying nonlinearity (Nagel and Doupe 2008; David, Mesgarani et al. 2009). In this example, increasing input amplitude leads to an increase in the linear slope. An experimenter might observe the separate fits and conclude that an expansive nonlinearity, as occurs in the threshold regime of a sigmoid, might explain the differences.

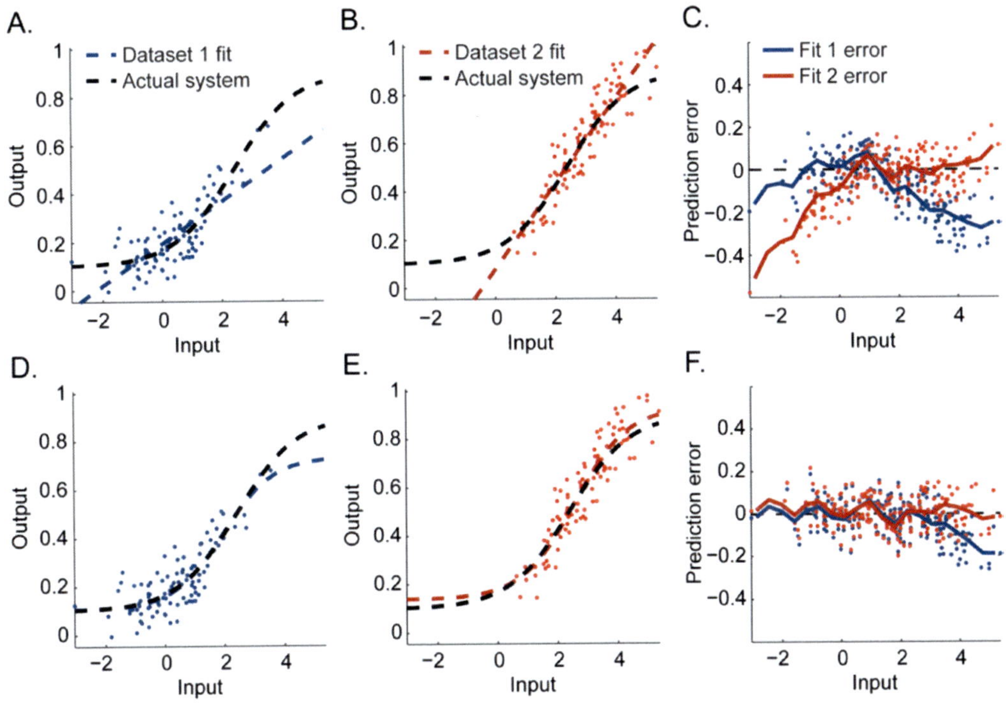

Figure 6. STRF stimulus domain comparison. A. Data and associated fit (blue dots and dashed lines) for the same one-dimensional system as in Fig. 1A. B. When stimuli are presented in a different range—in this case centered around higher input values (red dots)—the nonlinear system produces a different linear fit (red dashed line). C. Prediction analysis confirms the stimulus-dependence, as the first fit predicts with smaller error in the lower input regime while the second fit predicts with smaller error in the higher regime. D,E. Nonlinear fits more accurately capture the input-ouput relationship of the underlying system. F. In this case, both fits predict with similar accuracy across all input values. In extreme cases, (eg, dataset 1 fit predicting large inputs), sufficient fit data may not be available so that the correct model may still not generalize completely to all stimulus regimes.

Fitting the nonlinear model that incorporates the sigmoid provides a more accurate fit to both datasets (Figure 6D-E). Moreover, the fits are qualitatively similar and predict data in both stimulus domains with about the same accuracy (Figure 6F). Thus a careful analysis of the piecewise linear fits can provide deeper insight into a new model that describes the system better. The performance of the new model can be compared directly to the first model using the classical model comparison (Section II. 1).

Although one might infer nonlinear properties of the system from the piece-wise linear fits, it may be impractical to fit the same dataset with a model that often requires more parameters than the original one due to sampling limitations. When sampling limitations prevent estimation of the more complex model, evidence for the new nonlinearity can be demonstrated by simulation. One can simulate a neuron with the relevant nonlinear property and then measure the simpler linear model from simulated responses in the different stimulus regimes. If the separate fits show the same pattern as observed in the data, this provides evidence that the stimulus-dependent differences could be produced by the proposed nonlinearity (Christianson, Sahani et al. 2008; David, Mesgarani et al. 2009; Schneider and Woolley 2011).

II.3. Behavior Comparison: One Model, One Stimulus, Two Behavioral States

A variant of the one model/two stimulus approach described in the previous section follows similar logic but extends to hypotheses about the influence of behavioral state on sensory processing. In this approach the behavioral state, or context, of an animal is controlled by some form of classical or instrumental conditioning. A fixed stimulus set is then presented in both of these controlled behavioral conditions, and the same model is fit to data collected in each condition. Because the stimulus and model are held constant, any differences between STRFs must reflect changes in the animal's internal state, providing insight into how internal behavioral states can modulate sensory representations (Figure 7).

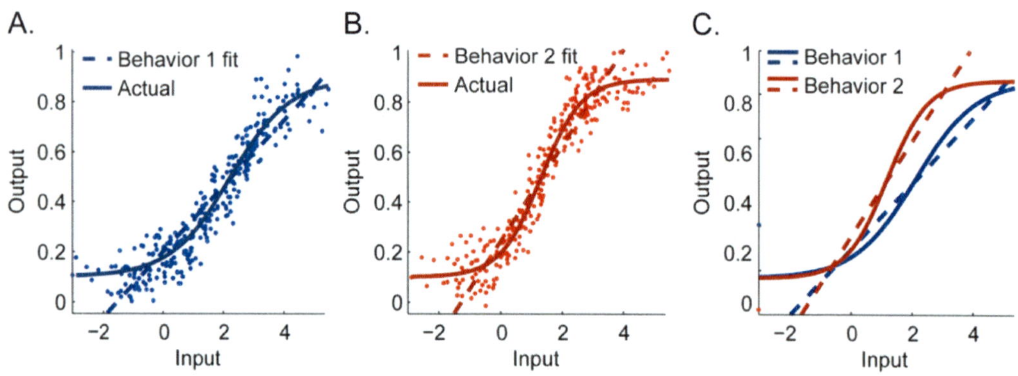

Figure 7. STRF dependence on behavioral state. A. Data and associated fit (blue dots and dashed lines) for the same one-dimensional system as in Fig. 1A. B. Data recorded using identical stimuli but when the input-output relationship has changed due to some change in behavioral state. C. Changes in the underlying system will be reflected in differences between fits under the two behavior conditions.

This approach has been used widely to study both long- and short-term tuning changes in both single neurons and non-invasive human recordings (Ohl and Scheich 1997; Fritz, Shamma et al. 2003; Fritz, Elhilali et al. 2005; David, Fritz et al. 2012; Ding and Simon 2012a).

III. STRFs and Physiological Mechanisms

Early experiments typically measured STRFs with a single stimulus, such as random chords (Eggermont, Aertsen et al. 1983; deCharms, Blake et al. 1998) or broadband modulated noise (Kowalski, Depireux et al. 1996; Klein, Depireux et al. 2000; Miller, Escabi et al. 2001), and the STRF was treated as a fixed property of an individual neuron. More recently, however, questions have been raised about the validity of using just a single stimulus regime, chosen somewhat arbitrarily from a number of possible stimuli. The statistical properties of a stimulus (temporal dynamics, density, bandwidth, dynamic range) vary across the diversity of acoustic environments, or contexts, that might be encountered in the real world. Studies using the one model/two dataset approach (Section II. 2) have shown repeatedly that STRFs estimated under one stimulus condition do not generalize across stimulus regimes. When these stimulus-dependent STRF changes are systematic, they can provide information about the nonlinear response properties that produce the changes. These functional nonlinearities can provide insight into underlying circuitry producing auditory responses and can be used to derive new, more general nonlinear models that can subsequently be evaluated using the two model/one dataset approach (Section II. 1).

III.1. STRF Dependence on Steady-state Stimulus Bandwidth, Level and Density

As reviewed earlier in this volume (see chapter by Schreiner and Atencio), the general approach of comparing STRFs estimated using stimuli with different steady-state statistics has an extensive history and continues be used across the auditory processing hierarchy in mammalian, avian, and amphibian auditory systems (Aertsen and Johannesma 1981; Blake and Merzenich 2002; Escabi, Miller et al. 2003; Reiss, Bandyopadhyay et al. 2007; Gourevitch, Norena et al. 2009).

III.2. Stimulus-dependent STRFs and Neuronal Gain Control Mechanisms

One area where comparing STRFs estimated from different stimuli has proven valuable recently has been in addressing contextual effects of stimulus dynamics that are explicitly factored out of steady-state models. The most frequently observed phenomenon excluded from steady-state models is the strong transient response to stimulus onset following a period of silence. In addition, however, a number of possibly related effects have been observed in auditory responses following abrupt changes in the statistical properties of complex noise and naturalistic stimuli. In many cases, open questions remain about how these phenomena can be incorporated into the SR model framework.

Depireux and colleagues (Depireux, Dobbins et al. 2012) performed an analysis of linear STRF properties of cortical neurons following the onset of rippled noise and found dynamic changes in spectro-temporal tuning between the onset and steady state. Generally, the STRF settled into a steady state after about 40 ms. These results provide evidence that auditory neurons encode different spectro-temporal features of the stimulus during these two stimulus epochs.

Onset responses can be interpreted as a specific example of more general changes in tuning following transitions in stimulus mean level and contrast (Dean, Robinson et al. 2008; Rabinowitz, Willmore et al. 2012). In experiments exploring this more general case, the level and/or contrast of a noise stimulus are held constant during fixed epochs lasting several seconds but then change randomly and rapidly between epochs. From this perspective, stimulus onset following silence represents a transition from a very weak stimulus to one with much higher level and contrast. Studies in both the inferior colliculus and auditory cortex revealed that increases in stimulus contrast lead to a reduction in the gain of auditory neurons. This phenomenon has the effect of normalizing the dynamic range of a neuron (i.e., minimum and maximum firing rate, which is limited by physiological circuit properties) to roughly span the dynamic range of the stimulus.

By comparing linear STRF estimates for A1 neurons during different stimulus contrast epochs, Rabinowitz et al. (Rabinowitz, Willmore et al. 2012) identified systematic gain changes in the STRF associated with changes in stimulus contrast. They then constructed a nonlinear model that incorporated a dynamic normalization term to scale the overall STRF gain by the recent stimulus contrast. The resulting model provided substantially improved predictive power over the linear model. Moreover, the contrast normalization term included a parameter that accounted for how quickly the normalization occurred. The normalization had a time constant averaging about 80 ms, which corresponds roughly to STRF changes associated with stimulus onsets (Depireux, Dobbins et al. 2012).

While the majority of this work has focused on the dynamics of neural responses immediately follow changes in stimulus statistics, other studies have identified slower changes in the STRF, taking up to many seconds (Shechter and Depireux 2006; Shechter and Depireux 2007; Pienkowski and Eggermont 2009). The mechanisms driving these changes and how they relate to the more rapid STRF changes remain open to future study.

Stimulus level and contrast transitions may be of particular importance to central auditory processing because natural stimuli, especially vocalizations, are characterized by large numbers of such transitions. In speech, for example, syllables are typically complex spectro-temporal patterns separated by many milleseconds of silence or background noise. Several studies have demonstrated clear differences between STRFs estimated using constant noise stimuli and natural sounds (Theunissen, Sen et al. 2000; Woolley, Gill et al. 2006; Nagel and Doupe 2008; David, Mesgarani et al. 2009).

Comparing STRFs estimated using noise and natural stimuli can be useful for identifying elements of the neural circuit that may be important for processing natural sounds. In their comparison of linear STRFs estimated from broadband rippled noise and continuous speech, David et al. (David, Mesgarani et al. 2009) identified systematic differences in the temporal response properties of STRFs estimated from the two stimulus sets. Speech STRFs tended to show more inhibition (i.e., negative STRF weights) at longer time lags than rippled noise

STRFs. These differences resulted from the temporal structure of the stimulus; STRFs estimated from a hybrid stimulus consisting of rippled noise modulated by a speech envelope were largely indistinguishable from speech STRFs. The authors hypothesized that a feedforward adaptation mechanism such as depression of synaptic inputs could produce the observed differences in STRFs. They simulated a neuron that underwent synaptic depression and found that STRFs estimated from the two stimulus categories for the simulated responses followed the same trends as the actual data. They concluded that a model accounting for synaptic depression or some other mechanism with similar nonlinear properties is necessary to fully characterize auditory representations of natural sounds. Mechanisms such as synaptic depression could play a role in the gain control mechanisms characterized by varying stimulus level and contrast (Depireux, Dobbins et al. 2012; Rabinowitz, Willmore et al. 2012).

Models incorporating nonlinear adaptation at the sensory periphery do show improved performance over linear models. Gill et al. (Gill, Zhang et al. 2006) used recordings from songbird midbrain and forebrain to compare a linear STRF to a model whose input first passed through a model of the auditory nerve that incorporated nonlinear adaptation and logarithmic compression (Lyon and Mead 1988). The nonlinear, biologically-derived model was better able to predict neural responses to birdsong stimuli than the linear STRF, indicating that nonlinear adaptation mechanisms do in fact capture important functional properties of the system.

III.3. Stimulus-dependent STRFs and Subthreshold Integration

Changes between STRFs estimated using different stimulus sets have also been used to gain insight into subthreshold excitatory and inhibitory inputs that influence neural responses, but that are not readily characterized by more traditional tuning curve analysis. Recent studies using whole cell recording techniques have determined that neurons in auditory cortex receive excitatory and inhibitory synaptic inputs with substantial overlap in their spectral tuning and that spiking output is regulated by the balance of excitatory and inhibitory inputs that are not apparent in the spiking output (Wehr and Zador 2003).

A number of studies, particularly in the songbird auditory system, have identified spectral tuning properties in STRFs estimated using natural vocalizations that are not observed in STRFs estimated using more traditional synthetic noise stimuli. Neurons in songbird areas Field L and MLd (homologous to mammalian auditory cortex and inferior colliculus, respectively) produce STRFs with different spectral bandwidth tuning, depending on whether they are estimated using random noise or conspecific birdsong (Theunissen, Sen et al. 2000; Woolley, Gill et al. 2006). Natural stimuli contain strong spectro-temporal correlations that are not present in synthetic noise stimuli, and these studies suggested that neural circuits may be activated specifically by patterns in natural stimuli in ways that cannot be observed with uncorrelated synthetic stimuli.

At first glance, the relationship between noise and song STRFs is not immediately obvious. Spectral tuning can be either broader or narrower in song STRFs compared to noise STRFs. In order to understand why tuning bandwidth might change in either direction, Schneider and Woolley (Schneider and Woolley 2011) completed a more detailed study in which they characterized nonlinear two-tone interactions in MLd neurons, in addition to measuring noise and song STRFs. They found "extra-classical" receptive field effects in which individual tones did not drive spiking responses but could either enhance or suppress responses when paired with a tone at a neuron's best frequency. These modulatory effects correlated with stimulus dependent changes in the STRF. Neurons whose STRFs had narrower bandwidth for songs tended to have inhibitory subthreshold sidebands, while those with a broader bandwidth STRFs tended to have excitatory sidebands. Birdsong, like other vocalizations, contains strong positive correlations between frequency bands, and the authors concluded these correlations produced correlated input into the subthreshold sidebands and best frequency band more often than the random noise stimuli. Thus the influence of the subthreshold inputs was stronger during the processing of natural sounds than could be observed from the responses to noise stimuli.

When linear STRFs were estimated for neurons in songbird Field L using song stimuli at different intensities, they revealed systematic changes in spectro-temporal tuning, largely consistent with a subthreshold extra-classical receptive field model (Nagel and Doupe 2008). At low sounds intensities, specto-temporal tuning was broad and contained little inhibition, consistent with neurons that acted as simple broadly-tuned detectors. At higher intensities, spectral and temporal tuning often narrowed, and inhibitory sidebands appeared, producing filters selective for more specific spectro-temporal patterns. The authors concluded that broadly tuned inhibitory inputs with high threshold are activated by the greater intensity stimuli, cancelling out broadly tuned excitation with a low threshold.

If excitation and inhibition combined linearly, they would simply cancel out, and STRFs would not depend on the spectro-temporal correlations in the stimulus. However, if excitation and inhibition combine nonlinearly, a nonlinear model accounting for subthreshold excitatory and inhibitory interactions should more accurately characterize neural response properties over a much wider range of stimuli than the linear STRF. Schinkel-Bielefeld et al. (Schinkel-Bielefeld, David et al. 2012) developed a nonlinear STRF based on the "generalized nonlinear model" approach previously used in the visual system (Butts, Weng et al. 2011) . This model fit separate linear spectro-temporal filters and static nonlinearities for excitatory and inhibitory inputs, conceptually similar to artificial neural networks (Prenger, Wu et al. 2004) and earlier models used to describe processing in the auditory periphery (Lewis and van Dijk 2003). Because the outputs of the linear filters were combined nonlinearly, the excitatory and inhibitory inputs did not simply cancel out. Instead, this architecture permitted modeling of excitatory and inhibitory inputs with different threshold and differential gain that varied across stimulus intensities.

When this excitatory/inhibitory model was applied to spiking activity recorded from ferret A1 during the presentation of speech stimuli, the resulting STRFs were able to predict neural responses to the speech stimuli better than linear STRFs estimated using the same data. Moreover, the STRFs showed several properties consistent with whole cell data (Wehr and Zador 2003) and predictions from other extracellular studies (Nagel and Doupe 2008; Schneider and Woolley 2011). Excitatory and inhibitory filters generally shared the same best frequency, and inhibitory tuning tended to be broader than excitatory tuning. Moreover, differences between the output nonlinearities for each filter lead to a recruitment of inhibition at high stimulus sound levels. The model even accounted for some unexpected phenomena. In some neurons, inhibitory gain substantially outweighed excitatory gain at high sound levels. This caused non-monotonic level tuning, with decreased response for very loud sounds (Pfingst and Oconnor 1981). Thus an STRF model that incorporated a circuit-level mechanism was better able to account for a diversity of functional properties observed throughout the auditory system.

III.4. STRF Dependence on Physiological Signal

Another question relevant to understanding the biological circuits underlying auditory processing is the relationship between single neuron activity and activity of the neural population on a larger scale. A greater understanding of these relationships can provide crucial links between single neuron data from animals and studies from humans where only the local field potential (LFP) or even coarser electroencephalographic (EEG) or magnetoencephalographic (MEG) signals can be measured (Pasley, David et al. 2012; Ding and Simon 2012a; Ding and Simon 2012b). To investigate these relationships, a few recent studies have used the LFP to measure large-scale synchronous neural activity in A1 and compared STRF estimates from LFP to those estimated from simultaneously recorded single neuron activity.

Different frequency bands of the LFP are hypothesized to represent activity of neural circuits spanning different spatial scales in the neural network. Lower frequency bands (alpha, beta, delta, 2-16 Hz) are typically attributed to large scale synchronous oscillations across or between brain areas (Pinto, Jones et al. 2003). The gamma band (16-40 Hz) is typically attributed to oscillating excitatory-inhibitory circuits within a cortical column (Borgers and Kopell 2003). The high gamma band is closely associated with the level of multi-unit activity (oscillatory or not) close to the recording site (Crone, Miglioretti et al. 1998).

The same fundamental analytical approaches used for STRF estimation with single unit data can be applied to LFP signals. However, because the LFP is thought to represent the combination of multiple physiological processes, the LFP signal can be pre-processed a variety of ways to produce the response vector, r (see above, section I), that captures activity on the scale of interest. For the analysis of low-frequency LFP, the response can simply be defined as the raw time-varying voltage trace recorded on the electrode. For higher frequencies (> 20 Hz), however, only very weak phase-locking is observed between the raw trace and the stimulus. Instead, the variance of the LFP, reflecting modulation of processes that are not perfectly stimulus-locked, is more often correlated with the stimulus envelope. In this case, the LFP is bandpass-filtered, selecting the frequency band of interest (e.g., 16-40 Hz for the gamma band), and the time-varying envelope amplitude of the bandpassed signal is used to define the response.

Eggermont et al (Eggermont, Munguia et al. 2011) found a rough agreement in the tuning of the LFP voltage trace and single neurons in A1, but that the LFP was generally much less selective for stimulus frequency, agreeing largely with earlier tuning curve analysis (Kayser, Petkov et al. 2007). When STRFs were computed for separate bands of the LFP envelope, the gamma band still showed relatively weak auditory tuning but had a much greater correspondence to the single neuron STRFs than the lower frequencies.

These results were largely replicated in a later study (Gaucher, Edeline et al. 2012) . This study also explored spectro-temporal tuning in higher gamma frequencies of the LFP (> 70 Hz) and found an even greater degree of similarity between the LFP in this band and single neuron STRFs. These findings add to growing evidence that high frequency LFP is closely related to nearby multi-unit activity.

Although the tuning of single low-frequency LFP channels tends to be quite broad, a recent study revealed that substantially finer-grained information can be extracted from LFP recorded simultaneously from multiple electrodes in A1 (de Cheveigne, Edeline et al. 2013) . This study adapted the denoising source separation algorithm (DSS, Sarela and Valpola 2005), originally developed for noninvasive human neurophysiology, into LFP analysis. The DSS algorithm linearly transforms the population LFP signal into a new space, each dimension defined by the LFP activity most correlated with a different stimulus frequency band (following the logic of input transformation described in Section I. 3). An STRF was then estimated between the transformed LFP signal for each band and the original stimulus. The resulting STRFs, surprisingly, showed spectral tuning bandwidths similar to those measured using multi-unit activity. Thus, although low sensory selectivity of low frequency LFP in A1 is sometimes attributed to a dominance of non-sensory inputs from other cortical areas, these findings suggest that sensory signals may also simply be degraded because low frequency LFP is pooled over neurons in a larger volume of cortex. If this pooling is relatively uniform, then more detailed stimulus information can be extracted by component analysis of LFP recorded simultaneously in multiple locations. Of course, the fact that more stimulus information may be available in the LFP does not rule out the possibility that intracortical inputs contribute substantially to the low frequency band. Further studies using simultaneous recordings from multiple brain areas will be necessary to completely characterize the neural activity that constitutes these signals.

Electrocorticographic (ECoG) recordings from human epilepsy patients produce signals similar to animal LFP. Because they are recorded subdurally, they can achieve greater anatomical resolution, preserving signals in the high gamma range that are not measurable with MEG or EEG. Understanding the relationship between high gamma signals and single units is of particular interest for interpreting data from these studies, and linking them to more invasive animal studies. High gamma ECoG recordings from the superior temporal gyrus (STG) of patients listening to speech have revealed tuned STRFs that roughly resemble STRFs measured from single neurons in animal cortex (Mesgarani and Chang 2012; Pasley, David et al. 2012). At high gamma frequencies (>100 Hz), the raw voltage trace is not phase-locked to the stimulus envelope. Instead, the envelope of the high gamma band is correlated with the stimulus. Because the STG is not a primary auditory area (rather one or two synapses downstream from A1) it is difficult to attribute any specific differences to properties of the physiological signals or to extra processing that may have taken place between primary auditory cortex and STG. Further analysis of high gamma in multiple areas of animal cortex promises to answer some of these open questions.

Additional questions remain about the relationship of low-frequency LFP signals and single neuron activity. The majority of the published work has been completed in anesthetized animals and has yet to be replicated in awake animals. Because the LFP is sensitive to the state of arousal and anesthesia, activity in awake animals may be qualitatively different than what has been observed thus far. Studies in awake animals have shown that the phase of low-frequency oscillations can reflect multi-modal or top-down feedback to auditory cortex that modulates neural response gain (Lakatos, Chen et al. 2007) . The relationship of these modulations to spectro-temporal filter properties remains largely unexplored.

III.5. STRF Dependence On Experience and Behavioral State

A final question of central importance to studies of auditory processing is the dependence of spectrotemporal filter properties on behavioral state. The basic role of the auditory system for an animal is to guide behavior. Thus at some level, auditory processing must extract behaviorally relevant features from the incoming stimulus, which can change rapidly between behavioral contexts. The influence of behavioral state on sensory representations can be characterized by comparing STRFs measured using identical stimuli while recording the same neural signal but controlling behavioral state (Section II. 3).

III.5.a. Long-term, Learning-dependent STRF Changes

Numerous studies using this approach have determined that the filter properties of neurons in the auditory system continue to change and adapt through adulthood. The brain changes as animals learn new sounds and sound categories (Bakin and Weinberger 1996; Ohl, Scheich et al. 2001; Blake, Strata et al. 2002). In a groundbreaking series of studies, Ohl and Scheich (Ohl and Scheich 1997) trained Mongolian gerbils on a number of behaviors in which stimuli were paired with rewards. Using chronic LFP recordings in auditory cortex, they observed systematic plasticity in STRFs. When animals were rewarded for a tone at a fixed frequency, the representation of that frequency was expanded. Subsequent experiments, which used similar behavior but required grouping stimuli across frequencies, produced responses that were invariant to the frequencies of sounds within a group. Thus the plastic changes observed in STRFs might reflect mechanisms that support the formation of new category representations.

III.5.b. Rapid, Reversible STRF Changes

In addition to long-term plasticity, the way sounds are processed can depend on short-term changes in behavioral state. A number of studies have taken this perspective in testing the hypothesis that the brain dynamically adjusts its auditory filtering properties in order to process sound features relevant to current task demands (Fritz, Elhilali et al. 2007) . A change in the STRF between controlled behavior conditions reflects the focus of selective attention or the influence of more general arousal or engagement during a particular task.

In a series of experiments, Fritz et al. (Fritz, Shamma et al. 2003; Fritz, Elhilali et al. 2005) set out to identify rapid changes in STRFs during tone detection tasks. The basic theory driving these studies is that when attention is directed toward a specific spectro-temporal feature or set of features, the selectivity of neurons in auditory cortex should shift to reflect differences between task-relevant categories (Mesgarani, Fritz et al. 2010).

In the initial study, ferrets were trained to discriminate between a reference sound, constructed from temporally orthogonal ripple combinations (TORCs, Klein, Depireux et al. 2000), and a target tone. Animals were trained by conditioned avoidance to cease licking a water spout after target offset in order to avoid a small tail shock. The carrier frequency of the target tone was fixed during a single behavioral block but was varied between experiments. By using TORC stimuli as reference sounds, this experimental design permitted the measurement of STRFs during behavior, which could then be compared to STRFs measured during passive listening immediately before and after behavior blocks. Thus the same stimulus was presented in two different behavioral conditions (Figure 7). When these STRFs were compared between passive and active states, the STRFs measured during behavior showed enhanced gain at the target frequency. This enhancement reverted back to baseline in the passive state, although the rate of return to baseline varied across cells (Fritz, Shamma et al. 2003).

In subsequent studies, the group used a similar behavior but with a two-tone discrimination task, in which the reference noise was concatenated with a second pure tone at a different frequency than the target (Fritz, Elhilali et al. 2005). Ferrets now had to discriminate between two tone frequencies. During this behavior, STRFs for A1 neurons underwent selective suppression at the reference tone frequency in addition to enhancement at the target frequency.

The initial studies by Fritz et al (Fritz, Shamma et al. 2003; Fritz, Elhilali et al. 2005) demonstrated that neurons in A1 change their spectro-temporal tuning properties so as to enhance differences between task-relevant sound features, in this case, the spectral differences between the broadband TORC reference and the narrowband, fixed frequency target. These changes made sense from the theoretical perspective of the matched filter (Mesgarani, Fritz et al. 2010), but the absolute direction of changes in tuning was not prescribed theoretically. Namely, if STRFs revealed a selective suppression rather than enhancement at the target frequency, the changes would be equally consistent with a matched filter. A later study determined that depending on the structure of the behavior, STRFs can change in the opposite direction with respect to the target (David, Fritz et al. 2012). When ferrets were trained to perform the identical noise versus tone detection, but were rewarded for licking a water spout after target onset (i.e., an approach, rather than avoidance, task), STRFs in A1 underwent opposite changes, namely selectively decreasing their gain at the target frequency. These results indicate that STRFs of single neurons in auditory cortex change their tuning not only to match task-relevant sound features, but also to reflect higher-order elements of the task structure, such as the required motor outputs or stimulus-related reward.

III.5.c. Rapid STRF Changes in Humans during Behavior

Behavioral studies with animals have opened up several exciting new avenues for exploring the interaction between behavioral state and spectro-temporal representations. However, studies so far have been limited to relatively simple behaviors, focusing on changes between a passive state and a single behavioral state. These limitations reflect the need for large datasets to measure accurate STRFs and the challenge of training animals to switch between auditory tasks. Recent studies in humans, while lacking the resolution of single-unit recordings, have produced several new findings that complement the animal studies.

In a study using noninvasive magnetoencephalography (MEG), human subjects were asked to selectively attend to one of two human speakers, presented either dichotically (Ding and Simon 2012a) or diotically (Ding and Simon 2012b). These behaviors modeled the more general process of streaming required to solve the classic "cocktail party" problem (Bregman 1990). Spectral tuning could only be measured very coarsely from the MEG signal, but the temporal response function (TRF), reflecting responses to the speech envelope averaged across stimulus frequencies could be recovered reliably. When TRFs were measured for the simultaneously presented speakers, they were found to reflect predominantly the influence of the attended speaker, in both dichotic and diotic conditions. Furthermore, the TRF measured for the attended speaker was invariant to level, with gain scaling reciprocally to the loudness of the attended speaker (Ding and Simon 2012b). These TRF changes were consistent with a decoding analysis, which revealed that the envelope of the attended speaker could be recovered more accurately than the envelope of the non-attended speaker.

Subdural electrocorticographic (ECoG) recordings from human neurosurgical patients provide access to finer spatial signals on the brain surface that permit measurement of more detailed spectro-temporal tuning (Mesgarani and Chang 2012; Pasley, David et al. 2012). Low-frequency ECoG signals, like LFP from animal recordings, tend to reveal STRFs with coarse spectral tuning and with strong correlations between recording channels. However, when the ECoG signal is filtered into the high-gamma band, STRFs reveal tighter spectro-temporal tuning which varies substantially, even between channels separated by as little as 0.4 mm. Although data limitations prevented the estimation of reliable STRFs during behavior, a decoding analysis reconstructed the spectrogram of the attended speaker with substantially greater fidelity than the non-attended speaker. These results are consistent with the MEG studies (Ding and Simon 2012a; Ding and Simon 2012b) and further show that the auditory system preserved lower-level spectral as well as temporal features of an attended sound while suppressing spectro-temporal information about the non-attended sound, even if the two sounds lie in overlapping spectral bands. Further studies in humans and animals will likely elucidate the mechanisms by which neurons dynamically adapt their spectro-temporal tuning properties to separate overlapping auditory streams and selectively enhance information about the attended stream.

IV. Discussion

The diversity of applications for STRF analysis continues to grow as new analytical and experimental methods are developed. As we have discussed, STRFs can be applied to a wide range of questions about the structure of neural circuits and the influence of behavioral context on sensory representation. Although the performance of more complex STRF models is often data-limited, this limitation is likely to become less problematic as new methods for chronic neurophysiological recording become more widely used.

Given the diversity of STRF models and methods, one of the biggest challenges facing the experimenter is the choice of which analytical approach is most appropriate to the scientific problem and data of interest. Critical to this decision is a clear understanding of the limitations of different STRF implementations and of the relationship between the STRF model and an underlying hypothesis about neural coding.

IV.1. Practical Considerations in STRF Estimation and Validation

The cross-validation framework for testing model predictive power provides a powerful tool for relatively unbiased comparison of models that might differ substantially in their underlying structure. It is important to keep in mind, however, that model complexity, taken roughly as the number of fit parameters, can still matter, especially when the amount of data available for model estimation is limited. These concerns are particularly relevant to studies of behavior, when data are often restricted to a relatively small number of behavioral trials. Finite estimation data fundamentally limits the accuracy of a model fit, which will then limit its performance in a cross-validation test (Sahani 2002; Hsu, Borst et al. 2004; David and Gallant 2005). When data are limited, a simpler, less physiologically accurate model may actually predict better than a more accurate model that requires many more parameters.

Additional concerns arise when comparing STRFs estimated using different stimulus sets. A model capable of capturing the relevant nonlinear properties of the system can fail to generalize across stimulus domains when those regimes are too narrowly sampled. For example, a nonlinear model may be able to explain gain adaptation to changes in stimulus contrast. If fit separately to stimuli sampling narrow but different stimulus contrast regimes, the model fits may appear substantially different that a single model fit to the combined stimulus sets. The example in Figure 6F illustrates this problem for the simpler regime of nonlinear gain. In this example, one sees a small disagreement between the fits, which is particularly evident in predictions for large inputs by the model fit using low-intensity inputs.

When estimation data are limited, model performance can often be improved by imposing prior assumptions on the fits, based on a broader understanding of the underlying neural circuit (Wu, David et al. 2006). Thus if frequency tuning curves in the auditory cortex tend to be smooth, one might impose a smooth prior on the STRF (Sahani and Linden 2003). Many regression methods contain implicit assumptions, for example, about the statistical properties of the input signal (Theunissen, David et al. 2001). While generally useful for improving performance in isolated conditions, these analytical biases may not generalize across data sets or systems and can confuse the interpretation of results. In general, simulations provide a useful way of testing how large a data set might be required for an experiment and of biases that might appear in model estimates when data are limited (David and Gallant 2005; David, Mesgarani et al. 2007).

IV.2. Stimulus Context and Spectro-temporal Filter Properties

Fundamentally, the brain is a nonstationary system, and STRFs represent a stationary model of that system. It has long been known that stimulus history, the pattern of auditory input (loudness, spectral bandwidth, temporal autocorrelation, etc) over the previous one to tens of seconds, can have dramatic influences on the response of a neuron, which largely cannot be modeled by the linear STRF, given its relatively short integration window. These effects become more profound as information travels more centrally into the nervous system. Classical implementations of the STRF have largely ignored this transient and focused instead on the "steady-state" period following the onset transient.

Creative adaptations of classical models have led to a number of useful strategies for incorporating contextual effects into STRF models. Recent studies have sought to address this limitation by accounting for dynamic aspects of stimulus context (Depireux, Dobbins et al. 2012; Rabinowitz, Willmore et al. 2012) or for differences in behavioral state (Ohl and Scheich 1997; Fritz, Shamma et al. 2003). Looking forward, STRF models that incorporate contextual influences directly into their structure promise new and exciting insight into the higher-order representation of auditory stimuli.

References

Abbott, L. F. and W. G. Regehr (2004). "Synaptic computation." *Nature* 431(7010): 796-803.

Aertsen, A. M. and P. I. Johannesma (1981). "The spectro-temporal receptive field. A functional characteristic of auditory neurons." *Biol. Cybern.* 42(2): 133-143.

Aertsen, A. M. H. J. and P. I. M. Johannesma (1981). "A comparison of the spectro-temporal sensitivity of auditory neurons to tonal and natural stimuli." *Biological Cybernetics* 42: 145-156.

Aguera y Arcas, B., A. L. Fairhall, et al. (2003). "Computation in a single neuron: Hodgkin and Huxley revisited." *Neural Comput.* 15(8): 1715-1749.

Atencio, C. A., T. O. Sharpee, et al. (2012). "Receptive field dimensionality increases from the auditory midbrain to cortex." *Journal of Neurophysiology* 107(10): 2594-2603.

Bakin, J. S. and N. M. Weinberger (1996). "Induction of a physiological memory in the cerebral cortex by stimulation of the nucleus basalis." *Proceedings of the National Academy of Sciences of the United States of America* 93(20): 11219-11224.

Blake, D. T. and M. M. Merzenich (2002). "Changes of AI receptive fields with sound density." *Journal of Neurophysiology* 88(6): 3409-3420.

Blake, D. T., F. Strata, et al. (2002). "Neural correlates of instrumental learning in primary auditory cortex." *Proceedings of the National Academy of Sciences of the United States of America* 99(15): 10114-10119.

Borgers, C. and N. Kopell (2003). "Synchronization in networks of excitatory and inhibitory neurons with sparse, random connectivity." *Neural Computation* 15(3): 509-538.

Bregman, A. (1990). *Auditory Scene Analysis.* Cambridge, Mass, MIT Press.

Brenner, N., W. Bialek, et al. (2000). "Adaptive rescaling maximizes information transmission." *Neuron* 26(3): 695-702.

Butts, D. A., C. Weng, et al. (2011). "Temporal precision in the visual pathway through the interplay of excitation and stimulus-driven suppression." *Journal of Neuroscience* 31(31): 11313-11327.

Calabrese, A., J. W. Schumacher, et al. (2011). "A generalized linear model for estimating spectrotemporal receptive fields from responses to natural sounds." *PLoS One* 6(1).

Christianson, G. B., M. Sahani, et al. (2008). "The consequences of response nonlinearities for interpretation of spectrotemporal receptive fields." *Journal of Neuroscience* 28(2): 446-455.

Clopton, B. M. and P. M. Backoff (1991). "Spectraltemporal receptive fields of neurons of cochlear nucleus of guinea pig." *Hear. Res.* 52: 410-422.

Crone, N. E., D. L. Miglioretti, et al. (1998). "Functional mapping of human sensorimotor cortex with electrocorticographic spectral analysis - I. Alpha and beta event-related desynchronization." *Brain* 121: 2271-2299.

David, S. V., J. B. Fritz, et al. (2012). "Task reward structure shapes rapid receptive field plasticity in auditory cortex." *Proceedings of the National Academy of Sciences of the United States of America* 109(6): 2144-2149.

David, S. V. and J. L. Gallant (2005). "Predicting neuronal responses during natural vision." *Network-Computation in Neural Systems* 16(2-3): 239-260.

David, S. V., N. Mesgarani, et al. (2009). "Rapid synaptic depression explains nonlinear modulation of spectro-temporal tuning in primary auditory cortex by natural stimuli." *Journal of Neuroscience* 29(11): 3374-3386.

David, S. V., N. Mesgarani, et al. (2007). "Estimating sparse spectro-temporal receptive fields with natural stimuli." *Network-Computation in Neural Systems* 18(3): 191-212.

de Boer, E. (1967). "Correlation studies applied to the frequency resolution of the cochlea." *Journal of Auditory Research* 7: 209-217.

de Boer, E. and P. Kuyper (1968). "Triggered correlation." *IEEE Transactions on Biomedical Engineering* 15: 159-179.

de Cheveigne, A., J.-M. Edeline, et al. (2013). "Component analysis reveals sharp tuning of the local field potential in the guinea pig auditory cortex." *Journal of Neurophysiology* 109(1): 261-272.

Dean, I., B. L. Robinson, et al. (2008). "Rapid neural adaptation to sound level statistics." *Journal of Neuroscience* 28(25): 6430-6438.

deCharms, R. C., D. T. Blake, et al. (1998). "Optimizing sound features for cortical neurons." *Science* 280(5368): 1439-1443.

Depireux, D. A., H. D. Dobbins, et al. (2012). "Dynamics of phase-independent spectro-temporal tuning in primary auditory cortex of the awake ferret." *Neuroscience* 214: 28-35.

Ding, N. and J. Z. Simon (2012a). "Neural coding of continuous speech in auditory cortex during monaural and dichotic listening." *Journal of Neurophysiology* 107(1): 78-89.

Ding, N. and J. Z. Simon (2012b). "Emergence of neural encoding of auditory objects while listening to competing speakers." *Proceedings of the National Academy of Sciences of the United States of America* 109(29): 11854-11859.

Dobson, A. (2002). *An Introduction to Generalized Linear Models.*, Chapman & Hall/CRC.

Egelhaaf, M. and W. Reichardt (1987). "Dynamic-response properties of movement detectors - theoretical-analysis and electrophysiological investigation in the visual-system of the fly." *Biological Cybernetics* 56(2-3): 69-87.

Eggermont, J. J., A. M. Aertsen, et al. (1983). "Quantitative characterisation procedure for auditory neurons based on the spectro-temporal receptive field." *Hear. Res.* 10(2): 167-190.

Eggermont, J. J., R. Munguia, et al. (2011). "Comparison of LFP-based and spike-based spectro-temporal receptive fields and cross-correlation in cat primary auditory cortex." *PLoS One* 6(5).

Escabi, M. A., L. M. Miller, et al. (2003). "Naturalistic auditory contrast improves spectrotemporal coding in the cat inferior colliculus." *J. Neurosci.* 23(37): 11489-11504.

Fitzgerald, J. D., L. C. Sincich, et al. (2011). "Minimal models of multidimensional computations." *Plos Computational Biology* 7(3).

Friedman, J. and B. Popescu (2003). "Gradient directed regularization for linear regression and classification." Technical Report, Statistics Department, Stanford University.

Fritz, J., S. Shamma, et al. (2003). "Rapid task-related plasticity of spectrotemporal receptive fields in primary auditory cortex." *Nature Neuroscience* 6(11): 1216-1223.

Fritz, J. B., M. Elhilali, et al. (2007). "Does attention play a role in dynamic receptive field adaptation to changing acoustic salience in Al?" *Hearing Research* 229(1-2): 186-203.

Fritz, J. B., M. Elhilali, et al. (2005). "Differential dynamic plasticity of A1 receptive fields during multiple spectral tasks." *Journal of Neuroscience* 25(33): 7623-7635.

Gabbiani, F., H. G. Krapp, et al. (2004). "Multiplication and stimulus invariance in a looming-sensitive neuron." *Journal of Physiology-Paris* 98(1-3): 19-34.

Gaucher, Q., J.-M. Edeline, et al. (2012). "How different are the local field potentials and spiking activities? Insights from multi-electrodes arrays." *Journal of Physiology-Paris* 106(3-4): 93-103.

Gill, P., J. Zhang, et al. (2006). "Sound representation methods for spectro-temporal receptive field estimation." *J. Comput. Neurosci.* 22: 22.

Gourevitch, B., A. Norena, et al. (2009). "Spectrotemporal receptive fields in anesthetized cat primary auditory cortex are context dependent." *Cerebral Cortex* 19(6): 1448-1461.

Hartline, H. K. (1940). "The receptive fields of optic nerve fibers." *Am. J. Physiol.* 130: 690-699.

Hermes, D. J., A. M. Aertsen, et al. (1981). "Spectro-temporal characteristics of single units in the auditory midbrain of the lightly anaesthetised grass frog (Rana temporaria L) investigated with noise stimuli." *Hear. Res.* 5(2-3): 147-178.

Hida, E. and K.-I. Naka (1983). "A new method for mapping spatio-temporal receptive fields using television snow stimulation." *Journal of Neuroscience Methods* 8: 225-230.

Hoerl, A. E. and R. W. Kennard (2000). "Ridge regression: Biased estimation for nonorthogonal problems." *Technometrics* 42(1): 80-86.

Hsu, A., A. Borst, et al. (2004). "Quantifying variability in neural responses and its application for the validation of model predictions." *Network* 15(2): 91-109.

Hunter, I. W. and M. J. Korenberg (1986). "The identification of nonlinear biological-systems - Wiener and Hammerstein cascade models." *Biological Cybernetics* 55(2-3): 135-144.

Karklin, Y. and M. S. Lewicki (2003). "Learning higher-order structures in natural images." *Network-Computation in Neural Systems* 14(3): 483-499.

Kay, K. N., T. Naselaris, et al. (2008). "Identifying natural images from human brain activity." *Nature* 452(7185): 352-355.

Kay, S. (1993). *Fundamentals of Statistical Signal Processing. Estimation Theory.* Englewood Cliffs, NJ, Prentice Hall.

Kayser, C., C. I. Petkov, et al. (2007). "Tuning to sound frequency in auditory field potentials." *Journal of Neurophysiology* 98(3): 1806-1809.

Klein, D. J., D. A. Depireux , et al. (2000). "Robust spectro-temporal reverse correlation for the auditory system: Optimizing stimulus design." *J. Comp. Neurosci.* 9(1): 85-111.

Korenberg, M. J. and I. W. Hunter (1999). "Two methods for identifying Wiener cascades having noninvertible static nonlinearities." *Annals of Biomedical Engineering* 27(6): 793-804.

Kouh, M. and T. O. Sharpee (2009). "Estimating linear-nonlinear models using Renyi divergences." *Network-Computation in Neural Systems* 20(2): 49-68.

Kowalski, N., D. A. Depireux, et al. (1996). "Analysis of dynamic spectra in ferret primary auditory cortex. I. Characteristics of single-unit responses to moving ripple spectra." *J. Neurophysiol.* 76(5): 3503-3523.

Lakatos, P., C.-M. Chen, et al. (2007). "Neuronal oscillations and multisensory interaction in primary auditory cortex." *Neuron* 53(2): 279-292.

Lewis, E. R. and P. van Dijk (2003). "New variations on the derivation of spectro-temporal receptive fields for primary auditory afferent axons." *Hearing Research* 186(1-2): 30-46.

Linden, J. F., R. C. Liu, et al. (2003). "Spectrotemporal structure of receptive fields in areas AI and AAF of mouse auditory cortex." *Journal of Neurophysiology* 90(4): 2660-2675.

Lyon, R. F. and C. Mead (1988). "An analog electronic cochlea." *Ieee Transactions on Acoustics Speech and Signal Processing* 36(7): 1119-1134.

Marmarelis, P.Z. and V.Z. Marmarelis (1978). *Analysis of Physiological Systems. The White Noise Approach*. New York, Plenum.

Mesgarani, N. and E. F. Chang (2012). "Selective cortical representation of attended speaker in multi-talker speech perception." *Nature* 485(7397): 233-236.

Mesgarani, N., J. Fritz, et al. (2010). "A computational model of rapid task-related plasticity of auditory cortical receptive fields." *Journal of Computational Neuroscience* 28(1): 19-27.

Miller, L. M., M. A. Escabi, et al. (2001). "Functional convergence of response properties in the auditory thalamocortical system." *Neuron* 32(1): 151-160.

Nagel, K. I. and A. J. Doupe (2008). "Organizing principles of spectro-temporal encoding in the avian primary auditory area field L." *Neuron* 58(6): 938-955.

Nemenman, I., W. Bialek, et al. (2004). "Entropy and information in neural spike trains: Progress on the sampling problem." *Physical Review E* 69(5): 056111.

Norena, A. J., B. Gourevitch, et al. (2008). "Increasing spectrotemporal sound density reveals an octave-based organization in cat primary auditory cortex." *Journal of Neuroscience* 28(36): 8885-8896.

Ohl, F. W. and H. Scheich (1997). "Learning-induced dynamic receptive field changes in primary auditory cortex of the unanaesthetized Mongolian gerbil." *Journal of Comparative Physiology a-Neuroethology Sensory Neural and Behavioral Physiology* 181(6): 685-696.

Ohl, F. W., H. Scheich, et al. (2001). "Change in pattern of ongoing cortical activity with auditory category learning." *Nature* 412(6848): 733-736.

Paninski, L. (2004). "Maximum likelihood estimation of cascade point-process neural encoding models." *Network: Computation in Neural Systems* 15(4): 243-262.

Paninski, L., J. W. Pillow, et al. (2004). "Maximum likelihood estimation of a stochastic integrate-and-fire neural encoding model." *Neural Computation* 16(12): 2533-2561.

Pasley, B. N., S. V. David, et al. (2012). "Reconstructing speech from human auditory cortex." *Plos Biology* 10(1).

Pena, J. L. and M. Konishi (2004). "Robustness of multiplicative processes in auditory spatial tuning." *Journal of Neuroscience* 24(40): 8907-8910.

Pfingst, B. E. and T. A. Oconnor (1981). "Characteristics of Neurons in Auditory-Cortex of Monkeys Performing a Simple Auditory Task." *Journal of Neurophysiology* 45(1): 16-34.

Pienkowski, M. and J. J. Eggermont (2009). "Effects of adaptation on spectrotemporal receptive fields in primary auditory cortex." *Neuroreport* 20(13): 1198-1203.

Pillow, J. W., L. Paninski, et al. (2005). "Prediction and decoding of retinal ganglion cell responses with a probabilistic spiking model." *Journal of Neuroscience* 25(47): 11003-11013.

Pinto, D. J., S. R. Jones, et al. (2003). "Analysis of state-dependent transitions in frequency and long-distance coordination in a model oscillatory cortical circuit." *Journal of Computational Neuroscience* 15(2): 283-298.

Prenger, R., M. C. K. Wu, et al. (2004). "Nonlinear V1 responses to natural scenes revealed by neural network analysis." *Neural Networks* 17(5-6): 663-679.

Rabinowitz, N. C., B. D. B. Willmore, et al. (2012). "Spectrotemporal contrast kernels for neurons in primary auditory cortex." *Journal of Neuroscience* 32(33): 11271-11284.

Reiss, L. A. J., S. Bandyopadhyay, et al. (2007). "Effects of stimulus spectral contrast on receptive fields of dorsal cochlear nucleus neurons." *Journal of Neurophysiology* 98(4): 2133-2143.

Richard, J. P., H. J. Leppelsack, et al. (1995). "A rapid correlation method for the analysis of spectro-temporal receptive fields of auditory neurons." *Journal of Neuroscience Methods* 61(1-2): 99-103.

Sahani, M. and J. Linden (2003). Evidence optimization techniques for estimating stimulus-response functions. *Advances in Neural Infomation Processing Systems*. S. Becker, S. Thrun and K. Obermeyer. Cambridge, MA, MIT Press. 15: 301-308.

Sahani, M., Linden, J (2002). "How linear are auditory cortical responses?" *Advances in Neural Infomation Processing Systems*. Vol. 15. Cambridge, MA, MIT Press..

Sarela, J. and H. Valpola (2005). "Denoising source separation." *Journal of Machine Learning Research* 6: 233-272.

Schinkel-Bielefeld, N., S. V. David, et al. (2012). "Inferring the role of inhibition in auditory processing of complex natural stimuli." *Journal of Neurophysiology* 107(12): 3296-3307.

Schneider, D. M. and S. M. N. Woolley (2010). "Discrimination of communication vocalizations by single neurons and groups of neurons in the auditory midbrain." *Journal of Neurophysiology* 103(6): 3248-3265.

Schneider, D. M. and S. M. N. Woolley (2011). "Extra-classical tuning predicts stimulus-dependent receptive fields in auditory neurons." *Journal of Neuroscience* 31(33): 11867-11878.

Sharpee, T., N. C. Rust, et al. (2004). "Analyzing neural responses to natural signals: maximally informative dimensions." *Neural Comput.* 16(2): 223-250.

Sharpee, T. O., K. D. Miller, et al. (2008). "On the importance of static nonlinearity in estimating spatiotemporal neural filters with natural stimuli." *Journal of Neurophysiology* 99(5): 2496-2509.

Shechter, B. and D. A. Depireux (2006). "Response adaptation to broadband sounds in primary auditory cortex of the awake ferret." *Hearing Research* 221(1-2): 91-103.

Shechter, B. and D. A. Depireux (2007). "Stability of spectro-temporal tuning over several seconds in primary auditory cortex of the awake ferret." *Neuroscience* 148(3): 806-814.

Singh, N. C. and F. E. Theunissen (2003). "Modulation spectra of natural sounds and ethological theories of auditory processing." *J. Acoust. Soc. Am.* 114(6 Pt 1): 3394-3411.

Theunissen, F. E., S. V. David, et al. (2001). "Estimating spatio-temporal receptive fields of auditory and visual neurons from their responses to natural stimuli." *Network: Comp. Neural Syst.* 12: 1-28.

Theunissen, F. E., K. Sen, et al. (2000). "Spectral-temporal receptive fields of nonlinear auditory neurons obtained using natural sounds." *J. Neurosci.* 20(6): 2315-2331.

Touryan, J., G. Felsen, et al. (2005). "Spatial Structure of Complex Cell Receptive Fields Measured with Natural Images." *Neuron* 45(5): 781-791.

Wehr, M. and A. M. Zador (2003). "Balanced inhibition underlies tuning and sharpens spike timing in auditory cortex." *Nature* 426(6965): 442-446.

Willmore, B. D. B., R. J. Prenger, et al. (2010). "Neural Representation of Natural Images in Visual Area V2." *Journal of Neuroscience* 30(6): 2102-2114.

Woolley, S. M., P. R. Gill, et al. (2006). "Stimulus-dependent auditory tuning results in synchronous population coding of vocalizations in the songbird midbrain." *J. Neurosci.* 26(9): 2499-2512.

Wu, M. C. K., S. V. David, et al. (2006). Complete functional characterization of sensory neurons by system identification. *Annual Review of Neuroscience*. 29: 477-505.

In: Handbook of Modern Techniques in Auditory Cortex ISBN: 978-1-62808-894-6
Editors: Didier A. Depireux and Mounya Elhailali

Chapter 7

Probabilistic Methods for Linear and Multilinear Models

***Maneesh Sahani*[1], *Ross S. Williamson*[1,2], *Misha B. Ahrens*[1] *and Jennifer F. Linden*[3]**
[1]Gatsby Computational Neuroscience Unit,
[2]Centre for Mathematics and Physics in the Life Sciences and Experimental Biology,
[3]Ear Institute and Department of Neuroscience, Physiology & Pharmacology
University College London, London, UK

1. Descriptive *versus* Predictive Characterisations of Sensory Neurons

A central goal of sensory neurophysiology is to identify those aspects of a stimulus that modulate the firing of individual neurons. There are at least two distinct but complementary conceptual approaches to this goal. Whilst both frequently converge on the same broad mathematical relationships, they differ subtly in their interpretation of the significance of those relationships; and those differences of interpretation may, in turn, lead to substantial differences in the details of the mathematical analyses adopted under each approach. One strategy, which we might call *receptive field characterisation*, seeks to describe the aspects of stimuli that increase or suppress firing probability in the neuron. The alternative, *response function identification*, attempts to construct a predictive model that mimics the true physiologically implemented function that maps an arbitrary stimulus to the resulting neuronal reponse.

The difference in the interpretations favoured by the two approaches appears even in consideration of the basic STRF, which plays a central role within both approaches either as the *spectrotemporal receptive field* or as the *spectrotemporally-linear response function*. Suppose an acoustic stimulus with spectrogram $s(i, k)$ evokes a neural response $r(i)$, where $i = 1 \dots T$ indexes time frames within the spectrogram and $k = 1 \dots K$ indexes spectral channel. For simplicity, we assume that the response is measured at the temporal precision of spectrogram timeframes, if necessary after oversampling one or the other signal. Thus, $r(i)$ might represent the number of action potentials produced by a neuron during stimulus timeframe i. This number is often averaged over multiple repetitions of the stimulus.

In the descriptive sense, the STRF may be defined in terms of the spike-triggered average (STA) of the stimulus spectrogram. The matched discretisation of response and stimulus makes the STA straightforward to compute. Each action potential falling in the ith frame is associated with the same section of the spectrogram, and so the STA is simply proportional to the sum of all spectrogram windows (chosen to be J frames long) weighted by the number of corresponding spikes:

$$\text{STA}(j, k) \propto \sum_{i=J-1}^{T} r(i) s(i - j + 1, k) \,, \tag{1}$$

where $j = 1 \dots J$ indexes time lag within the STA. As a description of the regions of spectrotemporal energy that either excite or suppress firing in a neuron, the STA suffers from possible confounding effects of correlations or other internal dependencies within the stimulus. For instance, suppose that a neuron were sensitive to energy in a frequency channel k, but not to energy in another channel k'. If energy in these two channels tended to co-occur in the stimulus then spikes induced by energy in channel k would also correlate with energy in channel k', and so the STA would incorrectly show an artifactual influence of that channel.

This confound can be lessened, and in some cases eliminated, by "correcting" the STA by the stimulus autocorrelation function. This correction takes a straightforward form once Eq. 1 is expressed in vector notation. Let us represent the stimulus spectrogram by a $T \times JK$ matrix $\mathbf{M}^{\mathtt{i(tf)}}$ (the origin of this notation will be explained below), in which the rows represent different times, and the column index ranges over all the frequency channels and time lags to be considered in the STRF. That is, $M_{il}^{\mathtt{i(tf)}} = s(i - j, k)$ for $i \geq J - 1$, $l = (k - 1) * J + j$, and $= 0$ when $i < J - 1$. If the response is now collected into a $1 \times T$ vector $\mathbf{r}$ then Eq. 1 can be written compactly in vector form $\mathbf{w}_{\text{STA}}^{\mathtt{(tf)}} \propto \mathbf{M}^{\mathtt{i(tf)}\top}\mathbf{r}$, where $\mathbf{w}_{\text{STA}}^{\mathtt{(tf)}}$ is a $JK \times 1$ column vector whose elements correspond to those of the STA and $^\top$ represents the matrix transpose.

In this notation, the stimulus autocorrelation is given by the $JK \times JK$ matrix $\mathbf{M}^{\mathtt{i(tf)}\top}\mathbf{M}^{\mathtt{i(tf)}}$ and so "correcting" the STA by premultiplying by the inverse autocorrelation matrix gives the STRF as a $JK \times 1$ vector

$$\mathbf{w}^{\mathtt{(tf)}} = (\mathbf{M}^{\mathtt{i(tf)}\top}\mathbf{M}^{\mathtt{i(tf)}})^{-1}\mathbf{M}^{\mathtt{i(tf)}\top}\mathbf{r} \,. \tag{2}$$

The elements of this vector can be rearranged to produce the familiar two-dimensional STRF, which depicts the spectrotemporal inputs that excite or suppress firing. It is important to note that although multiplication by the inverse of the autocorrelation matrix lessens the effects of internal dependence within the stimulus in many cases, it does not necessarily eliminate these effects entirely. In particular, if the neuron's response is a nonlinear function of the stimulus, and the energy at different points in the stimulus spectrogram is not statistically independent, then even the "corrected" STRF may substantially overestimate the true extent of the neuron's receptive field (Christianson et al., 2008).

The predictive approach takes a different route to the same expression. Here, we seek a mathematical model that generates stimulus-driven firing rate predictions that are linear in the spectrogram of the sound stimulus, and that approximates the true stimulus-response function of the neuron as well as possible. If the range of spectrogram time-frames used to predict the firing rate at time step i is restricted to $i - J + 1 \ldots i$, then the firing rate $\hat{\mathbf{r}}$ predicted by a spectogram-linear model can be written in terms of a weight vector $\widehat{\mathbf{w}}^{(\mathbf{tf})}$ and the stimulus matrix $\mathbf{M}^{\mathbf{i}(\mathbf{tf})}$ as

$$\widehat{\mathbf{r}} = \mathbf{M}^{\mathbf{i}(\mathbf{tf})}\widehat{\mathbf{w}}^{(\mathbf{tf})}. \tag{3}$$

The predictive goal is then to find an estimate $\widehat{\mathbf{w}}^{(\mathbf{tf})}$ such that $\widehat{\mathbf{r}} \approx \mathbf{r}$, ideally for as wide a range of input stimuli as possible. As perfect prediction is unlikely to be achieved for all stimulus values, the estimated weights will depend on the measure by which the closeness of $\widehat{\mathbf{r}}$ and $\mathbf{r}$ is defined. One common choice is to estimate $\widehat{\mathbf{w}}^{(\mathbf{tf})}$ such that the total squared difference between $\widehat{\mathbf{r}}$ and the measured $\mathbf{r}$ is minimised. This leads to the Wiener filter estimate, which, in our discrete-time setting is identical to least-squares linear regression and is solved by the Moore-Penrose pseudo-inverse (indicated by †):

$$\widehat{\mathbf{w}}^{(\mathbf{tf})} = (\mathbf{M}^{\mathbf{i}(\mathbf{tf})})^{\dagger}\mathbf{r} = (\mathbf{M}^{\mathbf{i}(\mathbf{tf})\top}\mathbf{M}^{\mathbf{i}(\mathbf{tf})})^{-1}\mathbf{M}^{\mathbf{i}(\mathbf{tf})\top}\mathbf{r}.$$

This result is identical to the STRF of Eq. 2. However, it is only one of many different possible choices for a predictive $\widehat{\mathbf{w}}^{(\mathbf{tf})}$. In particular, statistical techniques for *regularisation* may yield estimates that predict firing rates for novel stimuli (that is, stimuli that were not used to generate the original measured response $\mathbf{r}$ on which the model estimate is based) more accurately than does the Wiener filter. Although motivated from a predictive viewpoint, such an estimate might arguably also provide a more accurate *description* of the neuron's spectrotemporal sensitivities than the naïve STRF. Thus, the tools of statistical regression that emerge naturally within the predictive view have proven to be valuable for sensory neuronal characterisation in general.

2. Noise and Overfitting

Cortical neuronal responses to repetitions of an identical external stimulus can be extremely variable. This variability in measured responses necessarily translates into variability in estimates of the parameters of any response model. Even the average response computed from an experimentally feasible number of trials using identical stimuli will exhibit some residual variability (Sahani and Linden, 2003b), and in most physiological experiments with limited available recording time the number of such repetitions must be balanced against the desire to explore a wider range of different stimuli. These variations in response may be biologically significant; they may, for example, reflect ongoing processing within the cortex. However, as each response is associated with an identical stimulus, the variation clearly cannot be predicted from the stimulus alone. Thus such variation must be regarded as a source of noise when considering models of the stimulus-response function of a neuron. We refer to the noisy responses evoked by the limited set of experimental stimuli on which the model estimate is to be based as the "training data."

The naïve STRF or Wiener filter estimate yields the smallest possible squared error in prediction on the training data. However, a side-effect of this optimal minimisation is that the variance in the training data may have a relatively large impact on the value of the estimated model. In a sense, the parameters fit the training data too well; the resulting prediction follows both the true response of the neuron and that part of the noise in the (finite-sized) training data that happens by chance to match an aspect of the high-dimensional stimulus. This phenomenon is known as overfitting. As overfit parameters reflect the noise in the training data, they often predict the response of the neuron to novel stimuli poorly; this can be assessed in practice by cross-validation, where some training data are held out during model estimation and then used to measure the ability of the estimated model to generalise to novel stimuli.

Although it is possible to estimate the relative scale of noise from repeated measurements (Sahani and Linden, 2003b), there is no way to distinguish the parts of the recording that arise from random variability from those that are systematically related to the stimulus. However, the effects of noise on the estimated weights may nonetheless be identifiable, and may consequently be reduced. As the noise is by definition unrelated to the stimulus, the apparent correlation of some portion of that noise with the stimulus in any particular experiment will tend to give rise to unstructured, seemingly random weights. These resultant weights may have large magnitudes but opposite signs even for neighbouring regions of spectrotemporal space, a pattern which might be biologically implausible.

Thus, overfitting can often be contained by adding to the objective function a new term that penalises any unstructured component in the weights. Depending on the exact context, and the form that this additional term takes, the resulting approach might be called *regularisation*, *shrinkage* or *maximum a posteriori (MAP) estimation*. (The term "shrinkage" also refers to a more technical phenomeon in the theory of estimation (James and Stein, 1961), but this more general usage has become common.) In the following we will adopt the third of these perspectives, which derives from the Bayesian probabilistic approach to estimation. To take this approach we must add to the model specification of Eq. 3 an explicit choice of distribution for the expected variation of the measured $\mathbf{r}$ around the model prediction. If that variation is assumed to follow a Normal distribution with constant variance σ^2, then the maximum-likelihood parameter estimate is that which maximises the Gaussian log-probability-density at the observed response or, equivalently, minimises $\frac{1}{\sigma^2}\sum_i(\widehat{r}(i) - r(i))^2$. This is the Wiener filter once again.

MAP linear regression instead minimises an augmented objective function, or penalised log-likelihood, for example $\frac{1}{\sigma^2}\sum_i(\widehat{r}(i) - r(i))^2 + \mathbf{w}^\top\mathbf{C}^{-1}\mathbf{w}$. In the MAP approach, the second term in this function is also interpreted as a (negative) log-probability-density; in this case, it would be (up to terms and factors that do not depend on $\mathbf{w}$) the negative log-density of a Gaussian distribution on $\mathbf{w}$ with zero mean and covariance matrix $\mathbf{C}$. This distribution expresses a "prior" expectation or belief about the likely weight values that might be encountered. In this case, it assumes that weights are unlikely to be very large (as the distribution is concentrated around zero), and may favour some patterns of weights more than others depending on the form of the assumed covariance matrix $\mathbf{C}$. The combination of the prior and the data-derived squared error leads to a "posterior distribution" and the estimated weights are taken to lie at the peak of the associated density. For linear regression with Gaussian noise and a Gaussian prior, the MAP solution (for regression based on a generic stimulus matrix $\mathbf{M}$) is

$$\widehat{\mathbf{w}}_{\text{MAP}} = (\mathbf{M}^\top \mathbf{M} + \sigma^2 \mathbf{C}^{-1})^{-1} \mathbf{M}^\top \mathbf{r} \,. \tag{4}$$

The choice of the prior covariance matrix $\mathbf{C}$ can have a significant impact on the form of the MAP estimate parameters, and on their preditive ability. In the simplest case $\mathbf{C}$ is proportional to the identity matrix, a choice that corresponds to statistical technique known as "ridge regression." The resulting prior distribution expresses a belief about the most likely magnitude of the STRF weights, which is equal for all spectrotemporal inputs as the diagonal entries of $\mathbf{C}$ are equal. Furthermore, the off-diagonal zeros imply that there is no prior expectation of coordination between weights; e.g., neighbouring weights in the STRF are as likely to be of opposite as congruent sign. A different diagonal matrix might allow for the expected magnitudes of the weights to differ; perhaps being larger at mid-latencies than at very long ones. Finally, non-zero off-diagonal entries might express an expected correlation or anti-correlation between weights. For instance, positive covariance values corresponding to adjacent weights would favour similar values for those weights, leading to a spectrotemporally smoother estimate of the STRF.

2.1. Evidence Optimization

Thus, the prior covariance $\mathbf{C}$ that appears in the regularised objective function can influence the scale and smoothness of the estimated STRF. But how should this "prior" expectation be determined? What sorts of magnitude are reasonable, and over what spectrotemporal extent should smoothness be anticipated?

One way to solve this problem is to tune the matrix $\mathbf{C}$ empirically, so as to optimise the cross-validation performance of the model. That is, a subset of the available data is used to obtain a number of different sets of linear parameters by minimising cost functions regularised by different choices of $\mathbf{C}$. Each set of parameters is then evaluated by measuring the (unpenalised) squared-error of its prediction on the remaining data. This process may be repeated with different divisions of the available data into "training" and "validation" subsets, and the errors achieved by each choice of regulariser averaged over the validation sets. The regulariser that yields parameters with the smallest average validation error is selected, and used to estimate a final set of parameters from all the available training data.

This procedure may be computationally expensive, requiring repeated model fits. Furthermore, it is generally necessary to choose a finite subset of possible regularisers to evaluate. This may be practical if the prior covariance is parameterised by a small number of parameters, say one to set the values of all the diagonal elements and another to set all the off-diagonal elements. In this case a range of plausible settings of $\mathbf{C}$ may be constructed using a 2-dimensional "grid" of values. However, if (say) each diagonal element of $\mathbf{C}$ were to be determined separately, the number of different regularisers to consider would be infeasibly large. Furthermore, as the number of different regularisers to be evaluated increases, the danger grows of "overfitting" the regularisation choice to the validation data.

An alternative is to employ the calculus of probabilities directly to find the choice of $\mathbf{C}$ which best fits the data themselves (Sahani and Linden, 2003a). In loose terms one tries to find, say, the optimal smoothing scale for the STRF, but without estimating a particular value for the STRF itself. More precisely, we consider a two-stage hierarchical model in which a random set of parameters is chosen from the "prior" distribution—here, a Gaussian distribution with mean 0 and covariance $\mathbf{C}$—and the probability assigned by these parameters to the training data is evaluated. The quality of a particular choice of covariance $\mathbf{C}$ is measured by the average such probability:

$$\int d\mathbf{w} P(\mathbf{r}|\mathbf{w}, \mathbf{M}, \sigma^2) P(\mathbf{w}|\mathbf{C}) = \int d\mathbf{w} P(\mathbf{r}, \mathbf{w}|\mathbf{M}, \mathbf{C}, \sigma^2) = P(\mathbf{r}|\mathbf{M}, \mathbf{C}, \sigma^2),$$

where $\mathbf{r}$ are the measured responses generated by the stimulus represented by $\mathbf{M}$ and σ^2 is a noise-level which may be fixed, or may be optimised along with $\mathbf{C}$. This quantity is known as the *marginal likelihood* or *evidence* for $\mathbf{C}$ (and σ^2). A suitable choice of $\mathbf{C}$ would be one that maximised this quantity; thus, this approach may be called "evidence optimisation".

For linear regression with Gaussian observation noise and a Gaussian prior on $\mathbf{w}$, the evidence also has the form of a joint Gaussian distribution on the vector of all observed rates. The Gaussian noise assumption gives:

$$P(\mathbf{r}|\mathbf{M}, \mathbf{w}, \sigma^2) \propto \exp\left(-\frac{1}{2}\frac{(\mathbf{r} - \mathbf{M}\mathbf{w})^\top(\mathbf{r} - \mathbf{M}\mathbf{w})}{\sigma^2}\right).$$

(Here and below we will drop the normalising constants of the Gaussians, focusing only on the functional forms that appear in the exponents.) Multiplication by the Gaussian prior on $\mathbf{w}$ with covariance $\mathbf{C}$ then gives the joint density on $\mathbf{r}$ and $\mathbf{w}$:

$$P(\mathbf{r}, \mathbf{w}|\mathbf{M}, \mathbf{C}, \sigma^2) \propto \exp\left(-\frac{1}{2}\left(\frac{(\mathbf{r} - \mathbf{M}\mathbf{w})^\top(\mathbf{r} - \mathbf{M}\mathbf{w})}{\sigma^2} - \mathbf{w}^\top\mathbf{C}^{-1}\mathbf{w}\right)\right).$$

This is the expression that must be integrated with respect to $\mathbf{w}$ to obtain the marginal likelihood. Now, as $\mathbf{w}$ only appears within the quadratic forms of the exponent, the functional dependence of this expression on $\mathbf{w}$ is Gaussian. With some manipulation, we find that this Gaussian form (which is, in fact, the "posterior" distribution on $\mathbf{w}$, given the observed $\mathbf{r}$ and $\mathbf{M}$, and the assumed $\mathbf{C}$ and σ^2) has variance $\Sigma = \left(\frac{\mathbf{M}^\top\mathbf{M}}{\sigma^2} + \mathbf{C}^{-1}\right)^{-1}$ and mean $\boldsymbol{\mu} = \Sigma\frac{\mathbf{M}^\top\mathbf{r}}{\sigma^2} = \left(\mathbf{M}^\top\mathbf{M} + \sigma^2\mathbf{C}^{-1}\right)^{-1}\mathbf{M}^\top\mathbf{r}$. Thus, the integral is easily evaluated by the standard Gaussian formula, and we arrive at an expression for the evidence:

$$P(\mathbf{r}|\mathbf{M}, \mathbf{C}, \sigma^2) \propto \exp\left(-\frac{1}{2}\mathbf{r}^\top\left(\frac{I}{\sigma^2} - \frac{\mathbf{M}\Sigma\mathbf{M}^\top}{\sigma^4}\right)\mathbf{r}\right).$$

This evidence can be maximised with respect to $\mathbf{C}$ by iterative, gradient-based methods. Consider a parametrised covariance matrix $\mathbf{C}(\theta)$ where the parameter vector θ may determine the expected scales of different weights, or the extent of the anticipated spectrotemporal smoothness. The gradient of the log-evidence with respect to the parameters θ is then given by:

$$\frac{\partial}{\partial\theta}\log P(\mathbf{r}|\mathbf{M}, \mathbf{C}(\theta), \sigma^2) = \frac{1}{2}\,\mathrm{Tr}\left[(\mathbf{C}(\theta) - \Sigma - \boldsymbol{\mu}\boldsymbol{\mu}^\top)\frac{\partial}{\partial\theta}\mathbf{C}(\theta)^{-1}\right]. \qquad (5)$$

By gradually changing θ in the direction of this gradient (or, in some cases, using the gradient to derive a fixed-point iteration) it is possible to find a covariance matrix $\mathbf{C}(\theta)$ which (locally) maximises the evidence. Similarly, the gradient of the evidence with respect to σ^2 can be used to determine the most suitable level of variability. These values of $\mathbf{C}$ and σ^2 may then be used to estimate the desired model parameters $\mathbf{w}$ according to Eq. 4.

The parameterisation of $\mathbf{C}(\theta)$ determines the properties of the regulariser that are optimised. In this scheme the covariance $\mathbf{C}$ is being chosen to maximise a (marginal) likelihood, and so there is a similar danger of overfitting $\mathbf{C}$ as when fitting $\mathbf{w}$ by maximum likelihood. This is apparent if each element of $\mathbf{C}$ is parametrised separately. In this case it can be shown that the optimal value of $\mathbf{C}$ is a unit rank matrix whose sole significant eigenvector is just the maximum likelihood setting of $\mathbf{w}$. In this case evidence optimisation achieves nothing.

However, other choices of parametrisation may constrain $\mathbf{C}$ in useful ways and, empirically, the parameters obtained by evidence optimisation often generalise relatively well to new ("test") data. One approach constrains $\mathbf{C}$ to be diagonal, individually optimising the diagonal entries. At the optimum of the evidence many of these diagonal entries are found to be zero. As the mean of the regularising Gaussian is also zero, this forces the corresponding weight to be zero as well, yielding a sparse estimate of the STRF. Since it selects inputs to the model that are "relevant" to predicting the output, this approach is known as Automatic Relevance Determination (ARD; MacKay, 1994; Sahani and Linden, 2003a). Another approach parameterises the off-diagonal terms of the matrix so that weights nearby in time or spectrum are preferentially similar, and adjusts the time- and spectral-lengths over which such similarity is preferred. This is known as Automatic Smoothness Determination (ASD; Sahani and Linden, 2003a). A combination of the two approaches yields estimates composed of a superposition of a small set of optimally smooth basis functions (ASD/RD; Sahani and Linden, 2003a). Finally, the parametrisation may also be selected to favour non-zero weights that concentrate within a local region of spectro-temporal space by Automatic Locality Determination (ALD; Park and Pillow, 2011). Each of these approaches has been shown to provide robust and predictive estimates of receptive field models.

3. Nonlinear Models

The STRF model, where the predicted firing rate is linear in the spectrogram of the sound, has proven to be a powerful tool for characterising auditory cortical neurons (for a seminal early review, see Eggermont et al. 1983). Linear models are computationally simple, and easy to estimate. Nonetheless, they reflect the significant spectrotemporal sensitivities of a neuron in an easily interpreted form (although care must be taken in interpreting STRFs derived from stimuli that are not spectrotemporally independent; see Christianson et al. 2008). STRFs have therefore been used to explore both properties of neuronal responses in the auditory cortex (Kowalski et al., 1996; Calhoun and Schreiner, 1998; deCharms et al., 1998; Depireux et al., 2001; Schnupp et al., 2001; Miller et al., 2002; Rutkowski et al., 2002; Linden et al., 2003; Elhilali et al., 2004; Tomita and Eggermont, 2005) and adaptive changes in those responses (Fritz et al., 2003; Atiani et al., 2009; Pienkowski and Eggermont, 2009; David et al., 2012).

However, when viewed as a predictive model of firing, the STRF has often been found wanting. In one study (Sahani and Linden, 2003b), linear models were observed to predict only about 30% of the maximum possible predictable response of cortical cells to dynamic random chord stimuli. Another study (Machens et al., 2004) reported a yet lower accuracy, although this result did not account fully for the unreliability of response measurements. These predictive failures have motivated the construction of nonlinear models, particularly models in which the structure of the nonlinearity may yield further biologically-interpretable insights into the structure of the true cortical response functions.

The general problem of nonlinear regression is vast and complex. There are two main difficulties. First, many nonlinear descriptions of the stimulus-response function contain a large number of parameters, which may be overfit to the noise in the training data, leading to poor generalization to new data ("test data", or "cross-validation data"). A by-product of overfitting is a poor description of the stimulus-response function. Second, identifying good parameters for nonlinear models may be computationally challenging; in particular, there may be many local optima in the objective function, making it hard to find the best-fitting parameters for the model class. Therefore, nonlinear regression involves a tradeoff between flexibility (number of parameters), ease of estimation, and risk of local optima.

One general approach to nonlinear modelling is based on a series expansion (known as a Volterra or Wiener expansion) of the functional mapping from stimulus to response. It is possible to see such methods as a form of expanded linear regression; each stimulus vector is mapped nonlinearly to a higher-dimensional space, from which the predicted firing rate is formed by linear regression. For instance, instead of regressing on the stimulus elements $\{x_{i,j}\}$ directly, the second-order Volterra model also includes quadratic functions of the stimulus elements, giving an expanded set of regression inputs: $(\{x_{i,j}\}, \{x_{i,j}x_{i',j'}\})$. The advantage of this nonlinear model is that not only additive, but also multiplicative interactions between the predictor variables are now possible, and can be explored in the neural data (e.g. Pienkowski et al., 2009; Pienkowski and Eggermont, 2010). However, the general series expansion does not necessarily yield models that are easy to interpret. Moreover, the number of weights increases significantly (for example, in the second-order Volterra model example above, from J to $J + J(J+1)/2$, if $j = 1 \dots J$). Thus the risk of overfitting increases, and one has to take measures to counteract this risk.

4. Nonlinear Cascade Models

Many interpretable nonlinear models can be written as *cascades* of simple stages combining one or more STRF-like linear integrative stages with one or more simple nonlinearity. Some cascade models have been built to explicitly echo known or presumed steps of biological processing (Fishbach et al., 2001; Schinkel-Bielefeld et al., 2012). Others have been more abstract, using the cascade structure not to mimic the physiological pathway but solely to separate the computational stages reflected in the response.

4.1. LN Cascades

The best-established such model in sensory neuroscience is the linear-nonlinear (LN) cascade, also known as the *Wiener cascade or system* (not to be confused with the Wiener series or Wiener filter). As the name suggests, this model first involves one or more linear filters applied to the stimulus. For auditory cortex models, these filters are usually spectrotemporal, implemented in the same way as the STRF; that is, they are finite-impulse-response multichannel filters applied to the spectrogram of the sound stimulus. The output of the filter(s) is then transformed by a nonlinear function to yield the predicted firing rate. As the number of linear filters is usually much smaller than the number of spectrotemporal weights within each filter, such models are often thought to implement a form of dimensionality reduction.

For most cascade models, the interpretable characterisation of the response rests on the spectrotemporal structure observed within the linear filtering stages. Thus, an LN cascade model with only a single filter does not usually offer any greater intrinsic representational range than an STRF. However, even in this case, the predictive accuracy of the LN model may be higher and the estimates of the spectrotemporal weights may be less susceptible to stimulus- or noise-driven bias (Atencio et al., 2008; Calabrese et al., 2011; Shechter and Depireux, 2010). Futhermore, models in which the nonlinear mapping takes on a fixed assumed form—which reduces the LN cascade to a type of model called "generalised linear", studied extensively in statistics—can be relatively easily extended to take into account history-dependent phenomena in the spike-generation process such as the refractory period, intrinsic oscillation, or a tendency towards bursting (Truccolo et al., 2005).

LN cascade models may also combine multiple linear filters that act in parallel, and whose outputs are combined nonlinearly to predict the firing rate. In this case, the multiple filters—or, more precisely, the stimulus subspace that is spanned by those filters—offers a response representation that might depend on multiple different stimulus features. Thus, if an auditory cortical neuron were responsive to a specific temporal modulation frequency within a particular spectral band, but not to the phase of that temporal modulation, an appropriate LN model might include two filters each responding to the optimal modulation frequency but at phases in quadrature to each other. Clearly, such multi-dimensional LN models do indeed expand the range of interpretable response properties that can be characterised (Atencio et al., 2009, 2012; Rabinowitz et al., 2011, 2012).

5. NL Cascades and Multilinear Models

The LN cascade and other models which assume a small number of initial linear spectrotemporal integration filters are not very well suited to describing response functions that reflect locally nonlinear (or, indeed, non-monotonic) level sensitivity, nor those that involve local nonlinear interactions between different spectral channels or in time within a single channel. The scale on which acoustic power is measured (e.g. pressure or intensity on a linear or logarithmic decibel scale) must be pre-determined, and whilst that power may be weighted by the filter in a way that depends on the relative time and the frequency, these weights cannot depend on the rest of the stimulus as might be desired to model channel-specific gain adaptation, for instance. The problem is that the nonlinearity is restricted to act in the low-dimensional space of the outputs of the linear filters.

On the face of it, allowing for a general nonlinearity to act in the high-dimensional space of all spectrotemporal inputs to which a neuron might respond would pose a daunting statistical problem. The number of parameters needed to describe such a model would be very large, and thus the model would be prone to significant overfitting. Furthermore, even if it could be estimated well, such a generic high-dimensional nonlinearity might prove very difficult to interpet.

Thus, the nonlinearity needs somehow to be restricted to yield a tractable and interpretable model. One approach, which accords with the biological intuition of time- and spectral-translation invariance in the population processing of sounds at subcortical stages, is to construct an NL or Hammerstein cascade. Here, a relatively simple (often one-dimensional) nonlinearity acts uniformly on each spectrotemporal input, before these are then combined. NL cascades have appeared in the neuroscience literature for many years (Hunter and Korenberg, 1986) but had gained little popularity because robust methods for parametrisation and fitting were not available. Fortunately, newer methods based on multilinear representations (Ahrens et al., 2008b,a; Englitz et al., 2010) now offer both efficient and robust approaches to fitting certain NL models. These methods will be discussed below.

5.1. Notation

For consistency, we will employ the notation introduced by Ahrens et al. (2008a). The models to be discussed here will typically be described in terms of multi-dimensional arrays derived from the stimulus (denoted by bold-faced letters such as $\mathbf{M}$ or $\mathbf{Q}$). Bold superscripts specify the physical stimulus properties to which the dimensions of the array pertain, and italicised subscripts denote specific elements within the array. In the auditory system, the relevant physical dimensions are time, frequency and level. A time-frequency array of weights (essentially, an STRF) is thus denoted by $\mathbf{w}^{\mathbf{tf}}$, whilst $w_{jk}^{\mathbf{tf}}$ is the jk^{th} element in the array. On occasion (as we have already seen), two or more physical dimensions might be grouped into a single array dimension. This is indicated by parentheses around the relevant superscripts, as in the stimulus matrix $\mathbf{M}^{\mathbf{i(tf)}}$ discussed above.

We will consider two types of generalised operator acting on these arrays. First, the tensor or generalised outer product is denoted by $\otimes$ such that, for example, given vectors $\mathbf{b}$, $\mathbf{c}$, and $\mathbf{d}$

$$\mathbf{A} = \mathbf{b} \otimes \mathbf{c} \otimes \mathbf{d}$$

is a three-dimensional array, with the elements

$$A_{ijk} = b_i c_j d_k \,.$$

Similarly, the symbol $\bullet$ generalises the vector inner product (or tensor multiplication with implied contraction), so that physical dimensions shared on the left and right hand sides of the operator are summed. For example, if we have a three-dimensional array $\mathbf{a}^{\mathbf{xyz}}$, and a two-dimensional array $\mathbf{b}^{\mathbf{yz}}$, then

$$\mathbf{c}^{\mathbf{x}} = \mathbf{a}^{\mathbf{xyz}} \bullet \mathbf{b}^{\mathbf{yz}}$$

is a vector (one-dimensional array) with elements

$$c_i^{\mathbf{x}} = \sum_{jk} a_{ijk}^{\mathbf{xyz}} b_{jk}^{\mathbf{yz}} \,.$$

5.2. Bilinear or Separable STRFs

The simplest model to describe the functional relationship between stimulus and response is, of course, the spectrotemporally linear STRF. In the notation we have adopted such a model can be written

$$\hat{r}(i) = \sum_{j=1}^{J} \sum_{k=1}^{K} w_{jk}^{\mathbf{tf}} s(i - j + 1, k), \tag{6}$$

where $\hat{r}(i)$ is the estimated instantaneous firing rate at time i, $w_{jk}^{\mathbf{tf}}$ is the jk^{th} element of the two-dimensional time-frequency STRF, and $s(i - j + 1, k)$ denotes an element from the stimulus spectrogram s at time-lag $j + 1$ relative to the spike rate being predicted, and frequency k. The summation limits run from 1 to some maximal value of time-lag J and frequency channel K. For simplicity, we will suppress summation limits throughout the rest of the chapter. Unless stated otherwise, all sums run from 1 to the maximum value of the relevant variable.

In Eq. 6 we have kept the STRF weights arranged as a two-dimensional array $\mathbf{w}^{\mathbf{tf}}$, rather than "unrolling" this array into a vector $\mathbf{w}^{(\mathbf{tf})}$ as we did above in Eq. 3. Thus, to write this expression more compactly, we need to define a *three-dimensional* stimulus array $\mathbf{M}^{\mathbf{itf}}$, which incorporates time-lag along the added dimension:

$$M_{ijk}^{\mathbf{itf}} = \begin{cases} s(i - j + 1, k), & i \leq I, j \leq J, i - j \geq 0, k \leq K \\ 0, & \text{otherwise}. \end{cases}$$

Now, Eq. 6 can be written

$$\hat{r}(i) = \sum_{jk} w_{jk}^{\mathbf{tf}} M_{ijk}^{\mathbf{itf}} \qquad \text{or} \qquad \widehat{\mathbf{r}} = \mathbf{w}^{\mathbf{tf}} \bullet M^{\mathbf{itf}}.$$

These equations assume an inseparable (or full-rank) representation of the receptive field $\mathbf{w}^{\mathbf{tf}}$. If we were to assume that the STRF was instead *separable* in time and frequency, we could write

$$\hat{r}(i) = \sum_{jk} w_j^{\mathbf{t}} w_k^{\mathbf{f}} M_{ijk}^{\mathbf{itf}}, \tag{7}$$

where the separable STRF is given by the outer product of a time vector and a frequency vector, $\mathbf{w}^{\mathbf{tf}} = \mathbf{w}^{\mathbf{t}} \otimes \mathbf{w}^{\mathbf{f}}$. The separability of STRFs has been investigated frequently (Depireux et al., 2001; Klein et al., 2006), and is particularly useful from a statistical perspective as it is associated with a substantial reduction in free parameters (from $J \times K$ to $J + K$). From a functional perspective, separability implies that the sensitivity of the neuron to tones of different frequencies is preserved across time. It may be biologically appropriate if temporal filtering in (say) the cortex happens after spectral integration is complete. Indeed the STRFs of many neurons in the core auditory cortices seem to be well-modelled as separable (Linden et al., 2003; Klein et al., 2006; Simon et al., 2007).

The separable model described by Eq. 7 is *bilinear*; it is individually linear in each of parameter vectors $\mathbf{w}^{\mathbf{t}}$ and $\mathbf{w}^{\mathbf{f}}$. Using the generalised outer and inner products defined in section 5.1 we can write the bilinear model compactly:

$$\widehat{\mathbf{r}} = (\mathbf{w}^{\mathbf{t}} \otimes \mathbf{w}^{\mathbf{f}}) \bullet \mathbf{M}^{\mathbf{itf}}.$$

In practice, an STRF model often also incorporates a background firing rate, so that the spectrotemporal sensitivity describes variations around a non-zero value. Mathematically, this introduces a constant offset, c. The separable STRF model is then

$$\hat{\mathbf{r}} = c + (\mathbf{w}^{\mathbf{t}} \otimes \mathbf{w}^{\mathbf{f}}) \bullet \mathbf{M}^{\mathbf{itf}} . \tag{8}$$

The constant offset c can be incorporated cleanly into the bilinear framework by augmenting the stimulus array and weight vector appropriately. Consider a new, slightly larger, array $\mathbf{Q}^{\mathbf{itf}}$ such that

$$Q_{ijk}^{\mathbf{itf}} = \begin{cases} M_{ijk}^{\mathbf{itf}} & i \leq I, j \leq J, i - j \geq 0, k \leq K \\ 1 & i \leq I, j = J+1, k = K+1 \\ 0 & \text{otherwise}, \end{cases} \tag{9}$$

as well as augmented $\mathbf{w}^{\mathbf{t}}$ and $\mathbf{w}^{\mathbf{f}}$ vectors with $J+1$ and $K+1$ elements respectively. Then Eq. 8 can be rewritten

$$\hat{\mathbf{r}} = (\mathbf{w}^{\mathbf{t}} \otimes \mathbf{w}^{\mathbf{f}}) \bullet \mathbf{Q}^{\mathbf{itf}} ,$$

where the background rate c is now represented by the product $w_{J+1}^{\mathbf{t}} w_{K+1}^{\mathbf{f}}$.

5.3. Multilinear Input Nonlinearity Models

The preceding section showed how a separable STRF could be cast into a multilinear (in this case, bilinear) framework. We shall see as the chapter progresses that this multilinear framework can be extended to incorporate a number of realistic nonlinearities, thus parametrising a broad family of NL cascade models. The general form for a multilinear model is

$$\hat{\mathbf{r}} = (\mathbf{a} \otimes \mathbf{b} \otimes \cdots \otimes \mathbf{z}) \bullet \mathbf{Q} , \tag{10}$$

where $\mathbf{a}, \mathbf{b}, \cdots, \mathbf{z}$ are arbitrary vectors of free parameters and $\mathbf{Q}$ is a fixed multidimensional array derived from the stimulus.

The time-frequency representation of a sound requires a choice of linear or nonlinear operation on the sound pressure waveform (Gill et al., 2006) and the scaling chosen for the stimulus representation may have a substantial impact on the predictions of a spectrotemporal model. Rather than assuming a fixed scaling, the multilinear framework makes it possible to define an *input nonlinearity* model to infer such a nonlinear transform directly from the data (Ahrens et al., 2008a,b). Building on the separable STRF model of Eq. 7, a general input nonlinearity model would take the form

$$\hat{r}(i) = c + \sum_{jk} w_j^{\mathbf{t}} w_k^{\mathbf{f}} g(s(i-j+1, k)) ,$$

where the mapping g is an input nonlinearity that acts to transform the arbitrary representation of a sound level in the spectrogram prior to (separable) spectrotemporal filtering. The mapping g can be parametrised for estimation by re-expressing it as a linear combination of a fixed set of basis functions $\{g_l\}$, so that $g(x) = \sum_l w_l^{\mathbf{l}} g_l(x)$, for some parameter vector $\mathbf{w}^{\mathbf{l}}$. This yields

$$\hat{r}(i) = c + \sum_{jkl} w_j^{\mathbf{t}} w_k^{\mathbf{f}} w_l^{\mathbf{l}} g_l(s(i-j+1, k)) . \tag{11}$$

The use of such a representation reduces the problem of inferring the nonlinear stimulus transform to that of estimating the coefficients $\mathbf{w}^{\mathrm{l}}$ of the basis function set $\{g_l\}$.

This model can be written in multilinear form. If we define a four-dimensional stimulus array $M^{\mathbf{itfl}}_{ijkl} = g_l(s(i-j+1,k))$ over the appropriate ranges of indices, then we can then write

$$\hat{r}(i) = c + \sum_{jkl} w^{\mathrm{t}}_j w^{\mathrm{f}}_k w^{\mathrm{l}}_l M^{\mathbf{itfl}}_{ijkl} \quad \text{or} \quad \hat{\mathbf{r}} = (\mathbf{w}^{\mathrm{t}} \otimes \mathbf{w}^{\mathrm{f}} \otimes \mathbf{w}^{\mathrm{l}}) \bullet \mathbf{Q}^{\mathbf{itfl}},$$

with the four-dimensional array $\mathbf{Q}^{\mathbf{itfl}}$ defined by augmenting $\mathbf{M}^{\mathbf{itfl}}$ in a manner analogous to Eq. 9.

This provides a multilinear formulation of the simplest form of NL cascade, where the nonlinearity g acts separately on each spectrotemporal input value. (It is also possible to adopt an inseparable set of spectrotemporal weights for this model, or indeed to consider inseparable level-frequency or level-time interactions; Ahrens et al. 2008a.) The multilinear form leads to a straightforward and robust method to estimate the input nonlinearity as well as the spectrotemporal integration filter. However, before discussing this parameter estimation technique, we first explore more sophisticated NL cascade models which can also be reduced to a similar multilinear form.

5.4. Local Contextual Modulation

5.4.1. The Separable Context Model

The input nonlinearity model defined in Eq. 11 describes a way in which the multilinear framework can be used to extend a simple linear neural encoding model, incorporating an arbitrary nonlinear transformation of the stimulus power. However, even here the interaction within the model of sound energy at different times and in different channels is still linear. That is, different stimulus features are never combined in anything other than a weighted, additive fashion.

The multilinear framework can also be used to describe local nonlinear interactions within the stimulus, where the neuronal sensitivity to a particular spectrotemporal input depends on the local context within which the input appears (Ahrens et al., 2008a). This *context model* extends the previous models by additionally allowing a limited set of second-order interactions through the influence of local gain factors. A contextual gain factor is computed for each spectrotemporal input by weighting and integrating the stimulus spectrogram within a neighborhood centred on the input. These gains modulate the weights of a linear filter (analagous to the STRF, but here called the *principal receptive field* or PRF to distinguish its role in the context model from the linear STRF model) which yields the final firing rate prediction.

Specifically, the stimulus at time i with frequency k is given a strength denoted by

$$g(s(i,k)) \cdot (c_2 + \text{Context}(i,k)),$$

where the first term $g(s(i,k))$ is that of the input nonlinearity model discussed earlier, which will infer the effective level of a given tone pulse within the stimulus. This inferred level is then multiplicatively modulated by a context term given by

$$\text{Context}(i,k) = \sum_{\substack{mnp \\ (m,n)\neq(1,\Phi)}} w^{\boldsymbol{\tau}}_m w^{\boldsymbol{\phi}}_n w^{\boldsymbol{\lambda}}_p h_p(s(i-m+1, k-\Phi-1+n)), \tag{12}$$

where $\Phi = (N-1)/2$ dictates the maximum difference in frequency between the contextual and modulated time-frequency elements. The condition that $(m,n) \neq (1,\Phi)$ is to ensure that a tone does not appear within its own context.

Again, this contextual modulation can be succinctly expressed in multilinear notation. We define a *contextual subunit* array

$$[\mathbf{M}^{\boldsymbol{\tau\phi\lambda}}(i,k)]_{mnp} = \begin{cases} 0 & (m,n) = (1,\Phi) \\ M^{\mathbf{itfl}}_{im(k-\Phi-1+n)p} & \text{otherwise}, \end{cases} \tag{13}$$

where $\mathbf{M}^{\boldsymbol{\tau\phi\lambda}}(i,k)$ is a stimulus array which depends on the ik^{th} position of the time-frequency element being modulated. Using this stimulus representation, we can now denote the contextual modulation of Eq. 12 as

$$\text{Context}(i,k) = (\mathbf{w}^{\boldsymbol{\tau}} \otimes \mathbf{w}^{\boldsymbol{\phi}} \otimes \mathbf{w}^{\boldsymbol{\lambda}}) \bullet \mathbf{M}^{\boldsymbol{\tau\phi\lambda}}(i,k). \tag{14}$$

This contextual term can be viewed as a second input nonlinearity model. In a vein similar to $\mathbf{w}^{\mathbf{l}}$ in Eq. 11, $\mathbf{w}^{\boldsymbol{\lambda}}$ transforms the contextual sound energy in terms of a set of P basis functions $h_p(s)$ (which may be identical to the set of basis functions $g_l(s)$, although this is not essential). These transformed values are then integrated within a time and frequency window anchored at the point (i,k) in the spectrogram according to the parameters $\mathbf{w}^{\boldsymbol{\tau}}$ and $\mathbf{w}^{\boldsymbol{\phi}}$ which express weights in relative time and frequency offset respectively. Putting this contextual modulation together with a separable input nonlinearity PRF model, this fully separated context model can be expressed (in component notation) as

$$\hat{r}(i) = c + \sum_{jkl} w^{\mathbf{t}}_j w^{\mathbf{f}}_k w^{\mathbf{l}}_l M^{\mathbf{itfl}}_{ijkl} \left(c_2 + \sum_{mnp} w^{\boldsymbol{\tau}}_m w^{\boldsymbol{\phi}}_n w^{\boldsymbol{\lambda}}_p [\mathbf{M}^{\boldsymbol{\tau\phi\lambda}}(i-j+1,k)]_{mnp} \right). \tag{15}$$

Again, we can write this fully separated model in multilinear form. To do so, we need to define a seven-dimensional array $\mathbf{Q}^{\mathbf{itfl}\boldsymbol{\tau\phi\lambda}}$ as follows

$$Q^{\mathbf{itfl}\boldsymbol{\tau\phi\lambda}}_{ijklmnp} = \begin{cases} M^{\mathbf{itfl}}_{ijkl} \times [\mathbf{M}^{\boldsymbol{\tau\phi\lambda}}(i-j+1,k)]_{mnp} & (j,k,l,m,n,p) \leq (J,K,L,M,N,P) \\ 1 & (j,k,l) = (J+1,K+1,L+1), \\ & \quad (m,n,p) = (M+1,N+1,P+1) \\ M^{\mathbf{itfl}}_{ijkl} & (j,k,l) \leq (J,K,L), \\ & \quad (m,n,p) = (M+2,N+2,P+2) \\ 0 & \text{otherwise}. \end{cases} \tag{16}$$

Then, with appropriate augmentation of the parameter vectors, we can write the model as

$$\hat{\mathbf{r}} = (\mathbf{w}^{\mathbf{t}} \otimes \mathbf{w}^{\mathbf{f}} \otimes \mathbf{w}^{\mathbf{l}} \otimes \mathbf{w}^{\boldsymbol{\tau}} \otimes \mathbf{w}^{\boldsymbol{\phi}} \otimes \mathbf{w}^{\boldsymbol{\lambda}}) \bullet \mathbf{Q}^{\mathbf{itfl}\boldsymbol{\tau\phi\lambda}}.$$

This context model is able to capture local non-linear interactions succinctly, its fully separable form meaning that it has fewer parameters than does a single STRF model.

5.4.2. The Inseparable Context Model

Thus far, the contextual modulation has been modelled by two separate vectors $\mathbf{w}^{\tau}$ and $\mathbf{w}^{\phi}$, resulting in fully separable contextual interactions. That is, the shape with which the contextual influence depends on relative frequency offset does not depend on relative time offset and *vice versa*. This is a restrictive assumption, and it is possible to relax it whilst still retaining the overall multilinear formulation. We will consider a generalisation to a full-rank or inseparable contextual field $\mathbf{w}^{\tau\phi}$, which we will call the *contextual gain field* or CGF. Functionally, this now implies that frequency-offset-dependent contextual modulations can now be time-offset-dependent. Similarly, we can also include a full-rank principal receptive field $\mathbf{w}^{\mathrm{tf}}$. In principle, these inseparable contextual gain and principal receptive fields could be combined with input nonlinearities as in Eq. 15. In practice, however, the additional parameters introduced by the inseparable fields makes overfitting a very real risk. Furthermore, the basic principles of the analysis are essentially the same with and without the added complexity of the nonlinear basis functions. Thus, here we will make the further simplification of disregarding the input nonlinearity, and restricting amplitude transformations to be linear in stimulus amplitude.

This inseparable context model (with a fixed input nonlinearity) takes on a bilinear form, denoted by

$$\hat{\mathbf{r}} = (\mathbf{w}^{\mathrm{tf}} \otimes \mathbf{w}^{\tau\phi}) \bullet \mathbf{Q}^{\mathrm{itf}\tau\phi} . \tag{17}$$

The stimulus array $\mathbf{Q}^{\mathrm{itf}\tau\phi}$ is analagous to that of Eq. 16, but lacks the sound-level basis function components. It is given by

$$Q^{\mathrm{itf}\tau\phi}_{ijkmn} = \begin{cases} M^{\mathrm{itf}}_{ijk} \times [\mathbf{M}^{\tau\phi}(i,k)]_{mn} & (j,k,m,n) \leq (J,K,M,N) \\ 1 & (j,k,m,n) = (J+1,K+1,M+1,N+1) \\ M^{\mathrm{itf}}_{ijk} & (j,k) \leq (J,K), (m,n) = (M+2,N+2) \\ 0 & \text{otherwise}, \end{cases}$$

where the contextual subunit array is now two-dimensional:

$$[\mathbf{M}^{\tau\phi}(i,k)]_{mn} = \begin{cases} 0 & \text{if } (m,n) = (1,\Phi) \\ M^{\mathrm{itf}}_{im(k-\Phi-1+n)} & \text{otherwise}. \end{cases}$$

Both context models have been shown to outperform the simple STRF in predicting central auditory neuronal responses to complex sounds (Ahrens et al., 2008a; Williamson et al., 2011).

6. Parameter Estimation in Multilinear Models

The preceding section showed how a range of NL cascade models can be cast within a multilinear framework, and suggested that this formulation would give rise to a family of robust estimation methods. Here, we examine these methods.

6.1. Alternating Least Squares

Parameter estimates are typically based on the minimisation of a cost or error function that measures the discrepancy between the model prediction and the measured stimulus. As we saw above, the most common approach to estimation in the linear STRF model is equivalent to minimising the mean squared error between the model prediction and firing rate. The same cost function leads to a simple and efficient estimation method for a multilinear model (Ahrens et al., 2008b).

For a general multilinear model, the squared error is

$$\begin{aligned} \mathcal{E} &= \|\mathbf{r} - \hat{\mathbf{r}}\|^2 \\ &= \|\mathbf{r} - ((\mathbf{a} \otimes \mathbf{b} \otimes \cdots \otimes \mathbf{z}) \bullet \mathbf{Q})\|^2 , \end{aligned} \tag{18}$$

where $\|\mathbf{x}\|^2$ represents the squared norm of the vector $\mathbf{x}$: *i. e.* the sum of squares of its elements. This function can be minimised by cycling through a set of update equations for each individual parameter vector, each of which resembles the ordinary least-squares solution to a classical linear regression problem. Differentiating Eq. 18 with respect to each parameter vector in turn, and solving for the zero of the derivatives, yields the following set of equations:

$$\begin{aligned} \mathbf{A} &= (\mathbf{b} \otimes \mathbf{c} \cdots \otimes \mathbf{z}) \bullet \mathbf{Q} & \mathbf{a} &= (\mathbf{A}^\top \mathbf{A})^{-1} \mathbf{A}^\top \mathbf{r} \\ \mathbf{B} &= (\mathbf{a} \otimes \mathbf{c} \cdots \otimes \mathbf{z}) \bullet \mathbf{Q} & \mathbf{b} &= (\mathbf{B}^\top \mathbf{B})^{-1} \mathbf{B}^\top \mathbf{r} \\ &\vdots & &\vdots \\ \mathbf{Z} &= (\mathbf{a} \otimes \mathbf{b} \cdots \otimes \mathbf{y}) \bullet \mathbf{Q} & \mathbf{z} &= (\mathbf{Z}^\top \mathbf{Z})^{-1} \mathbf{Z}^\top \mathbf{r} . \end{aligned} \tag{19}$$

These equations are applied iteratively, alternating between the different updates. Thus, this approach may be called Alternating Least Squares or ALS. Since each iteration of the algorithm will decrease the squared error and since $\mathcal{E}$ is non-negative, the iterations are guaranteed to converge to an optimum within the parameter space.

6.2. Update Equations for the Context Model

The ALS updates can be applied to find iterative estimates of $\mathbf{w}^{\mathbf{tf}}$ and $\mathbf{w}^{\boldsymbol{\tau\phi}}$ in the inseparable context model of Eq. 17.

6.2.1. Update for $\mathbf{w}^{\mathbf{tf}}$

In component notation, the full predictive equation of the inseparable context model is given by

$$\hat{r}(i) = c_1 + \sum_{j=1}^{J} \sum_{k=1}^{K} w_{jk}^{\mathbf{tf}} s(i-j+1,k) \left(1 + \sum_{m=0}^{M} \sum_{n=-N}^{N} w_{mn}^{\boldsymbol{\tau\phi}} s(i-j+1-m, k+n)\right) , \tag{20}$$

where the the summation limits have been altered to simplify the subsequent algebra. The j and k summations are identical to those before. The summations over m and n are subtly different. The m summation begins at 0 (rather than 1), in order to incorporate a contextual time-lag of 0 into the model (thus the CGF $\boldsymbol{\tau}$ dimensionality will be $(M+1)$). The subscript n corresponds to frequency deviation and thus can be either positive or negative, with N denoting the maximum allowed deviation, leading to a CGF $\boldsymbol{\phi}$ dimensionality of $(2\times N+1)$.

Collecting all the factors that do not depend on $\mathbf{w}^{\mathbf{tf}}$ in Eq. 20, we define a new three-dimensional array A_{ijk} such that

$$A_{ijk} = s(i-j+1,k) + s(i-j+1,k)\sum_{mn} w_{mn}^{\boldsymbol{\tau\phi}} s(i-j+1-m,k+n)\,,$$

and obtain the simple linear form

$$\hat{r}(i) = c_1 + \sum_{jk} w_{jk}^{\mathbf{tf}} A_{ijk}\,,$$

where it is important to recall that $\mathbf{A}$ depends on the other parameter vector $\mathbf{w}^{\boldsymbol{\tau\phi}}$. If we now introduce "unrolled" versions of the arrays as we did for the STRF above, this expression for a matrix $\mathbf{w}^{\mathbf{tf}}$ is transformed into an equivalent one for the vector $\mathbf{w}^{(\mathbf{tf})}$, which can be solved by the familiar least-squares linear regression:

$$\widehat{\mathbf{r}} = c_1 + \mathbf{w}^{(\mathbf{tf})} \bullet \mathbf{A}^{\mathbf{i}(\mathbf{tf})}\,.$$

6.2.2. Update for $\mathbf{w}^{\boldsymbol{\tau\phi}}$

To derive the update equation for $\mathbf{w}^{\boldsymbol{\tau\phi}}$ we begin by rearranging the terms of Eq. 20 to obtain:

$$\hat{r}(i) = c_1 + \sum_{jk} w_{jk}^{\mathbf{tf}} s(i-j+1,k) + \sum_{mn} w_{mn}^{\boldsymbol{\tau\phi}} \sum_{jk} w_{jk}^{\mathbf{tf}} s(i-j+1,k) s(i-j+1-m,k+n)\,.$$

Again, we regard $\mathbf{w}^{\mathbf{tf}}$ as fixed, and attempt to solve for the $\mathbf{w}^{\boldsymbol{\tau\phi}}$ which gives minimum squared error. This leads, with further rearrangment and the definition of an array B_{imn}, to the expression

$$\begin{aligned}\hat{r}(i) - \sum_{jk} \mathbf{w}_{jk}^{\mathbf{tf}} s(i-j+1,k) &= c_1 + \sum_{mn} \mathbf{w}_{mn}^{\boldsymbol{\tau\phi}} \times \sum_{jk} \mathbf{w}_{jk}^{\mathbf{tf}} s(i-j+1,k) s(i-j+1-m,k+n) \\ &= c_1 + \sum_{mn} \mathbf{w}_{mn}^{\boldsymbol{\tau\phi}} B_{imn}\,. \end{aligned} \tag{21}$$

Thus, in order to update $\mathbf{w}^{\boldsymbol{\tau\phi}}$, we hold $\mathbf{w}^{\mathbf{tf}}$ fixed and regress according to

$$\widehat{\mathbf{r}} - \mathbf{w}^{\mathbf{tf}} \bullet \mathbf{M}^{\mathbf{itf}} = \mathbf{w}^{(\boldsymbol{\tau\phi})} \bullet \mathbf{B}^{\mathbf{i}(\boldsymbol{\tau\phi})}\,, \tag{22}$$

where $M_{ijk}^{\mathbf{itf}} = s(i-j+1,k)$ as before.

6.2.3. Implementation Issues

Although the multilinear notation (through the use of high-dimensional stimulus arrays) has allowed us to formulate a number of models in an elegant way, in its most naïve form it raises a number of computational issues. In practice, storing even a five-dimensional stimulus tensor can require substantial memory resources. Consider, for example, the extended context model detailed in Eq. 17. If we were to consider 3000 data points ($T = 3000$), a PRF of dimension $(J = 15) \times (K = 48)$, and a CGF of dimension $(M = 13) \times (N = 25)$, values which are typical in our own experiments, then the full five-dimensional stimulus tensor $\mathbf{Q}^{\text{itf}\tau\phi}$ would need to contain $(3000 \times 15 \times 48 \times 13 \times 25 = 702,000,000)$ elements. If these numbers are to be stored with 8-byte double precision this could pose resource challenges on a contemporary desktop computer. Thus, implementations may not generally reflect the full multidimensional formulae.

Many experimental stimuli, such as the dynamic random chord, are designed to be spectrotemporally-sparse, with $s(i, k)$ being mostly zero. In this case, the vast majority of entries in (say) $\mathbf{Q}^{\text{itf}\tau\phi}$ will also be zero—a greater proportion, in fact, than in the stimulus spectrogram itself due to the effects of multiplying different sparse components. Thus, such arrays may be maintained as compact lists of non-zero entries and corresponding indices, and sparse multiplication algorithms can greatly speed computation. In the general case of a spectrotemporally-dense stimulus such as a ripple or temporally orthogonal ripple combination (TORC; Klein et al. 2000), or a natural sound, it may be necessary to compute the arrays $\mathbf{A}$ and $\mathbf{B}$ directly from the spectrogram as they were defined above, without introducing the intermediate high-dimensional array.

6.3. Control of Overfitting

Overfitting is a particular concern when dealing with a large number of parameters. Depending on exactly how the parameters are separated multilinear context models may contain upwards of 1000 parameters, which can result in the incorrect "explanation" of noise within the data. As was the case for linear models, this effect can be discouraged by statistical regularisation.

The ALS algorithm for multilinear models minimises the squared error on the training data through a series of ordinary least-squares regression steps. It might therefore seem straightforward to carry over the techniques of regularisation developed for linear regression to this case. Indeed, if the form and strength of the regularisation penalties are fixed, or are to be determined by cross-validation, then the penalties can legitimately be introduced separately to each linear-regression weight update. This reduces regularised fitting of a multilinear model to a series of regularised linear regression steps.

However, as in the case of linear regression, determining appropriate values for the regularisation penalties by cross-validation may be overly expensive. Indeed, the difficulty is more severe for multilinear models as we have more regularisers to set (one for each component vector) and each regularised objective must be minimised by a relatively costly iterative process rather than by a single matrix equation. Thus, evidence optimisation methods are particularly attractive in this case.

A straightforward application of evidence optimisation might seem to be to replace each linear regression stage of ALS with a corresponding evidence optimisation stage. Thus, when updating $\mathbf{w}^{\text{tf}}$, say, we would first optimise a corresponding parametrised weight-covariance $\mathbf{C}^{\text{tf}}$ and then estimate a new value of $\mathbf{w}^{\text{tf}}$ under the optimal such covariance. The computational cost of the evidence optimisation could be reduced by initialising the search for the optimal covariance from the parameters determined at its last update.

However, whilst practical, this approach is not well-founded. The evidence being optimised in each case pertains only to a particular linear regression problem. As other weight vectors in the model are changed, the linear regression problem for a particular set of weights must be revised. Although this can indeed be done at the next iteration, there is no guarantee that a consistent solution will ever be found. Indeed, we observe empirically that this process often fails to converge. A practical but suboptimal solution may be to update the weight covariances only on the first few iterations of ALS, thereafter holding them fixed and making simple MAP updates; this has been observed to provide reasonable results in many situations.

Ideally, however, the covariances would be chosen to maximise the evidence derived from the complete multilinear model, rather than each separate evidence associated with the individual linear stages. Unfortunately, there is no closed form for the total evidence in this case, and so it cannot be optimised exactly. However, it is amenable to a robust form of approximation which does provide guarantees of convergence.

6.4. Approximate Variational Evidence Optimisation

Consider a full-rank bilinear context model given by

$$\widehat{\mathbf{r}} = (\mathbf{w}^{\mathbf{tf}} \otimes \mathbf{w}^{\boldsymbol{\tau\phi}}) \bullet \mathbf{Q}^{\mathbf{itf}\boldsymbol{\tau\phi}}.$$

It will be convenient to represent the weights as vectors rather than as two-dimensional arrays. Thus, as when we first discussed the STRF model, we express the model in terms of "unrolled" spectrotemporal vectors of both PRF and CGF. Using the notation introduced in section 5.1, this is written:

$$\widehat{\mathbf{r}} = (\mathbf{w}^{(\mathbf{tf})} \otimes \mathbf{w}^{(\boldsymbol{\tau\phi})}) \bullet \mathbf{Q}^{\mathbf{i}(\mathbf{tf})(\boldsymbol{\tau\phi})}.$$

.

6.4.1. Derivative-based Smoothing

Evidence optimisation schemes for receptive-field determination have most often been specified by parametrisation of the covariance matrix $\mathbf{C}$, as described in the section above. In the multilinear case, the resulting matrices seem often to become ill-conditioned, making their inversion numerically unstable. Thus, it has proven more robust to instead parametrise directly the *inverse covariance* (or *precision*) matrix $\mathbf{D} = \mathbf{C}^{-1}$. Consider first a linear regression problem. The augmented log-likelihood objective function is

$$\mathcal{E} = \frac{1}{2\sigma^2}\|\mathbf{r} - \widehat{\mathbf{r}}\|^2 + \mathbf{w}^\top \mathbf{D}\mathbf{w}.$$

How might one choose a suitable form for $\mathbf{D}$? One approach is to penalise derivatives of the weight vector (or equally, to adopt a prior belief that this derivative should be small—a different form of smoothness to that assumed in ASD). For example, to penalise large first derivatives $\mathbf{D}$ could be chosen such that $\mathbf{w}^\top\mathbf{D}\mathbf{w} = \alpha\sum_j(w_{j+1} - w_j)^2$, with α setting the relative strength of regularisation, or equivalently the expected scale of the derivative. This leads to a form in which a tri-diagonal matrix with main diagonal entries all equal to 2 and adjacent off-diagonal elements equal to -1 is scaled by α. More generally, if we define Z to be the difference matrix:

$$\mathbf{Z} = \begin{pmatrix} 1 & -1 & 0 & \cdots & 0 & 0 \\ 0 & 1 & -1 & & 0 & 0 \\ 0 & 0 & 1 & \ddots & 0 & 0 \\ \vdots & & & \ddots & & \vdots \\ 0 & 0 & 0 & & 1 & -1 \\ 0 & 0 & 0 & \cdots & 0 & 0 \end{pmatrix},$$

then a first derivative penalty is achieved by setting $\mathbf{D}$ proportional to $\mathbf{D}_1 = \mathbf{Z}^\top\mathbf{Z}$. A second derivative penalty is achieved by setting $\mathbf{D}$ proportional to $\mathbf{D}_2 = \mathbf{D}_1^\top\mathbf{D}_1$. A direct penalty on the scale of $\mathbf{w}$ is achieved by taking $\mathbf{D}$ proportional to $\mathbf{D}_0 = I$ (which is equivalent to ridge regression). More generally, we can mix all three forms of derivative, with unknown relative weights. If the vector $\mathbf{w}$ reflects an pair of unrolled dimensions (as does $\mathbf{w}^{(\mathrm{tf})}$, for example), then we would define two separate difference matrices $\mathbf{Z}^{\mathrm{t}/(\mathrm{tf})}$ and $\mathbf{Z}^{\mathrm{f}/(\mathrm{tf})}$, each taking differences of weights along the time or frequency dimensions alone, and $\mathbf{D}_1^{\mathrm{t}} = \mathbf{Z}^{\mathrm{t}/(\mathrm{tf})\top}\mathbf{Z}^{\mathrm{t}/(\mathrm{tf})}$, $\mathbf{D}_2^{\mathrm{t}} = \mathbf{D}_1^{\mathrm{t}\top}\mathbf{D}_1^{\mathrm{t}}$ (and similarly for $\mathbf{D}_1^{\mathrm{f}}$ and $\mathbf{D}_2^{\mathrm{f}}$) and define

$$\mathbf{D}^{(\mathrm{tf})}(\boldsymbol{\alpha}^{(\mathrm{tf})}) = \alpha_0^{(\mathrm{tf})}\mathbf{D}_0 + \alpha_1^{(\mathrm{tf})}\mathbf{D}_1^{\mathrm{t}} + \alpha_2^{(\mathrm{tf})}\mathbf{D}_2^{\mathrm{t}} + \alpha_3^{(\mathrm{tf})}\mathbf{D}_1^{\mathrm{f}} + \alpha_4^{(\mathrm{tf})}\mathbf{D}_2^{\mathrm{f}}. \tag{23}$$

Evidence optimisation can then be used to select suitable values for the parameters $\boldsymbol{\alpha}^{(\mathrm{tf})}$.

6.4.2. The Variational Approximation

For the multilinear model, the goal is to select both parameters $\boldsymbol{\alpha}^{(\mathrm{tf})}$ as defined in Eq. 23 and an analagously defined $\boldsymbol{\alpha}^{(\tau\phi)}$ which determines the regulariser for $\mathbf{w}^{(\tau\phi)}$. Ideally, these would be chosen to maximise the joint (log) evidence:

$$\log P(\mathbf{r}|\hat{\sigma}^2, \boldsymbol{\alpha}^{\mathrm{tf}}, \boldsymbol{\alpha}^{\tau\phi}) = \log \int d\mathbf{w}^{(\mathrm{tf})} d\mathbf{w}^{(\tau\phi)} P(\mathbf{r}|\mathbf{w}^{(\mathrm{tf})}, \mathbf{w}^{(\tau\phi)}, \hat{\sigma}^2) P(\mathbf{w}^{(\mathrm{tf})}|\boldsymbol{\alpha}^{\mathrm{tf}}) P(\mathbf{w}^{(\tau\phi)}|\boldsymbol{\alpha}^{\tau\phi}),$$

but there is no closed form expression for this (or for its gradients). Instead, we use a variational approximation to the evidence (Jordan et al., 1999; Beal, 2003), in which a lower bound that depends on an unknown distribution over $\mathbf{w}^{\mathrm{tf}}$ and $\mathbf{w}^{\tau\phi}$ is maximised iteratively with respect to this distribution and with respect to the precision parameters. Maximisation of this lower bound, known as the free energy, becomes tractable if the distribution on $\mathbf{w}^{\mathrm{tf}}$ and $\mathbf{w}^{\tau\phi}$ is assumed to factor; that is, it has the form $q^{(\mathrm{tf})}(\mathbf{w}^{(\mathrm{tf})})q^{(\tau\phi)}(\mathbf{w}^{(\tau\phi)})$. Although maximisation of such a lower bound does not guarantee that the parameters also maximise the evidence, many empirical studies have suggested that the approximation can yield good results (Beal 2003; but see Turner and Sahani 2011). This section provides an outline of the resulting algorithm. Further details are provided in section 8.

The lower bound is defined by way of Jensen's inequality for the log expectation of a concave function (the third step below — we suppress the superscripts to the distributions

q where the identity of the distribution is clear from its argument):

$$
\begin{aligned}
&\log P(\mathbf{r}|\hat{\sigma}^2, \boldsymbol{\alpha}^{\mathrm{tf}}, \boldsymbol{\alpha}^{\tau\phi}) \\
&= \log \int d\mathbf{w}^{(\mathrm{tf})} d\mathbf{w}^{(\tau\phi)} P(\mathbf{r}|\mathbf{w}^{(\mathrm{tf})}, \mathbf{w}^{(\tau\phi)}, \sigma^2) P(\mathbf{w}^{(\mathrm{tf})}|\boldsymbol{\alpha}^{\mathrm{tf}}) P(\mathbf{w}^{(\tau\phi)}|\boldsymbol{\alpha}^{\tau\phi}) \\
&= \log \int d\mathbf{w}^{(\mathrm{tf})} d\mathbf{w}^{(\tau\phi)} \frac{q(\mathbf{w}^{(\mathrm{tf})}) q(\mathbf{w}^{(\tau\phi)})}{q(\mathbf{w}^{(\mathrm{tf})}) q(\mathbf{w}^{(\tau\phi)})} P(\mathbf{r}|\mathbf{w}^{(\mathrm{tf})}, \mathbf{w}^{(\tau\phi)}, \sigma^2) P(\mathbf{w}^{(\mathrm{tf})}|\boldsymbol{\alpha}^{\mathrm{tf}}) P(\mathbf{w}^{(\tau\phi)}|\boldsymbol{\alpha}^{\tau\phi}) \\
&\geq \int d\mathbf{w}^{(\mathrm{tf})} d\mathbf{w}^{(\tau\phi)} q(\mathbf{w}^{(\mathrm{tf})}) q(\mathbf{w}^{(\tau\phi)}) \log \left(P(\mathbf{r}|\mathbf{w}^{(\mathrm{tf})}, \mathbf{w}^{(\tau\phi)}, \sigma^2) P(\mathbf{w}^{(\mathrm{tf})}|\boldsymbol{\alpha}^{\mathrm{tf}}) P(\mathbf{w}^{(\tau\phi)}|\boldsymbol{\alpha}^{\tau\phi}) \right) \\
&\qquad - \int d\mathbf{w}^{(\mathrm{tf})} q(\mathbf{w}^{(\mathrm{tf})}) \log \left(q(\mathbf{w}^{(\mathrm{tf})} \right) - \int d\mathbf{w}^{(\tau\phi)} q(\mathbf{w}^{(\tau\phi)}) \log \left(q(\mathbf{w}^{(\tau\phi)}) \right) \\
&= \int d\mathbf{w}^{(\mathrm{tf})} d\mathbf{w}^{(\tau\phi)} q(\mathbf{w}^{(\mathrm{tf})}) q(\mathbf{w}^{(\tau\phi)}) \log \left(P(\mathbf{r}|\mathbf{w}^{(\mathrm{tf})}, \mathbf{w}^{(\tau\phi)}, \sigma^2) P(\mathbf{w}^{(\mathrm{tf})}|\boldsymbol{\alpha}^{\mathrm{tf}}) P(\mathbf{w}^{(\tau\phi)}|\boldsymbol{\alpha}^{\tau\phi}) \right) \\
&\qquad + H(q^{(\mathrm{tf})}) + H(q^{(\tau\phi)}) \\
&\equiv \mathcal{F}(q^{(\mathrm{tf})}, q^{(\tau\phi)}, \sigma^2, \boldsymbol{\alpha}^{\mathrm{tf}}, \boldsymbol{\alpha}^{\tau\phi}) \,.
\end{aligned}
$$

Here $\mathcal{F}$ is the free energy, and the two H terms are entropies. The free energy is optimised alternately with respect to $q^{(\mathrm{tf})}$, $q^{(\tau\phi)}$, $\boldsymbol{\alpha}^{(\mathrm{tf})}$, $\boldsymbol{\alpha}^{(\tau\phi)}$ and σ^2. The updates can be divided into two groups.

6.4.3. Distributional Updates

Goal: optimise $\mathcal{F}$ with respect to $q^{(\mathrm{tf})}$ and $q^{(\tau\phi)}$ (by setting the variational derivatives in $q^{(\mathrm{tf})}$ and $q^{(\tau\phi)}$ to zero).

Differentiating and setting equal to zero yields

$$
q^{(\mathrm{tf})}(\mathbf{w}^{(\mathrm{tf})}) \propto \exp \left\langle \log \left(P(\mathbf{r}|\mathbf{w}^{(\mathrm{tf})}, \mathbf{w}^{(\tau\phi)}, \sigma^2) \right) \right\rangle_{q^{(\tau\phi)}} P(\mathbf{w}^{(\mathrm{tf})}|\boldsymbol{\alpha}^{\mathrm{tf}}) \,,
$$

where the angle brackets $\langle\rangle_q$ represent an expected value with respect to the distribution q. The constant of proportionality is set by the requirement that $q^{(\mathrm{tf})}$ be a normalised density. The update for $q^{(\tau\phi)}$ is written similarly.

It should be reasonably evident that $\log P(\mathbf{r}|\mathbf{w}^{(\mathrm{tf})}, \mathbf{w}^{(\tau\phi)}, \sigma^2)$ will be quadratic in $\mathbf{w}^{(\mathrm{tf})}$, and remains quadratic after averaging with respect to $q^{(\tau\phi)}$. Thus, if the prior $P(\mathbf{w}^{(\mathrm{tf})}|\boldsymbol{\alpha}^{\mathrm{tf}})$ is Gaussian, then $q^{(\mathrm{tf})}$ will also be Gaussian (and likewise for $q^{(\tau\phi)}$). Let $q^{(\mathrm{tf})} = \mathcal{N}(\boldsymbol{\mu}^{(\mathrm{tf})}, \boldsymbol{\Sigma}^{(\mathrm{tf})})$, and $q^{(\tau\phi)} = \mathcal{N}(\boldsymbol{\mu}^{(\tau\phi)}, \boldsymbol{\Sigma}^{(\tau\phi)})$. We note that $\boldsymbol{\mu}^{(\mathrm{tf})}$ and $\boldsymbol{\Sigma}^{(\mathrm{tf})}$ depend on $\boldsymbol{\mu}^{(\tau\phi)}$ and $\boldsymbol{\Sigma}^{(\tau\phi)}$ (and vice-versa). Thus, the parameters of these two Gaussians must be found iteratively, but it is possible to prove that this iteration must converge under weak regularity conditions. Futhermore, this interaction is precisely the element that would be missing if evidence optimisation were to be carried out separately at each stage of ALS. The detailed iterations are provided in section 8.

6.4.4. Parameter Updates

Goal: with $q^{(\mathrm{tf})}$ and $q^{(\tau\phi)}$ held fixed, $\mathcal{F}$ is maximised with respect to the precision parameters $\boldsymbol{\alpha}^{\mathrm{tf}}$,$\boldsymbol{\alpha}^{\tau\phi}$, and the noise scale σ^2. The optimal noise scale σ^2 can be found in closed form, but the optimisation of the precision must be numerical, as for evidence optimisation for linear regression. The gradients are given in section 8.

6.4.5. Scheduling

The various updates are then repeated in a nested form:

Assume initial values for $\boldsymbol{\mu}^{(\tau\phi)}$ and $\boldsymbol{\Sigma}^{(\tau\phi)}$.
while not converged **do**
    while not converged **and** max iterations not reached **do**
        Update the values of $\boldsymbol{\mu}^{(\mathrm{tf})}$ and $\boldsymbol{\Sigma}^{(\mathrm{tf})}$.
        Update the values of $\boldsymbol{\mu}^{(\tau\phi)}$ and $\boldsymbol{\Sigma}^{(\tau\phi)}$.
    end while
    Update the noise scale σ^2.
    Maximise $\mathcal{F}$ with respect to the $\boldsymbol{\alpha}^{\mathrm{tf}}$ and $\boldsymbol{\alpha}^{\tau\phi}$ by gradient ascent.
end while

7. Conclusion

The fundamental question of how sensory stimuli are encoded by the neurons of the sensory pathways is of central importance to neuroscience. This chapter has investigated the *predictive* probabilistic approach to answering this question. We have seen how this approach allows us to adopt statistical tools so as to minimise the impact of noise on estimates of systematic stimulus representation. For the spectrogram-linear auditory representation embodied by the STRF, variants of these tools can provide optimally smoothed, sparsified or localised estimates of neurons' spectrotemporal selectivities.

The same predictive approach and similar statistical techniques extend to studies of nonlinear auditory representations and models. In particular, we have investigated a *multilinear* formulation, in which representations that contain both nonlinear transforms of the input and spectrotemporally local contextual interactions can be studied.

In our discussion of both linear and nonlinear models, we have focused on the mathematical methods that underlie the predictive probabilistic approach, and on the motivations behind the approach overall and behind various choices of model structure or regulariser. We have not considered the conclusions that have been reached by applying these methods to data from the auditory system; for these, we refer the interested reader to the primary publications cited above.

8. Appendix: Variational EM for Bilinear Systems

In section 6.4.2 we outlined a variational Bayesian algorithm for performing approximate evidence optimisation in a bilinear system. For brevity, only key results were presented. The full derivation of the variational algorithm follows here.

The (log) evidence of the bilinear model is

$$\log P(\mathbf{r}|\sigma^2, \boldsymbol{\alpha}^{\mathrm{tf}}, \boldsymbol{\alpha}^{\tau\phi}) = \log \int d\mathbf{w}^{(\mathrm{tf})} d\mathbf{w}^{(\tau\phi)} P(\mathbf{r}|\mathbf{w}^{(\mathrm{tf})}, \mathbf{w}^{(\tau\phi)}, \sigma^2) P(\mathbf{w}^{(\mathrm{tf})}|\boldsymbol{\alpha}^{\mathrm{tf}}) P(\mathbf{w}^{(\tau\phi)}|\boldsymbol{\alpha}^{\tau\phi}) \tag{24}$$

We use a factorised distribution $q^{(\mathrm{tf})}(\mathbf{w}^{(\mathrm{tf})})\ q^{(\tau\phi)}(\mathbf{w}^{(\tau\phi)})$ and Jensen's inequality to lower bound this evidence. (To improve readability, we have omitted the superscripts for the distributions q when the identity of the distribution is clear from its argument).

$$
\begin{aligned}
&\log P(\mathbf{r}|\sigma^2, \boldsymbol{\alpha}^{\mathrm{tf}}, \boldsymbol{\alpha}^{\tau\phi}) \\
&= \log \int d\mathbf{w}^{(\mathrm{tf})}\, d\mathbf{w}^{(\tau\phi)}\ P(\mathbf{r}|\mathbf{w}^{(\mathrm{tf})}, \mathbf{w}^{(\tau\phi)}, \sigma^2)\ P(\mathbf{w}^{(\mathrm{tf})}|\boldsymbol{\alpha}^{\mathrm{tf}})\ P(\mathbf{w}^{(\tau\phi)}|\boldsymbol{\alpha}^{\tau\phi}) \\
&= \log \int d\mathbf{w}^{(\mathrm{tf})}\, d\mathbf{w}^{(\tau\phi)}\ \frac{q(\mathbf{w}^{(\mathrm{tf})})q(\mathbf{w}^{(\tau\phi)})}{q(\mathbf{w}^{(\mathrm{tf})})q(\mathbf{w}^{(\tau\phi)})}\ P(\mathbf{r}|\mathbf{w}^{(\mathrm{tf})}, \mathbf{w}^{(\tau\phi)}, \sigma^2)\ P(\mathbf{w}^{(\mathrm{tf})}|\boldsymbol{\alpha}^{\mathrm{tf}})\ P(\mathbf{w}^{(\tau\phi)}|\boldsymbol{\alpha}^{\tau\phi}) \\
&\geq \int d\mathbf{w}^{(\mathrm{tf})}\, d\mathbf{w}^{(\tau\phi)}\ q(\mathbf{w}^{(\mathrm{tf})})\ q(\mathbf{w}^{(\tau\phi)}) \log \left(\frac{P(\mathbf{r}|\mathbf{w}^{(\mathrm{tf})}, \mathbf{w}^{(\tau\phi)}, \sigma^2)\ P(\mathbf{w}^{(\mathrm{tf})}|\boldsymbol{\alpha}^{\mathrm{tf}})\ P(\mathbf{w}^{(\tau\phi)}|\boldsymbol{\alpha}^{\tau\phi})}{q(\mathbf{w}^{(\mathrm{tf})})\ q(\mathbf{w}^{(\tau\phi)})} \right) \\
&= \int d\mathbf{w}^{(\mathrm{tf})}\, d\mathbf{w}^{(\tau\phi)}\ q(\mathbf{w}^{(\mathrm{tf})})\ q(\mathbf{w}^{(\tau\phi)})\ \log \left(P(\mathbf{r}|\mathbf{w}^{(\mathrm{tf})}, \mathbf{w}^{(\tau\phi)}, \sigma^2) P(\mathbf{w}^{(\mathrm{tf})}|\boldsymbol{\alpha}^{\mathrm{tf}}) P(\mathbf{w}^{(\tau\phi)}|\boldsymbol{\alpha}^{\tau\phi}) \right) \\
&\qquad - \int d\mathbf{w}^{(\mathrm{tf})}\, d\mathbf{w}^{(\tau\phi)}\ q(\mathbf{w}^{(\mathrm{tf})})\ q(\mathbf{w}^{(\tau\phi)})\ \log \left(q(\mathbf{w}^{(\mathrm{tf})})\ q(\mathbf{w}^{(\tau\phi)}) \right) \\
&= \int d\mathbf{w}^{(\mathrm{tf})}\, d\mathbf{w}^{(\tau\phi)}\ q(\mathbf{w}^{(\mathrm{tf})})\ q(\mathbf{w}^{(\tau\phi)})\ \log \left(P(\mathbf{r}|\mathbf{w}^{(\mathrm{tf})}, \mathbf{w}^{(\tau\phi)}, \sigma^2)\ P(\mathbf{w}^{(\mathrm{tf})}|\boldsymbol{\alpha}^{\mathrm{tf}})\ P(\mathbf{w}^{(\tau\phi)}|\boldsymbol{\alpha}^{\tau\phi}) \right) \\
&\qquad - \int d\mathbf{w}^{(\mathrm{tf})}\ q(\mathbf{w}^{(\mathrm{tf})})\ \log \left(q(\mathbf{w}^{(\mathrm{tf})}) \right) - \int d\mathbf{w}^{(\tau\phi)}\ q(\mathbf{w}^{(\tau\phi)})\ \log \left(q(\mathbf{w}^{(\tau\phi)}) \right) \\
&= \int d\mathbf{w}^{(\mathrm{tf})}\, d\mathbf{w}^{(\tau\phi)}\ q(\mathbf{w}^{(\mathrm{tf})})\ q(\mathbf{w}^{(\tau\phi)})\ \log \left(P(\mathbf{r}|\mathbf{w}^{(\mathrm{tf})}, \mathbf{w}^{(\tau\phi)}, \sigma^2)\ P(\mathbf{w}^{(\mathrm{tf})}|\boldsymbol{\alpha}^{\mathrm{tf}})\ P(\mathbf{w}^{(\tau\phi)}|\boldsymbol{\alpha}^{\tau\phi}) \right) \\
&\qquad + H(q^{(\mathrm{tf})}) + H(q^{(\tau\phi)}) \\
&\equiv \mathcal{F}(q^{(\mathrm{tf})}, q^{(\tau\phi)}, \sigma^2, \boldsymbol{\alpha}^{\mathrm{tf}}, \boldsymbol{\alpha}^{\tau\phi})
\end{aligned} \tag{25}
$$

Here $\mathcal{F}$ is the free energy, and the two H terms are entropies.

8.1. Distributional Updates

Goal: optimise $\mathcal{F}$ w.r.t. $q^{(\mathrm{tf})}$ and $q^{(\tau\phi)}$ (by taking variational derivatives w.r.t. $q^{(\mathrm{tf})}$ and $q^{(\tau\phi)}$ and setting these to zero).

The derivation that follows will focus on $q^{(\mathrm{tf})}$ only. $q^{(\tau\phi)}$ follows in a very similar fashion. We start by adding a Lagrange multiplier to $\mathcal{F}$ to constrain $q^{(\mathrm{tf})}$ to be normalised

$$
\begin{aligned}
&\frac{\delta}{\delta q^{(\mathrm{tf})}} \left(\mathcal{F} + \lambda \left(\int d\mathbf{w}^{(\mathrm{tf})}\ q(\mathbf{w}^{(\mathrm{tf})}) - 1 \right) \right) \\
&\qquad = \int d\mathbf{w}^{(\tau\phi)}\ q(\mathbf{w}^{(\tau\phi)})\ \log \left(P(\mathbf{r}|\mathbf{w}^{(\mathrm{tf})}, \mathbf{w}^{(\tau\phi)}, \sigma^2)\ P(\mathbf{w}^{(\mathrm{tf})}|\boldsymbol{\alpha}^{\mathrm{tf}})\ P(\mathbf{w}^{(\tau\phi)}|\boldsymbol{\alpha}^{\tau\phi}) \right) \\
&\qquad\quad - \log \left(q(\mathbf{w}^{(\mathrm{tf})}) \right) - 1 + \lambda
\end{aligned} \tag{26}
$$

Setting this to zero yields

$$
q^{(\mathrm{tf})}(\mathbf{w}^{(\mathrm{tf})}) = \exp(\lambda - 1) \exp \left\langle \log \left(P(\mathbf{r}|\mathbf{w}^{(\mathrm{tf})}, \mathbf{w}^{(\tau\phi)}, \sigma^2) \right) \right\rangle_{q^{(\tau\phi)}} P(\mathbf{w}^{(\mathrm{tf})}|\boldsymbol{\alpha}^{\mathrm{tf}}) \tag{27}
$$

(although the term $P(\mathbf{w}^{(\mathrm{tf})}|\boldsymbol{\alpha}^{\mathrm{tf}})$ also appears inside an $\exp\langle\log(\ldots)\rangle_{q^{(\tau\phi)}}$, it is independent of $\mathbf{w}^{(\tau\phi)}$ and so reduced to $P(\mathbf{w}^{(\mathrm{tf})}|\boldsymbol{\alpha}^{\mathrm{tf}})$.) Here λ is a constant that serves to normalise $q^{(\mathrm{tf})}$.

Now $\log P(\mathbf{r}|\mathbf{w}^{(\mathrm{tf})}, \mathbf{w}^{(\tau\phi)}, \sigma^2)$ is quadratic in $\mathbf{w}^{(\mathrm{tf})}$ and this gets preserved in the average $\langle\ldots\rangle_{q^{(\tau\phi)}}$, so that if the prior $P(\mathbf{w}^{(\mathrm{tf})}|\boldsymbol{\alpha}^{\mathrm{tf}})$ is Gaussian, then $q^{(\mathrm{tf})}$ is also Gaussian. We can now give the parameters of these Gaussians a name: let $q^{(\mathrm{tf})} = \mathcal{N}(\boldsymbol{\mu}^{(\mathrm{tf})}, \boldsymbol{\Sigma}^{(\mathrm{tf})})$ and

$q^{(\tau\phi)} = \mathcal{N}(\boldsymbol{\mu}^{(\tau\phi)}, \boldsymbol{\Sigma}^{(\tau\phi)})$. The algorithm is iterative, so we can assume we have values for $\boldsymbol{\mu}^{(\tau\phi)}$ and $\boldsymbol{\Sigma}^{(\tau\phi)}$ and use these to update the values of $\boldsymbol{\mu}^{(\mathrm{tf})}$ and $\boldsymbol{\Sigma}^{(\mathrm{tf})}$. To find these, we first ignore the prior and look at the likelihood term (absorbing the log-determinant in the constant),

$$\begin{aligned}
&\left\langle \log\left(P(\mathbf{r}|\mathbf{w}^{(\mathrm{tf})}, \mathbf{w}^{(\tau\phi)}, \sigma^2)\right)\right\rangle_{q^{(\tau\phi)}} \\
&\quad = \mathrm{const} - \frac{1}{2\sigma^2}\left\langle (\mathbf{r} - (\mathbf{w}^{(\mathrm{tf})} \otimes \mathbf{w}^{(\tau\phi)}) \bullet Q)^2 \right\rangle_{q^{(\tau\phi)}} \\
&\quad = \mathrm{const} - \frac{1}{2\sigma^2}\langle \mathbf{r}^2 - 2\mathbf{r}^\top \left((\mathbf{w}^{(\mathrm{tf})} \otimes \mathbf{w}^{(\tau\phi)}) \bullet Q\right) \\
&\qquad + \left((\mathbf{w}^{(\mathrm{tf})} \otimes \mathbf{w}^{(\tau\phi)}) \bullet Q\right)^\top \left((\mathbf{w}^{(\mathrm{tf})} \otimes \mathbf{w}^{(\tau\phi)}) \bullet Q\right)\rangle_{q^{(\tau\phi)}}
\end{aligned} \tag{28}$$

We can now simplify the quadratic term. Ignoring the $\frac{1}{2\sigma^2}$ for the moment and writing in component notation, the quadratic term is

$$\left\langle \sum_{iaa'bb'} w_a^{\mathrm{tf}} w_{a'}^{\mathrm{tf}} w_b^{\tau\phi} w_{b'}^{\tau\phi} Q_{iab} Q_{ia'b'} \right\rangle_{q^{(\tau\phi)}} = \sum_{iaa'bb'} w_a^{\mathrm{tf}} w_{a'}^{\mathrm{tf}} \left\langle w_b^{\tau\phi} w_{b'}^{\tau\phi} \right\rangle_{q^{(\tau\phi)}} Q_{iab} Q_{ia'b'} \tag{29}$$

The term in angle brackets is the $(b, b')^{\mathrm{th}}$ element of $\left\langle \mathbf{w}^{(\tau\phi)} \mathbf{w}^{(\tau\phi)\top} \right\rangle_{q^{(\tau\phi)}}$, which equals $\boldsymbol{\mu}^{(\tau\phi)} \boldsymbol{\mu}^{(\tau\phi)\top} + \boldsymbol{\Sigma}^{(\tau\phi)}$. We shrink this expression, and reintroduce $\frac{1}{\sigma^2}$, by setting

$$C_{aa'}^{\mathrm{tf}} = \frac{1}{\sigma^2} \sum_{ibb'} \left(\mu_b^{\tau\phi} \mu_{b'}^{\tau\phi} + \Sigma_{bb'}^{\tau\phi}\right) Q_{iab} Q_{ia'b'} \tag{30}$$

to get the quadratic term

$$\sum_{aa'} w_a^{\mathrm{tf}} w_{a'}^{\mathrm{tf}} C_{aa'}^{\mathrm{tf}} = \mathbf{w}^{(\mathrm{tf})\top} \mathbf{C}^{\mathrm{tf}} \mathbf{w}^{(\mathrm{tf})} \tag{31}$$

In order to establish the covariance of $q^{(\mathrm{tf})}$, we simply need to multiply by the prior, or equivalently, add the log-prior to the above expression. The log-prior is

$$\log P(\mathbf{w}^{(\mathrm{tf})} | \boldsymbol{\alpha}^{\mathrm{tf}}) = -\frac{1}{2} \mathbf{w}^{\mathrm{tf}T} D^{\mathrm{tf}} \mathbf{w}^{(\mathrm{tf})} \tag{32}$$

therefore the entire quadratic term is $-\frac{1}{2}\mathbf{w}^{(\mathrm{tf})\top}\left(C^{\mathrm{tf}} + D^{\mathrm{tf}}\right)\mathbf{w}^{(\mathrm{tf})}$ and so the covariance of $q^{(\mathrm{tf})}$ is:

$$\boldsymbol{\Sigma}^{(\mathrm{tf})} = \left(C^{\mathrm{tf}} + D^{\mathrm{tf}}\right)^{-1} \tag{33}$$

The mean of $q^{(\mathrm{tf})}$ is found similarly and is defined via the vector:

$$v_a^{\mathrm{tf}} = \sum_i r_i Q_{iab} \mu_b^{\tau\phi}, \tag{34}$$

and equals:

$$\boldsymbol{\mu}^{(\mathrm{tf})} = \frac{1}{\sigma^2} \boldsymbol{\Sigma}^{(\mathrm{tf})} v^{\mathrm{tf}}. \tag{35}$$

This is the update for $q^{(\mathrm{tf})}$. The update for $q^{(\tau\phi)}$ is exactly the same except the averaging is over $q^{(\mathrm{tf})}$, and $\boldsymbol{\mu}^{(\tau\phi)}$ and $\boldsymbol{\Sigma}^{(\tau\phi)}$ get defined in terms of $\boldsymbol{\mu}^{(\mathrm{tf})}$ and $\boldsymbol{\Sigma}^{(\mathrm{tf})}$.

8.2. Parameter updates

Goal: with $q^{(\mathbf{tf})}$ and $q^{(\boldsymbol{\tau\phi})}$ held fixed, $\mathcal{F}$ is maximised with respect to the hyperparameters $\boldsymbol{\alpha}^{\mathbf{tf}}$,$\boldsymbol{\alpha}^{\boldsymbol{\tau\phi}}$, and the noise scale σ^2.

The noise scale σ^2 has an exact update, but the hyperparameter optimisation needs to be done through the use of gradient ascent, since there is no closed-form solution. The gradient is obtained by differentiating $\mathcal{F}$ w.r.t. $\boldsymbol{\alpha}^{\mathbf{tf}}$ and $\boldsymbol{\alpha}^{\boldsymbol{\tau\phi}}$. Since we are differentiating with respect to the hyperparameters, only the terms in $\mathcal{F}$ that depend on $\boldsymbol{\alpha}^{\mathbf{tf}}$ and $\boldsymbol{\alpha}^{\boldsymbol{\tau\phi}}$ need to be considered; namely, the log-priors averaged over the $q^{(\mathbf{tf})}$ and $q^{(\boldsymbol{\tau\phi})}$. Note that the hyperparameters also appear implicitly in the distributions $q^{(\mathbf{tf})}$ and $q^{(\boldsymbol{\tau\phi})}$, but since these are being held fixed they do not contribute here. For notational purposes, we call the α-dependent terms $\bar{\mathcal{F}}$ and thus

$$\begin{aligned}\bar{\mathcal{F}} &= \int d\mathbf{w}^{(\mathbf{tf})}\, d\mathbf{w}^{(\boldsymbol{\tau\phi})}\, q(\mathbf{w}^{(\mathbf{tf})})\, q(\mathbf{w}^{(\boldsymbol{\tau\phi})})\, \log\left(P(\mathbf{w}^{(\mathbf{tf})}|\boldsymbol{\alpha}^{\mathbf{tf}})\, P(\mathbf{w}^{(\boldsymbol{\tau\phi})}|\boldsymbol{\alpha}^{\boldsymbol{\tau\phi}})\right)\\ &= \left\langle \log P(\mathbf{w}^{(\mathbf{tf})}|\boldsymbol{\alpha}^{\mathbf{tf}})\right\rangle_{q^{(\mathbf{tf})}} + \left\langle \log P(\mathbf{w}^{(\boldsymbol{\tau\phi})}|\boldsymbol{\alpha}^{\boldsymbol{\tau\phi}})\right\rangle_{q^{(\boldsymbol{\tau\phi})}}\\ &= \frac{1}{2}\log\det\mathbf{D}^{(\mathbf{tf})} + \frac{1}{2}\log\det\mathbf{D}^{(\boldsymbol{\tau\phi})} - \frac{1}{2}\text{trace}\left((\boldsymbol{\mu}^{(\mathbf{tf})}\boldsymbol{\mu}^{(\mathbf{tf})^\top} + \boldsymbol{\Sigma}^{(\mathbf{tf})})\mathbf{D}^{(\mathbf{tf})}\right)\\ &\quad - \frac{1}{2}\text{trace}\left((\boldsymbol{\mu}^{(\boldsymbol{\tau\phi})}\boldsymbol{\mu}^{(\boldsymbol{\tau\phi})^\top} + \boldsymbol{\Sigma}^{(\boldsymbol{\tau\phi})})\mathbf{D}^{(\boldsymbol{\tau\phi})}\right)\end{aligned} \tag{36}$$

(using $\det X^{-1} = \frac{1}{\det X}$ for the first two terms). Now we differentiate w.r.t. the parameters that specify the D's, e.g. $\alpha_i^{(\mathbf{tf})}$. The derivative can be taken inside the trace, and for the log terms, we use $\frac{\partial}{\partial\theta}\log\det X(\theta) =^\top \left(X^{-1}\frac{\partial}{\partial\theta}X\right)$. Thus

$$\frac{\partial}{\partial\alpha_i^{(\mathbf{tf})}}\bar{\mathcal{F}} = \frac{1}{2}\,\text{Tr}\left(\mathbf{D}^{(\mathbf{tf})^{-1}}\frac{\partial}{\partial\alpha_i^{(\mathbf{tf})}}\mathbf{D}^{(\mathbf{tf})}\right) - \frac{1}{2}\,\text{Tr}\left((\boldsymbol{\mu}^{(\boldsymbol{\tau\phi})}\boldsymbol{\mu}^{(\boldsymbol{\tau\phi})^\top} + \boldsymbol{\Sigma}^{(\boldsymbol{\tau\phi})})\frac{\partial}{\partial\alpha_i^{(\mathbf{tf})}}\mathbf{D}^{(\mathbf{tf})}\right) \tag{37}$$

With the form of $\mathbf{D}^{(\mathbf{tf})}$ above, i.e. $\mathbf{D}^{(\mathbf{tf})}(\boldsymbol{\alpha}^{\mathbf{tf}}) = \sum_i \alpha_i^{(\mathbf{tf})}\mathbf{D}_i^{(\mathbf{tf})}$, this becomes:

$$\frac{\partial}{\partial\alpha_i^{(\mathbf{tf})}}\bar{\mathcal{F}} = \frac{1}{2}\,\text{Tr}\left(\mathbf{D}_i^{(\mathbf{tf})}\left(\mathbf{D}^{(\mathbf{tf})^{-1}} - (\boldsymbol{\mu}^{(\boldsymbol{\tau\phi})}\boldsymbol{\mu}^{(\boldsymbol{\tau\phi})^\top} + \boldsymbol{\Sigma}^{(\boldsymbol{\tau\phi})})\right)\right). \tag{38}$$

The gradients over all $\boldsymbol{\alpha}_i^{\mathbf{tf}}$'s and all $\boldsymbol{\alpha}_i^{\boldsymbol{\tau\phi}}$'s can then be used in a gradient ascent to maximise $\bar{\mathcal{F}}$ and thus to maximise $\mathcal{F}$.

The noise scale σ^2 is also considered a hyperparameter, and must be optimised too. This parameter is found in the likelihood term, and implicitly in the Σ's and μ's. Again we consider the Σ's and μ's fixed because $q^{(\mathbf{tf})}$ and $q^{(\boldsymbol{\tau\phi})}$ are fixed during the M step of EM. Thus, only the likelihood term contributes here, and we define $\hat{\mathcal{F}}$ to be the part of $\mathcal{F}$ containing σ^2. Thus

$$\begin{aligned}\hat{\mathcal{F}} &= \int d\mathbf{w}^{(\mathbf{tf})}\, d\mathbf{w}^{(\boldsymbol{\tau\phi})}\, q(\mathbf{w}^{(\mathbf{tf})})\, q(\mathbf{w}^{(\boldsymbol{\tau\phi})})\, \log P(\mathbf{r}|\mathbf{w}^{(\mathbf{tf})}, \mathbf{w}^{(\boldsymbol{\tau\phi})}\}, \sigma^2)\\ &= \text{const} - \frac{T}{2}\log(\sigma^2) - \frac{1}{2\sigma^2}\left\langle\left(\mathbf{r} - (\mathbf{w}^{(\mathbf{tf})}\otimes\mathbf{w}^{(\boldsymbol{\tau\phi})})\bullet Q\right)^2\right\rangle_{q^{(\mathbf{tf})},q^{(\boldsymbol{\tau\phi})}}\end{aligned} \tag{39}$$

Differentiating w.r.t. σ^2 yields

$$\frac{\partial}{\partial\sigma^2}\hat{\mathcal{F}} = -\frac{T}{2\sigma^2} + \frac{1}{2\sigma^4}\left\langle\left(\mathbf{r} - (\mathbf{w}^{(\mathbf{tf})}\otimes\mathbf{w}^{(\boldsymbol{\tau\phi})})\bullet Q\right)^2\right\rangle_{q^{(\mathbf{tf})},q^{(\boldsymbol{\tau\phi})}} \tag{40}$$

The optimum lies at $\frac{\partial}{\partial \sigma^2}\hat{\mathcal{F}} = 0$, which can be solved as

$$\sigma^2 = \frac{1}{T}\left\langle \left(\mathbf{r} - (\mathbf{w}^{(\mathbf{tf})} \otimes \mathbf{w}^{(\tau\phi)}) \bullet Q\right)^2 \right\rangle_{q^{(\mathbf{tf})}, q^{(\tau\phi)}}$$

$$= \frac{1}{T}\left(\mathbf{r}^\top \mathbf{r} - 2t_1 + t_2\right) \tag{41}$$

where T is the number of time points and

$$t_1 = \mathbf{r}^\top \left(\boldsymbol{\mu}^{(\mathbf{tf})} \otimes \boldsymbol{\mu}^{(\tau\phi)}\right) \bullet Q = \sum_{iab} r_i \mu_a^{\mathbf{tf}} \mu_b^{\tau\phi} Q_{iab}$$

$$t_2 = \sum_{iaa'bb'} \left(\mu_a^{\mathbf{tf}} \mu_{a'}^{\mathbf{tf}} + \Sigma_{aa'}\right)\left(\mu_b^{\tau\phi} \mu_{b'}^{\tau\phi} + \Sigma_{bb'}^{\tau\phi}\right) Q_{iab} Q_{ia'b'} \tag{42}$$

References

M. B. Ahrens, J. F. Linden, and M. Sahani. Nonlinearities and contextual influences in auditory cortical responses modeled with multilinear spectrotemporal methods. *J Neurosci*, 28(8):1929–1942, 2008a.

M. B. Ahrens, L. Paninski, and M. Sahani. Inferring input nonlinearities in neural encoding models. *Network*, 19(1):35–67, 2008b.

C. A. Atencio, T. O. Sharpee, and C. E. Schreiner. Cooperative nonlinearities in auditory cortical neurons. *Neuron*, 58(6):956–66, 2008.

C. A. Atencio, T. O. Sharpee, and C. E. Schreiner. Hierarchical computation in the canonical auditory cortical circuit. *Proc Natl Acad Sci USA*, 106(51):21894–9, 2009.

C. A. Atencio, T. O. Sharpee, and C. E. Schreiner. Receptive field dimensionality increases from the auditory midbrain to cortex. *J Neurophysiol*, 107(10):2594–603, 2012.

S. Atiani, M. Elhilali, S. V. David, J. B. Fritz, and S. A. Shamma. Task difficulty and performance induce diverse adaptive patterns in gain and shape of primary auditory cortical receptive fields. *Neuron*, 61(3):467–80, 2009.

M. J. Beal. *Variational algorithms for approximate Bayesian inference*. PhD thesis, University College London, 2003.

A. Calabrese, J. W. Schumacher, D. M. Schneider, L. Paninski, and S. M. N. Woolley. A generalized linear model for estimating spectrotemporal receptive fields from responses to natural sounds. *PLoS ONE*, 6(1):e16104, 2011.

B. M. Calhoun and C. E. Schreiner. Spectral envelope coding in cat primary auditory cortex: linear and non-linear effects of stimulus characteristics. *Eur J Neurosci*, 10(3):926–940, 1998.

G. B. Christianson, M. Sahani, and J. F. Linden. The consequences of response nonlinearities for interpretation of spectrotemporal receptive fields. *J Neurosci*, 28(2):446–455, 2008.

S. V. David, J. B. Fritz, and S. A. Shamma. Task reward structure shapes rapid receptive field plasticity in auditory cortex. *Proc Natl Acad Sci USA*, 109(6):2144–9, 2012.

R. C. deCharms, D. T. Blake, and M. M. Merzenich. Optimizing sound features for cortical neurons. *Science*, 280(5368):1439–1443, 1998.

D. A. Depireux, J. Z. Simon, D. J. Klein, and S. A. Shamma. Spectro-temporal response field characterization with dynamic ripples in ferret primary auditory cortex. *J Neurophysiol*, 85(3):1220–1234, 2001.

J. J. Eggermont, P. M. Johannesma, and A. M. Aertsen. Reverse-correlation methods in auditory research. *Q Rev Biophys*, 16:341–414, 1983.

M. Elhilali, J. B. Fritz, D. J. Klein, J. Z. Simon, and S. A. Shamma. Dynamics of precise spike timing in primary auditory cortex. *J Neurosci*, 24(5):1159–1172, 2004.

B. Englitz, M. Ahrens, S. Tolnai, R. Rübsamen, M. Sahani, and J. Jost. Multilinear models of single cell responses in the medial nucleus of the trapezoid body. *Network*, 21(1-2): 91–124, 2010.

A. Fishbach, I. Nelken, and Y. Yeshurun. Auditory edge detection: a neural model for physiological and psychoacoustical responses to amplitude transients. *J Neurophysiol*, 85(6):2303–23, 2001.

J. Fritz, S. Shamma, M. Elhilali, and D. Klein. Rapid task-related plasticity of spectrotemporal receptive fields in primary auditory cortex. *Nat Neurosci*, 6(11):1216–23, 2003.

P. R. Gill, J. Zhang, S. M. N. Woolley, T. Fremouw, and F. E. Theunissen. Sound representation methods for spectro-temporal receptive field estimation. *J Comput Neurosci*, 21 (1):5–20, 2006.

I. W. Hunter and M. J. Korenberg. The identification of nonlinear biological systems: Wiener and Hammerstein cascade models. *Biol Cybern*, 55(2-3):135–144, 1986.

W. James and C. Stein. Estimation with quadratic loss. In *Proceedings of the Fourth Berkeley Symposium on Mathematical Statistics and Probability*, volume 1, pages 1–379, 1961.

M. I. Jordan, Z. Ghahramani, T. S. Jaakkola, and L. K. Sau l. An introduction to variational methods for graphical models. *Mach Learning*, 37(2):183–233, 1999.

D. J. Klein, D. A. Depireux, J. Z. Simon, and S. A. Shamma. Robust spectrotemporal reverse correlation for the auditory system: optimizing stimulus design. *J Comput Neurosci*, 9(1):85–111, 2000.

D. J. Klein, J. Z. Simon, D. A. Depireux, and S. A. Shamma. Stimulus-invariant processing and spectrotemporal reverse correlation in primary auditory cortex. *J Comput Neurosci*, 20(2):111–136, 2006.

N. Kowalski, D. A. Depireux, and S. A. Shamma. Analysis of dynamic spectra in ferret primary auditory cortex. I. Characteristics of single-unit responses to moving ripple spectra. *J Neurophysiol*, 76(5):3503–3523, 1996.

J. F. Linden, R. C. Liu, M. Sahani, C. E. Schreiner, and M. M. Merzenich. Spectrotemporal structure of receptive fields in areas AI and AAF of mouse auditory cortex. *J Neurophysiol*, 90(4):2660–2675, 2003.

C. K. Machens, M. S. Wehr, and A. M. Zador. Linearity of cortical receptive fields measured with natural sounds. *J Neurosci*, 24(5):1089–100, 2004.

D. J. C. MacKay. Bayesian non-linear modelling for the prediction competition. *ASHRAE Transactions*, 100(2):1053–1062, 1994.

L. M. Miller, M. A. Escabí, H. L. Read, and C. E. Schreiner. Spectrotemporal receptive fields in the lemniscal auditory thalamus and cortex. *J Neurophysiol*, 87:516–527, 2002.

M. Park and J. W. Pillow. Receptive field inference with localized priors. *PLoS Comput Biol*, 7(10):e1002219, 2011.

M. Pienkowski and J. J. Eggermont. Effects of adaptation on spectrotemporal receptive fields in primary auditory cortex. *Neuroreport*, 20(13):1198–203, 2009.

M. Pienkowski and J. J. Eggermont. Nonlinear cross-frequency interactions in primary auditory cortex spectrotemporal receptive fields: a Wiener-Volterra analysis. *J Comput Neurosci*, 28(2):285–303, 2010.

M. Pienkowski, G. Shaw, and J. J. Eggermont. Wiener-Volterra characterization of neurons in primary auditory cortex using Poisson-distributed impulse train inputs. *J Neurophysiol*, 101(6):3031–3041, 2009.

N. C. Rabinowitz, B. D. B. Willmore, J. W. H. Schnupp, and A. J. King. Contrast gain control in auditory cortex. *Neuron*, 70(6):1178–91, 2011.

N. C. Rabinowitz, B. D. B. Willmore, J. W. H. Schnupp, and A. J. King. Spectrotemporal contrast kernels for neurons in primary auditory cortex. *J Neurosci*, 32(33):11271–84, 2012.

R. G. Rutkowski, T. M. Shackleton, J. W. H. Schnupp, M. N. Wallace, and A. R. Palmer. Spectrotemporal receptive field properties of single units in the primary, dorsocaudal and ventrorostral auditory cortex of the guinea pig. *Audiol Neurotol*, 7(4):214–227, 2002.

M. Sahani and J. F. Linden. Evidence optimization techniques for estimating stimulus-response functions. In S. Becker, S. Thrun, and K. Obermayer, editors, *Advances in Neural Information Processing Systems*, volume 15, pages 301–308, Cambridge, Massachusetts, 2003a. MIT Press.

M. Sahani and J. F. Linden. How linear are auditory cortical responses? In S. Becker, S. Thrun, and K. Obermayer, editors, *Advances in Neural Information Processing Systems*, volume 15, pages 109–116, Cambridge, Massachusetts, 2003b. MIT Press.

N. Schinkel-Bielefeld, S. V. David, S. A. Shamma, and D. A. Butts. Inferring the role of inhibition in auditory processing of complex natural stimuli. *J Neurophysiol*, 107(12): 3296–307, 2012.

J. W. Schnupp, T. D. Mrsic-Flogel, and A. J. King. Linear processing of spatial cues in primary auditory cortex. *Nature*, 414(6860):200–204, 2001.

B. Shechter and D. A. Depireux. Nonlinearity of coding in primary auditory cortex of the awake ferret. *Neuroscience*, 165(2):612–20, 2010.

J. Z. Simon, D. A. Depireux, D. J. Klein, J. B. Fritz, and S. A. Shamma. Temporal symmetry in primary auditory cortex: implications for cortical connectivity. *Neural Comput*, 19(3): 583–638, 2007.

M. Tomita and J. J. Eggermont. Cross-correlation and joint spectro-temporal receptive field properties in auditory cortex. *J Neurophysiol*, 93(1):378–392, 2005.

W. Truccolo, U. T. Eden, M. R. Fellows, J. P. Donoghue, and E. N. Brown. A point process framework for relating neural spiking activity to spiking history, neural ensemble, and extrinsic covariate effects. *J Neurophysiol*, 93(2):1074–89, 2005.

R. E. Turner and M. Sahani. Two problems with variational expectation maximisation for time-series models. In D. Barber, A. T. Cemgil, and S. Chiappa, editors, *Inference and Learning in Dynamic Models*. Cambridge University Press, 2011.

R. S. Williamson, L. A. Anderson, G. B. Christianson, M. Sahani and J. F. Linden Auditory thalamic neurons show nonlinear sensitivity to stimulus context *Society for Neuroscience Annual Meeting Abstracts*. 2011.

Index

D

E

F

G

H

I

J

L

M

N

O

P

R

S

T

U

V

W

Y